EL CERRITO HIGH SCHOOL EL CERRITO, CALIFORNIA				NO.14
DATE RECD.	DATE RET.	COND.	TEACHER	PUPIL

RUTH BENNETT WHITE has for many years taught courses in foods, nutrition, and general home economics at all levels of education, both in the United States and in Turkey and Nigeria. She has served as adviser to 4-H Clubs and lectures widely to educational and professional groups. Mrs. White has done research in nutrition and the chemistry of foods, as well as in biochemistry, human physiology, and embryology, at the University of Iowa, Cornell University, and Columbia University. A member of local, state, and national home economics associations, she was a delegate to the Eleventh International Congress of Home Economics at the University of Bristol, England, in 1968 and to the International Permanent Council meeting of the International Federation of Home Economists in Königstein, Germany, in 1970. She was a member of the Official Publications Committee of the California Home Economics Association from 1967 to 1970, serving as its chairman in 1969–70, and has been chairman of International Relations for the California unit for 1970–72. Mrs. White is a member of the American Association of University Women and of the National League of American Pen Women, Inc., and contributes articles to both scientific and popular publications.

RUTH BENNETT WHITE

food and your future

PRENTICE-HALL, INC., ENGLEWOOD CLIFFS, N.J.

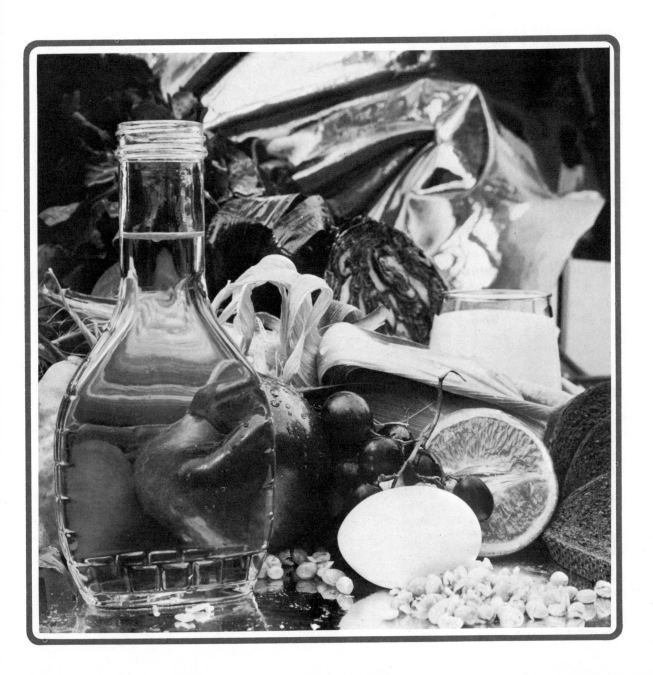

FOOD AND YOUR FUTURE by RUTH BENNETT WHITE

RELATED PRENTICE-HALL BOOKS

BUILDING YOUR LIFE
by Judson T. Landis and Mary G. Landis

EXPLORING HOME AND FAMILY LIVING
by Henrietta Fleck and Louise Fernandez

LIVING WITH YOUR FAMILY
by Henrietta Fleck, Louise Fernandez, and Elizabeth Munves

PERSONAL ADJUSTMENT, MARRIAGE, AND FAMILY LIVING
by Judson T. Landis and Mary G. Landis

UNDERSTANDING AND GUIDING YOUNG CHILDREN
by Katherine Read Baker and Xenia F. Fane

YOU AND YOUR FOOD
by Ruth Bennett White

Design by Celine Alvarez. Illustrations by Gary Schuermann. Technical Assistance by John Brandes.

Cover photograph by John Brandes

ISBN 0–13–322982–3
10 9 8 7 6 5 4 3 2

PRENTICE-HALL INTERNATIONAL, INC., *London*
PRENTICE-HALL OF AUSTRALIA, PTY. LTD., *Sydney*
PRENTICE-HALL OF CANADA, LTD., *Toronto*
PRENTICE-HALL OF INDIA PRIVATE LTD., *New Delhi*
PRENTICE-HALL OF JAPAN, INC., *Tokyo*

The science of nutrition is one of the most remarkable breakthroughs of the twentieth century. The knowledge it affords puts in our hands the power to help every human being to reach his hereditary potential. No other century has enjoyed this insight. Man has always eaten for survival and for enjoyment, but only recently have we come to understand fully the importance of food—how it undergirds our health and enhances our appearance.

We cannot derive benefits from this knowledge unless we use it. Although we are the richest nation in the world, with the most abundant food supply, more than one hundred million of us eat a diet that is less than good. Even people on a low budget can eat well, if they make wise choices of food. We fail to get the benefits that sound nutrition can give us, not so much because we lack money or food, as because we do not know what to eat. This is true of people of all age groups. They need to know more about foods and nutrition, and how to apply the information they acquire.

Young people have the most to gain by establishing good eating habits. You stand on the threshold of life, getting ready to launch your career and establish your own home. Your future will be enriched by good eating habits or impoverished by poor ones. The trend in America in this century has been toward poorer diets. Of the entire population, young people are the ones most in need of a better understanding of what to do, for teen-age girls and young adults of both sexes are at the bottom of the totem pole nutritionally.

This book brings you the significant findings of the latest scientific and clinical studies. It interprets these findings simply but accurately, to help you personally to reach immediate and long-term goals. But you must make the effort to learn what has been presented. The book is designed to help you absorb this newer knowledge and make it part of your way of life.

Part I, "Building a Better Life with an Understanding of Food," analyzes the practical significance of the new research on food and nutrition. It explains why your present and future fitness, good appearance, mental alertness, emotional stability, and continuing vigor are all dependent on the food you eat. It also shows you how you can use this information in planning meals, shopping for food, and preparing and serving meals on low, moderate, and liberal food budgets.

Part II, "Nutrition and the Beginning of Life," focuses on feeding a young family. It traces the influence of the mother's nutrition on a baby, from conception to birth and on into the future. It shows the great contribution of both mother and father in producing a healthy child and helping it establish good eating habits in the preschool years.

Part III turns to the important problems of "The Consumer and Food Protection." Although consumer education is integrated in the study of every food discussed in Part I, special attention is given here to food contamination, food fads and fallacies, convenience foods in modern life, the responsibility of government in protecting the consumer, the responsibility of the food industry, and what we can do to protect ourselves.

Part IV, "The Science and Art of Meal Management," draws together the major ideas on managing meals and on managing food to prevent and correct overweight and some types of heart disease. It emphasizes the rewards in store for those who develop and maintain good eating habits—the major reward being a longer, happier, more vigorous life. The text ends with a chapter devoted to the gourmet style of preparing meals, through the use of imagination and careful attention to details. It is a technique that can be mastered even by a beginner.

The low-calorie, low-fat Cookbook features basic recipes with gourmet variations. It is an essential part of the text. It applies the principles taught in the text, converting them into concrete action, first in the school laboratory and then in the home kitchen.

Teaching-learning aids are an integral part of each chapter. They are designed to stimulate the student to think over the text material, evaluate it, and apply it in planning and preparing balanced meals and snacks to meet the nutritional needs of the entire day. They encourage the student to share with the family the new knowledge and insights gained in the study of the chapter. In addition, new vocabulary is defined, with pronunciation, as it occurs, and is listed at the end of each chapter.

The Appendix includes the Recommended Daily Dietary Allowances, the Nutritive Values in Common Portions of Food, Weight-Height Tables, and a comprehensive Bibliography. By using these materials, you can learn simple research techniques and calculate the nutrients in your own diet at specified intervals.

The visual aids—photographs, artwork, charts, and tables—are designed to highlight the text matter and quicken your interest. These are not purely decorative, but are an important supplement to the text.

It is hoped that you will catch the spirit of the inquiring scientist and the enlightened homemaker, and feel the thrill of stretching your mind. Then you will be on your way to mastering what many consider the most rewarding of all pursuits— making a good family life.

Ruth Bennett White

acknowledgments

It is a pleasure to express my appreciation to the many colleagues and friends who have contributed to the preparation of this book.

To the teachers, supervisors, and others in the field of foods and nutrition who read and commented on the proposed content: Mrs. Elizabeth Brysiewicz, Orinda, California; Mrs. Patricia Chambers, Abilene, Texas; Mrs. Grace Coleman, New York City; Mrs. Elizabeth Denham, Rutgers, The State University, New Brunswick, New Jersey; Dr. Mary Durrett, University of Texas, Austin, Texas; Mrs. Velma Farrand, St. Louis, Missouri; Mrs. Cedona Kendall, Ferguson, Missouri; Dr. Flemmie P. Kittrell, Howard University, Washington, D.C.; Mrs. Martha Thompson, Nacona, Texas; Mrs. Beverly Ritter, Liberty, Missouri; Mrs. Helen S. Poulsen, Oakland, California; Mrs. Lois Rogers, Oklahoma City, Oklahoma; Miss Suzanne Sickler, West Orange, New Jersey; Mrs. Maurice Silk, Abilene, Texas; Mrs. Jean S. Taylor, Arlington, Virginia; Miss Ethel Leh, South Orange, New Jersey; Mrs. Helen Wuester, Beattie, Kansas; Miss Katherine Young, San Jose State College, San Jose, California; Mrs. Barbara Trumble, Winnetka, Illinois; and Mr. A. Daniel Trumble, Winnetka, Illinois.

To the teachers who taught parts of the manuscript: Mrs. Velma Farrand, St. Louis, Missouri; Mrs. Virginia Fowler, San Diego, California; Mrs. Audrey Hallett, San Diego, California; Mrs. Cedona Kendall, Ferguson, Missouri; and Mrs. Elizabeth Tillman, San Diego, California.

To the many who have taught *You and Your Food* and have encouraged me to write this book, and to the young married couples, college and high school students, educators, teachers, physicians, and homemakers who have read all or part of the manuscript.

I cannot thank by name all of the Prentice-Hall staff who have joined in producing this book, but wish to thank with special warmth Mrs. Fanny S. Mach, Production Editor, with whom I have worked so closely.

I would like to express my continuing gratitude to my parents, Sarah and A. L. Bennett, who taught me by example that being a responsible partner in making a good home is of first importance in life; and to my husband, Carl, who with our children, Sherril and Caroline, has made life so worthwhile.

R. B. W.

contents

(T = top; B = bottom; L = left; R = right)

Ac'cent International, 161 (T), 426; Aluminum Assn., 361; American Dry Milk Inst., 108, 118, 353, 401; American Heart Assn., 382, 383; American Meat Inst., 75 (R), 211, 349 (R), 411 (L), 413; American Spice Trade Assn., 45 (L), 49, 76 (B), 77, 99, 194, 215, 217, 222 (T & B), 234, 237, 334, 343 (T), 373, 377, 394 (T), 412, 414, 425 434 437; Armstrong/Rapho-Guillumette, 136 (B), 244, 252, 312, 340, 344, 357 (T & B); Beame/DPI, 42; Marion Bernstein, 156, 231, 284; Bijur/Monkmeyer, 347; California Raisin Advisory Bd., 153; Camera Press/Pix, 43; Campbell Soup, 40 (B), 348, 350, 402; Cereal Inst., 199, 352 (R), 390; Walter Chandoha, 286; Cline Advertising Service, 130; Conklin/Pix, 261; Corning Ware, 349 (L); Corry/DPI, 22; Dairymen's League Cooperative Assn., 109; Davis/DPI, 54; De Wys, 9, 142, 150, 204, 275, 282, 326, 369; Diamond Walnuts 235 (B); Dudley-Anderson-Yutzy, 332 (T), 419; Ekco Products, 358, 359; Engh/Photo Researchers, 196; Esso Research & Engineering, 301; Falk/Monkmeyer, 13 (T); Florida Citrus Comm., 26, 30, 137, 151, 191, 193, 246, 310, 320, 421, 422, 436; Food & Drug Admin., 294, 295, 297, 304, 319; Frank/DPI, 128 (R); French Govt. Tourist Office, 52, 157, 394 (B); Charles Gatewood, 175 (B); General Mills, 197; Gould/Pix, 299; Granitsas/Photo Researchers, 178; Grant Heilman, 106, 172 (T), 296, 298; Heron/Monkmeyer, 258; Jell-O Pudding & Pie Filling, 431; Kellogg Co., 177, 352 (L); Betty Crocker/General Mills, 218; Knox Gelatine, 374, 389; Koch/Rapho-Guillumette, 29, 329, 399 (T); Kraft Foods, 101; Levy/Photo Researchers, 128 (L); Jane Latta, 5, 6, 188; Madagascar Vanilla Growers, 111 (L); Mannheim/DPI, 249; Martin/DPI, 107; McIlhenny Co., 40 (T), 54, 79 (L), 82, 116, 162, 165, 196 (T), 420; Molasses, 229; Molnar, 41; Monsanto Co., 308; National Broiler Council, 23 (T), 68, 75 (L), 386, 405; National Canners Assn., 95 (B), 152; National Dairy Council, 17, 76 (T), 96, 100 (B) 253, 260, 327, 343 (B), 418; National Film Board of Canada, 97; National Fisheries Inst., 45 (R); National Live Stock & Meat Bd., 60 (L), 62, 64, 65, 66, 67; National Macaroni Inst., 198; National Medical Audiovisual Center, 92, 93; National Presto Industries, 100 (T), 135, 213; Nestlé, 442; *The New York Times*, 8 (B); Nova Scotia Information Service, 69; Peace Corps, 94; Pepperidge Farm, 175 (T); Pet Milk, 95 (T); Photo Researchers, 128 (L); Processed Apples Inst., 136 (T), 235, 332 (B), 439; Ralston Purina, 180, 219; Reeberg/DPI, 189 (B); Revere Copper & Brass, 360; Reynolds Metals, 331, 411 (R); Rogers/Monkmeyer, 155, 311, 368; St. Louis *Post Dispatch*/Black Star, 321; San Diego City Schools, 154, 160; Scandinavian Airlines System, 403; Schreiber/Rapho-Guillumette, 272, 281, 292; Shackman/Monkmeyer, 15; Shelton/Monkmeyer, 10, 11; Sirkis/Pix, 13 (B), 31; Smith/Rapho-Guillumette, 38, 354; Stephanus/DPI, 24; Swans Down Cake Flour, 441 (T & B); Suzanne Szasz, 28, 60 (R), 173, 228, 277, 283, Swedish National Travel Office, 404; Tucson Public Schools, 131; Tuna, 330, 388; Union Tribune Publishing, 16; United Fresh Fruit & Vegetable Assn., 111 (R), 124, 127, 139, 159, 161 (B), 164, 166, 230, 232, 263, 266, 333, 341, 371, 372, 395, 400, 415, 423, 424, 429, 430; United Nations, 208; Upjohn Co., 133; USDA, 23 (B), 63, 79 (R), 126, 141, 149, 150, 314, 316, 342, 432; USDA, Food & Nutrition Bd., 281, 370; Westinghouse, 356 (B); Westvaco, 132; Carl M. White, 50, 148, 172 (B), 273; Wilkinson/National Film Board of Canada, 8; Zalon/DPI, 384.

CHAPTER OPENING PHOTO CREDITS *Chapters* 1–12, 14, 16–21, and *Cookbook*, John Brandes; 13, Eugene Anthony/Black Star; 15, Suzanne Szasz; 22, Scandinavian Airlines System.

COLOR PHOTO CREDITS Ac'cent International, 54d; B. Altman & Co., 374d (T); Aluminum Assn., 374b (BL); American Dairy Assn., 22c (T), 246a (T), 342a (T), 342d (R); American Spice Trade Assn., 22d (B), 54b (B), 150c (TL); Anderson-Clayton Co., 22c (B), 182c (T); California Strawberry Advisory Bd., 150d (L); Chicken of the Sea, 278b (C); CPC International, 182b and 182c (B); Del Monte, 22b (T), 150b, 182b (TR), 278c (T); Diamond Walnuts, 182d (T); Florida Citrus Comm., 54a (T), 150d (TR), 342d (L); Florida Fruit & Vegetable Assn., 150a (T & B); Frigidaire, 374b (BR); Knox Gelatine, 246d (T), 342d (L); Kohn & Hass Co., 182b (TL); Land O' Lakes, 278a; McIlhenny Co., 22d (T), 150c (B); Monsanto Co., 278c (B); National Fisheries Inst., 54c (T), 54b and 54c (B), 278b (BR); National Live Stock & Meat Bd., 246a (T); National Macaroni Inst., 182d (B), 246b (BR), 278b (T), 342b (T); Pepperidge Farm, 182a; Processed Apples Inst., 54b (TR), 342a (B); Regal Ware, 374a (T); Revere Copper & Brass, 374b (T); Reynolds Metals, 22a, 54b (TL), 150c (TR), 182b (BL), 246c, 374c; Rice Council, 22b (B), 54a (B), 246b (T), 246d (B), 278d (B); Tupperware, 374a (B); United Fresh Fruit & Vegetable Assn., 150d (BR), 278d (T), 342b (BR); Universal Oil Products Co., 246b (BL), 342c; Westinghouse, 374d (B).

part i

building
a better life
with an
understanding of food

eating habits, mirror of the future

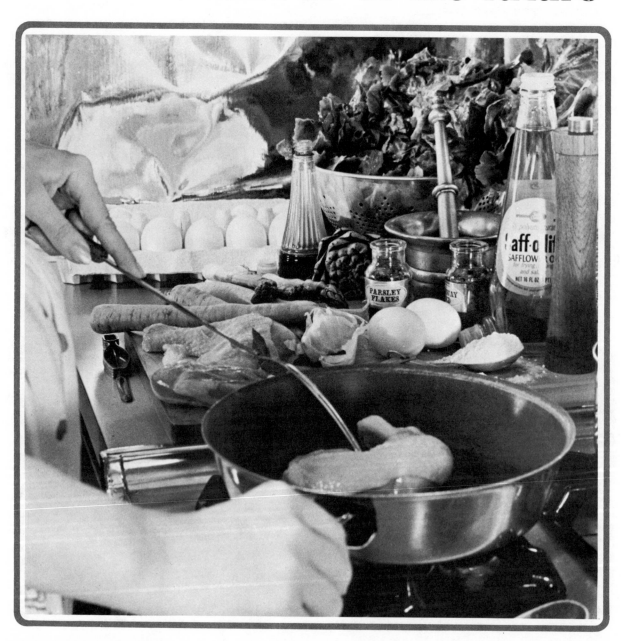

Your mirror reflects your eating habits

If you want to see how food helps form you year by year, stand in front of a full-length mirror and study the image it reflects.

Is your figure trim—or too fat or too thin?

Your posture—is it straight or sagging, with a curved back or round shoulders?

Are your legs straight—or bowed or knock-kneed?

What about your complexion—is it smooth and clear, with a good color, or sallow, rough, dry, or too oily?

The tissue beneath the skin—is it firm or flabby?

How about your teeth and gums—are they firm, well formed, with few or no cavities or fillings, or do you have trouble with them?

Your eyes—are they clear and do they sparkle with vitality, or are they bloodshot, dull, and listless?

If your mirror answers "Yes" to the first part of each question, you are a well-nourished person and off to a good start in life. If not, your mirror is telling you that you are not well-nourished and it is time for a change.

Food and heredity

All human life begins with the union of two tiny cells. The new life that is created develops according to a "genetic blueprint." With this basic structure, nature uses food like modeling clay to mold us, over the years, into what we are. Food in no way determines that we shall have a face, eyes, hair, and other physical features—these are part of our biological inheritance—but food does de-termine how well these features develop. What we have to bear in mind is that it takes good eating habits to make us achieve our full inherited potential. For more examples of how physical characteristics reflect eating habits, see Table 1–1.

This concept is still so new that you will find people who believe, or seem to believe, that the whole purpose of food is merely "to keep body and soul together." If this were all—if food did nothing but satisfy hunger and prevent starvation—it would make no difference what you eat so long as you eat enough to satisfy your appetite.

Modern science has taught us better. Good nutrition enhances the condition of all the features that go into the making of an attractive physique. What is more, these effects go more than skin deep. Indeed, you will find as the story of the effects of food unfolds in these pages that our whole life—beginning with the physical normality of the unborn babe straight through to later years—our mental alertness, physical attractiveness, and emotional stability are all bound up with the quality of our diet.

Forecast of the future

While today's image in your mirror reflects the cumulative effect of food choices made by you or for you since your life began, you are standing on the doorstep of adult life and are looking ahead. What will the image look like 20 years from now? Forty years from now? That image is as plastic as modeling clay, it can and will be shaped by you. Happily, the science of nutrition has advanced far enough to guide you as you give it the form it will have when the future becomes the present. You need only the understanding of what to do and the will to do it.

table 1–1   Characteristics of Good Nutrition and Poor Nutrition

	GOOD NUTRITION	POOR NUTRITION
EYES	Bright and clear; sparkle	Bloodshot; with dark circles under them; puffy; hollow
BODY	Well-developed; attractive; bones straight and strong; weight normal for height and age. Flat abdomen.	Defects; underweight or overweight; undersize; bones misshapen in one or more places; weak; sagging abdomen.
MUSCLES	Firm, well-developed	Flabby, soft, small
TEETH	Enamel—hard and smooth; tooth and root structure—sound	Many cavities; poor root structure
GUMS	Firm; resistant to sores or bleeding; pink color	Spongy; subject to sores and bleeding; too red or too pale
COLOR	Skin—healthy, pinkish tone; mucous membrane of mouth and eyelids pink inside	Skin—pale; mucous membrane of eyelids and mouth pale
SKIN	Firm, smooth; healthy color	Loose; sallow or waxy
HAIR	Glossy, soft	Rough, dry, or oily; lacking luster
DISPOSITION	Good-natured, happy attitude	Irritable, listless; poor ability to concentrate
ENERGY	Full of life, ability to get work done without undue fatigue; recovers from fatigue quickly	Tires easily and quickly; recovers slowly
GENERAL HEALTH	Excellent; disease and infections not severe; recovers quickly	Susceptible to infections; recovers more slowly from disease or infections
APPETITE	Good	Poor to fair
MENTAL HEALTH	Alert, good concentration; able to reach intellectual potential; cooperative; emotionally stable	Listless, restless, careless, inattentive, depressed, moody, sullen; uncooperative; less able to reach intellectual potential; less emotional stability

This book aims to help you understand what to do and why you need to select and manage your food wisely, what to do to gain buoyant vitality, physical attractiveness, and other personal triumphs to which a balanced diet holds the key. It focuses on young people, especially young women and young men who are thinking of marriage and their future happiness.

Your study of food and its effect on your future is going to reward you. It will help you bridge the wide gap between the abundance of food knowledge available today and the poor use that is often made of it. You will find out for yourself that, when you reach the peak state of nutrition, you have more personal vigor, better physical appearance, and sounder health. You will develop self-confidence and enthusiasm for managing the family's meals. Your rewards will go beyond yourself. Your family will admire your competence, but they will thank you most for helping them form eating habits that give them the same benefits you seek.

Why some are poorly fed

There are four main reasons why some people miss the advantages of being well-fed: (1) lack of an adequate national food supply, (2) lack of money to buy food, (3) improper eating habits, and (4) inadequate knowledge of what constitutes a balanced diet and inability to select or prepare it.

Food Supply

In man's long climb upward, he has had to fight the threat of hunger all the way. The struggle explains why some chose to be farmers and live in fertile valleys, and why others became nomads and moved with the seasons to find food. It is the story of countless wars, floods, famines, and migrations of large populations. Our mobile society expresses the same age-old search, for many a family may move to a new community in search of "a better living." One of man's deepest longings, the desire to survive, finds utterance in the ancient prayer "Give us this day our daily bread."

An international study of 61 nations has shown that 69 percent of the people of the world are hungry or poorly fed—roughly, two out of every three. The battle has gained intensity in our time because of a world-wide population explosion

At every stage in our lives, our choice of diet affects our health and appearance.

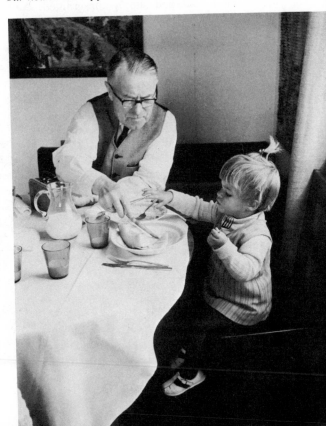

which requires more food production on the one hand and ever more land for housing on the other.

Acutely concerned about this global battle for food, in his last speech to Congress President John F. Kennedy said:

> So long as freedom from hunger is only half-achieved, so long as two-thirds of the nations of the world have food deficits, . . . no citizen, no nation can afford to feel satisfied or secure. We have the ability, we have the means, and we have the capacity to eliminate hunger from the face of the earth in our lifetime. We need only the will.

Money and the diet

Most of us who were born and grew up in America take an abundant food supply for granted. And the standard of living has risen to the point where the average family can buy the food it needs.

Is this enough? Does an abundance of food and money assure us a proper diet? No. If the person responsible for managing the family's food—usually the wife or mother—does not know her job, these are not sufficient. You will see repeatedly as we progress through this book that the only sure way to a balanced diet is through informed selection and preparation of foods—through understanding of nutrition.

This is contrary to the mistaken belief, held by many people, that when a family is poorly fed it is due to lack of money. Sometimes it is, but according to O. V. Wells of the Food and Nutrition Board of the National Academy of Sciences-National Research Council:

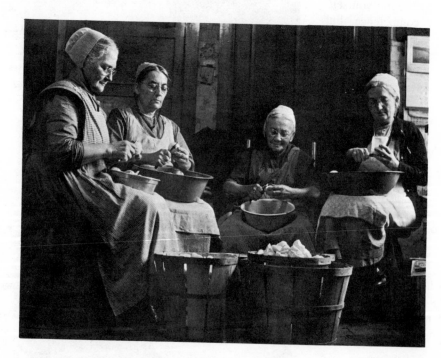

The Pennsylvania Dutch have a hearty, substantial diet, consisting mainly of home-grown foods. Women work together (as in this "snitz" party) preparing food for winter use.

Poor diets today are due as much to lack of knowledge about nutrition as to low income. Some families in every income level have diets that could be improved nutritionally. Also, most families with such diets, even those at lower income levels, could make better choices of food and so achieve better nourishment at the same cost.

How eating habits are formed

Up to this point, we have discussed the relation of food to your personal development and that of the family for which you are to be responsible, when you marry. Your choices will determine whether food will be beneficial or harmful. Your first requirement will be an understanding of foods. The next is a willingness to change your eating habits, if necessary.

Psychologists tell us that habits may rest on a rational or irrational basis and that, once established, they resist change. This is true of eating habits. They may be formed simply by indifference to what food we eat or by enlightened self-interest, on the basis of what food can do for us. They are formed sometimes by accidental circumstances, sometimes by conscious acts of will. They may be based on unexamined tradition, on unreasoning prejudice, or on reliable scientific knowledge.

Upbringing

Anthropologists have studied the eating habits of both primitive and sophisticated cultures. They find that food tastes or preferences are not inborn, that children can and do learn to like the foods their elders teach them to eat. They also learn to like the way these foods are prepared. As a result, some people learn to consider snake meat a delicacy, while others find it repulsive. Some learn to like fish raw and meat "blood rare," and others like foods well done. The wide range of food likes and dislikes is remarkable, and sometimes amusing, but food preferences are acquired by cultivation and can be changed by cultivation.

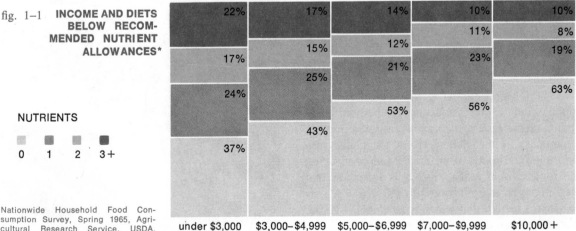

fig. 1–1 **INCOME AND DIETS BELOW RECOMMENDED NUTRIENT ALLOWANCES***

NUTRIENTS

0   1   2   3+

*Nationwide Household Food Consumption Survey, Spring 1965, Agricultural Research Service, USDA.

	under $3,000	$3,000–$4,999	$5,000–$6,999	$7,000–$9,999	$10,000+
	22%	17%	14%	10%	10%
				11%	8%
	17%	15%	12%	23%	19%
		25%	21%		
	24%		53%	56%	63%
		43%			
	37%				

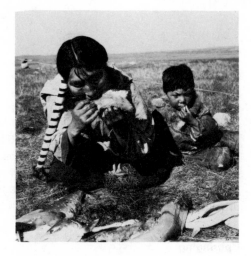

Eskimos enjoy raw fish. It is a delicacy to these natives of the Northwest Territories in Canada.

Food prejudices

Food prejudice is one of the most common obstacles to good eating habits. Some people have quite narrow food likes, and their feelings may be so strong that they prefer doing without food to eating what they dislike. We see even in times of disaster the damaging effect of food prejudice. After World War I, America sent corn to starving Europeans. Accustomed to using corn for feeding animals, some preferred malnourishment to eating "animal fodder." A similar thing happened in Japan after World War II. We have no surplus

Japanese children grow tall and healthy on a balanced American diet.

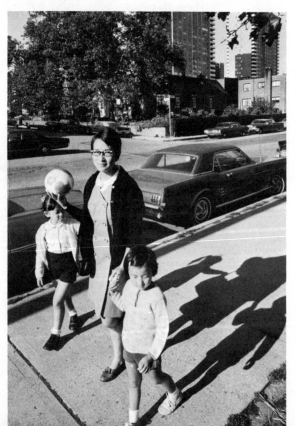

Cultural and religious taboos

Some cultural and religious groups are forbidden to eat certain foods. These prohibitions have no relationship to the nutritional value of the foods involved, but are part of traditions that have existed for generations. For example, the devout Hindu eats no beef, because cows are sacred in India. Observance of such taboos does not necessarily mean a poor diet. If wise choices of substitute foods are made, a balanced diet can still be achieved.

Availability of foods

The food a person can obtain is another factor influencing eating habits. By accident of geography the Eskimo eats blubber, the Chinese has rice as his basic food, and the Frenchman drinks wine rather than water or milk. Food production in any given region depends on terrain, sunshine, water supply, climate, soil, seeds, and methods of cultivation. Such geographic factors as proximity to mountains, oceans, lakes, rivers, or plains also determine the foods of an area. Man survives on the foods within reach, thus it is fortunate that food preferences are acquired, not inborn. A person learns to like that which is available, whether it means a good diet or a poor one.

rice, a staple Japanese food, but sent over some wheat. Some refused to eat it. Studies show that those who learned to like it and the other foods introduced were healthier and grew better than those on a rice diet. For instance, on the average, six-year-olds were found to be 3½ inches taller in 1968 than the same age group in 1938, and young adults were taller and better-formed.

Prejudices apply not only to foods but to the way they are prepared and cooked. For example, hominy, seasoned with salt, pepper, and fat, is a popular dish in the South. In the armed services it was found that men from other sections of the country did not like this dish. A quick-thinking cook hit upon the idea of preparing it like macaroni and cheese. Then all the men ate it.

Superstition and folk beliefs

Superstition and folk beliefs often encourage poor food habits the world over. For example, ancient beliefs among certain West African tribes are that "He who eats an egg will become a thief," and that oranges and mangoes cause yellow fever. Many still believe such nonsense.

A scientific journal reports that Yugoslavia, with a population of about 19,000,000, has 400,000 alcoholics, and explains that "drinking extends to the children, whose parents still hold to the old superstition that slivovitz [a potent alcoholic beverage] is good for the blood."

Food superstitions in our country are just as ridiculous. Recently a professional journal reported that some women eat "starch and clay" during pregnancy, in the belief that this is good for the unborn child. The same practice is found among some rural women in Nigeria.

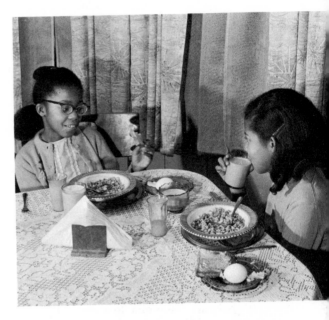

Advertising for cereals and some other foods is directed at children and teen-agers. Alert parents can help their families choose balanced meals like this one.

Food advertising

Commercial advertising may contribute to poor eating habits in our country. Some advertising is reliable. Some spreads misleading half-truths, twisted information, and even deliberate inaccuracies. Highly paid experts are skilled in the proper psychological approach to persuade us to buy the product they have to sell. The propaganda they create is especially persuasive to those—including the educated—whose knowledge of foods and nutrition is limited. Appeals are made to children and teen-agers, because the seller knows that parents like to please their children.

The Council on Food and Nutrition of the American Medical Association cites one technique in misleading the public through advertising:

> XYZ product made with hot milk is not only delicious but nourishing. It is rich in proteins, fats, carbohydrates, and minerals children should have.

What makes this food so rich in these nutrients? If you think it is XYZ, the advertising has misled you. The product would not be so nutritious were it not "made with hot milk." Thus it is not XYZ, but milk, that deserves the credit for the good effects.

Food as status symbol

Status symbols are important to some people in selecting their food. Caviar and pâté de foie gras (a paste of goose liver and truffles) are delicacies that symbolize good taste or indicate that a family can afford the rare and expensive. Round steak is leaner and less costly than T-bone steak, but the latter is a status meat for some people. White bread, white rice, and white sugar were first available to royalty and the wealthy, and thus became status symbols around the world, though the refining of these products reduces their nutritive value. Certain brand names and imported foods are preferred by some because they are expensive, and to them this implies the best.

Good eating habits

Good eating habits are those which include in the daily diet the amount and variety of foods required by the body for energy, growth, and the functioning and repair of all types of body tissues. They must

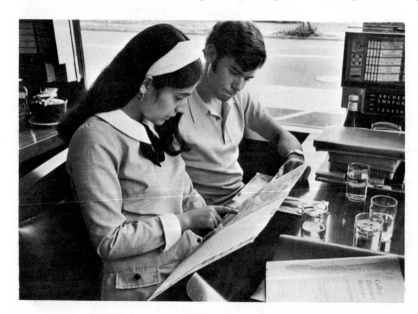

Good eating habits mean wise selection of food, both at home and in public eating places.

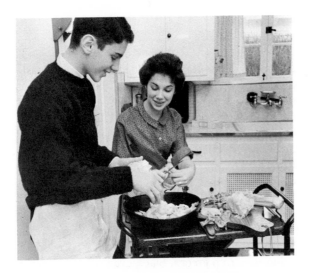

also provide for reproduction and for lactation, if the mother breast-feeds her baby. If these needs are met, one has a diet considered "normal."

Pioneer work by Dr. H. C. Sherman at Columbia University, confirmed later by others, indicates that characteristics of vigor and appearance that we associate with youth can, through good eating habits, be prolonged into middle age and beyond. The life span can be increased by about 10 percent by a daily diet that is superior to the so-called normal diet.

Some people choose only the foods that satisfy their momentary whims, personal tastes, or prejudices, to the neglect of foods required to round out their total nutritional needs. These are poor eating habits.

Studies show that the person with poor eating habits may think it doesn't matter whether meals are eaten regularly or skipped completely. He may also believe that hunger is a sufficient guide as to when to eat and his personal taste the only criterion as to what to eat. He is indifferent to the fact that his body has requirements that can be met only by an intelligent meal-and-snack plan for a balance of nutrients each day.

Eating habits developed in youth affect future appearance and vitality.

Role of the mother

The mother is the strongest force in molding good eating habits. It is she who manages the family's daily food. If she is ignorant or indifferent, she surrenders her family's interests to prejudices, advertising, or chance likes and dislikes. But when she is educated to buy the foods the family needs, and when she knows how to prepare and serve them well, her family develops good eating habits. It is such women who dignify the fine art of homemaking.

This is an art that requires not only depth of understanding of food, but time and thought as well. The stresses of modern living often rob it of the attention it deserves. The result is poor meal planning, hurried meal preparation, rushed meals, skipped meals, irregular meal schedules, poor selection of snacks and meals away from home, misguided dieting to control weight, and overdependence on some types of convenience foods. The wise mother avoids these situations.

Role of the father

Marriage is a partnership, and the homemaker especially needs the cooperation of her husband in developing the family's eating habits. Studies show that it is the father, as a rule, whose tastes are most influential in deciding a family's food preferences. If he has food prejudices, his children are quick to adopt them. Psychologists observe that his influence stems not only from what he does, but also from what he says. One young father who habitually asked, "Is this margarine or butter?" was horrified to hear his four-year-old son use the same words and even the same tone when the family was dining with friends.

National conditions that favor good eating habits

Variety of backgrounds

American food customs have been enriched by contact with many cultures. The constant intermingling of families from different cultures for generations has made the development of sound eating habits easier.

First, we have a wider variety of favorite foods that have become part of our national inheritance. The English brought with them their prized roast beef and mutton; the Scots, their oatmeal porridge; the Irish, corned beef and cabbage, boiled white potatoes, and Irish stew. The Germans introduced sauerkraut, sauerbraten, red cabbage, and sausage. From the French and the Swiss we got cheeses of

Cheese and sausage are found in great variety and abundance in Italian food stores. Many foods introduced by Italians have become American favorites.

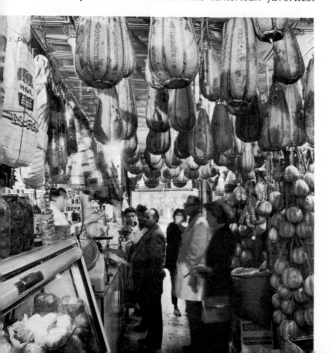

all sorts. The Italians added numerous pasta dishes, broccoli, antipasto, escarole, and various types of sausage. The Russians contributed sour cream, caviar, and beet borscht to our national cuisine. All over the country, these foods are used and enjoyed today.

REGIONAL FOODS. In many sections of the country, regional favorites have been developed. Some derive from the cultural backgrounds of their people, and some use the foods typical of their areas in special ways. For example, the South has fried chicken, hot biscuits, corn bread, collards, turnip greens, black-eyed peas, and pecan pie. New England has its baked beans, Boston brown bread, New England boiled dinner, fish and seafood chowders, codfish cakes, baked squash, cranberry sauce, and steamed clams. The Gulf Coast enjoys its Creole dishes, such as shrimp jambalaya, bouillabaise, French bread, chicken gumbo, crawfish pie, and filé-seasoned soups and stews. The Southwest developed the art of barbecuing meat, and adopted a number of Mexican dishes, including chili con carne, tacos, enchiladas, and frijoles (beans). The West Coast has its lush variety of fruits, huge green salads, seafood, and many Mexican and Oriental dishes adopted from the people from these areas who came to live there.

A varied and balanced diet can easily be achieved with the foods that are brought to us from these different sources. The homemaker who understands the values of each food gets an opportunity to choose favorite foods in working out the family's menus and at the same time can avoid a dull and monotonous diet.

The cultural interchanges in our national life have fostered a flexible attitude towards new foods. This open-mindedness is a great asset. It is too much to expect any food, or even a few foods, to provide all the nutrients the body needs.

The individual or family that enjoys variety has already won half the battle for good eating habits.

Travel

Our cosmopolitan attitude toward food has been stimulated by travel. Each country has its special food ways, and part of the excitement of visiting

Travel has stimulated the interest of Americans in foreign food habits. This street in Hong Kong is teeming with people, most of them buying food.

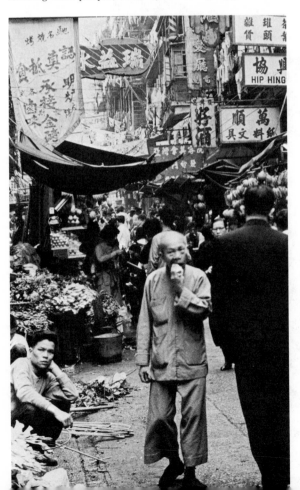

the people of another land is to try out the foods they like best. Since World War II, Americans have become the foremost travelers of the world. This has broadened our tastes, and partly explains the popularity of gourmet cooking. It has also meant thriving business for restaurants that specialize in foreign foods—Chinese, Russian, Swedish, Italian, French, and others. We are becoming a nation that welcomes the opportunity to try out new foods and that seeks both to benefit from and to enjoy the best they have to offer.

Food abundance

The food supply is a national asset that encourages the formation of healthful eating habits. One of the notable achievements of more advanced nations is illustrated by America's organization of food production, processing, and distribution. Ours is a remarkable success story of how a nation has learned to take full advantage of its climate, land, and water, and to use the labor of only a fraction of its population to provide all the people with the food they need to be well fed.

How good are the eating habits of American families?

Nationwide studies give the following picture of America's food habits:

1/About half of our families chose "good" diets in 1965, as compared with 60 percent in 1955 (Figure 1–2, page 14), a drop of 10 percent. A good diet is one that meets or surpasses the Recommended Daily Dietary Allowances given in the table on pages 446–447 and hereafter re-

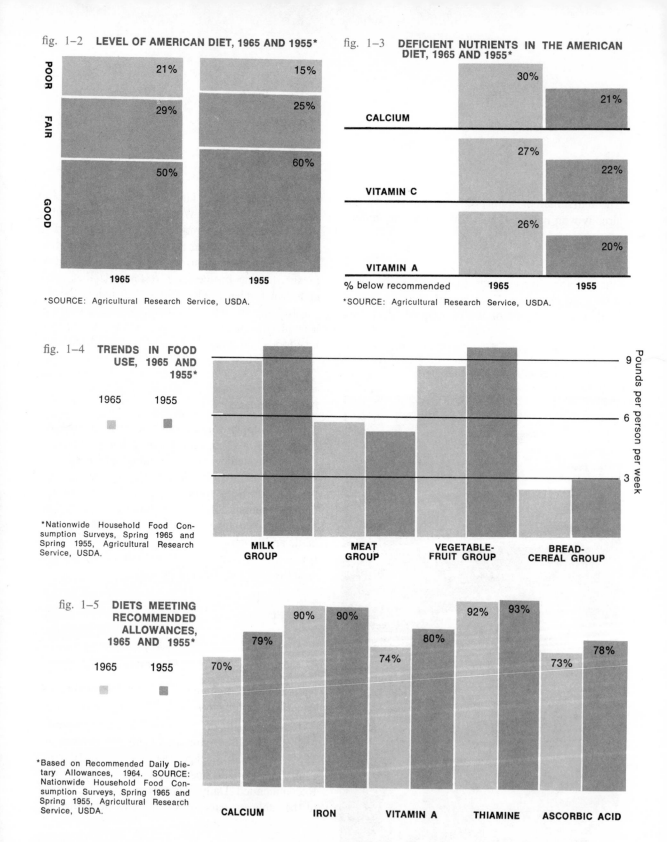

fig. 1–2 **LEVEL OF AMERICAN DIET, 1965 AND 1955***

POOR
FAIR
GOOD

21%   15%
29%   25%
50%   60%

1965   1955

*SOURCE: Agricultural Research Service, USDA.

fig. 1–3 **DEFICIENT NUTRIENTS IN THE AMERICAN DIET, 1965 AND 1955***

CALCIUM   30%   21%
VITAMIN C   27%   22%
VITAMIN A   26%   20%

% below recommended   1965   1955

*SOURCE: Agricultural Research Service, USDA.

fig. 1–4 **TRENDS IN FOOD USE, 1965 AND 1955***

1965   1955

*Nationwide Household Food Consumption Surveys, Spring 1965 and Spring 1955, Agricultural Research Service, USDA.

Pounds per person per week

9
6
3

MILK GROUP   MEAT GROUP   VEGETABLE-FRUIT GROUP   BREAD-CEREAL GROUP

fig. 1–5 **DIETS MEETING RECOMMENDED ALLOWANCES, 1965 AND 1955***

1965   1955

*Based on Recommended Daily Dietary Allowances, 1964. SOURCE: Nationwide Household Food Consumption Surveys, Spring 1965 and Spring 1955, Agricultural Research Service, USDA.

CALCIUM   70% 79%
IRON   90% 90%
VITAMIN A   74% 80%
THIAMINE   92% 93%
ASCORBIC ACID   73% 78%

CALCIUM   IRON   VITAMIN A   THIAMINE   ASCORBIC ACID

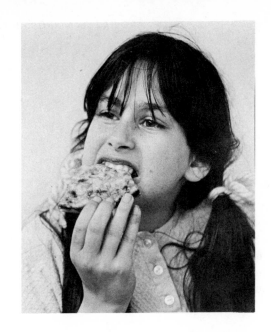

Snacks are important in the day's diet. A glass of milk with this pizza would make it a nourishing snack.

ferred to as RDA. The food actually eaten was perhaps less, because the U.S. Department of Agriculture (hereafter referred to as USDA), which made the study, took no account of food wasted in preparation or thrown away when not used.

2/The nutrients in which American diets are most deficient are calcium, vitamin C, and vitamin A. The decline in use from 1955 to 1965 is illustrated in Figure 1–3.

3/There is a downward trend in the use of milk and milk products, vegetables and fruits, and bread-cereal, as shown in Figure 1–4. We eat more meat today than in 1955.

4/With the downward trend in the use of these important foods, the nutrient content of our diet, as indicated in Figure 1–5, is lower in calcium, vitamins A and C (ascorbic acid), and thiamine.

5/Enough time has elapsed to permit the 1955 dietary survey to be thoroughly analyzed. The percentage of eight essential nutrients that were below the RDA is listed by regions. This ranged, for example, from 18 to 25 percent in riboflavin, 26 to 34 percent in calcium, and 17 to 37 percent in vitamin C. Since we ate fewer foods in 1965 from the groups that provide all of the nutrients listed (except meat, which provides iron and protein especially), it follows that the percentage of the nutrients in which there were deficiencies is lower in 1965 than 1955.

The studies indicate that having the most abundant food supply in the world and the highest per capita income does not assure a good diet for our nation's families. The future homemaker has a challenge: to do a better job in feeding herself and her family.

There is no substitute for a knowledge of food and nutrition, if one is to be well-fed. This knowledge must be applied every day in the choice of foods.

Teen-age diets tend to be poorest

The quality of the average teen-agers' diet tends to conform to the pattern of their families. About 50 percent of teen-agers have good eating habits, thanks to the early guidance of their parents and to their own success in maintaining these habits.

But research shows that on the whole people tend to have the poorest eating habits when they are in their teens—the very years when they need the greatest help that food can give them in developing into the adults they are to be.

The Departments of Health of the States of New York and Pennsylvania have made independent studies of the diets of a cross section of young people. The New York study covered those aged 12 to 20, while that of Pennsylvania surveyed those from 11 to 19. The results were similar. While girls and boys both ate too few green leafy and yellow vegetables and citrus fruits, the diets of the girls "were much less satisfactory than those of the boys in providing recommended amounts of nutrients." Girls 13 to 15 had the poorest diets of all. Laboratory tests showed their nutritional state to be even lower than the record of food eaten had revealed. Dental examinations disclosed that, out of 2536 students, only 7 girls and 12 boys had perfect teeth.

Nutrients lacking

Dr. A. F. Morgan of the University of California at Berkeley, who summarized the national regional studies of 1955, points out that "40 to 60 percent of the teen-age girls' diets were lacking in calcium, iron, and vitamin C; 20 to 40 percent were lacking in thiamine, vitamin A, and riboflavin." This discovery gains added importance when we realize that the quality of American eating habits has declined since 1955.

Some older girls do little better in choosing their food than teen-agers. This is illustrated by a study at Cornell University, where college girls chose diets that were too low by 30 percent in calcium, iron, and thiamine. The girls chose diets, not because they disliked foods that provide good nutrition, but because they simply "did not know the importance of milk, eggs, bread, and cereal." There is a growing consciousness of the need to know more about the foods we eat. Had they known, the Cornell girls could have balanced their diet by including one egg, two additional glasses of milk, three slices of bread (whole wheat or enriched), and a serving of potato.

MEAL SKIPPING. A study made of the 18–24 age group in 1969* reveals that 16 percent skipped breakfast, 11 percent skipped dinner, and 19 percent of the women and 22 percent of the men skipped lunch. This meal skipping is, without doubt, a big factor in the lowered state of our nutrition.

Peace Corps volunteers must first become familiar with the diet of the country in which they work, before they can try to improve that diet.

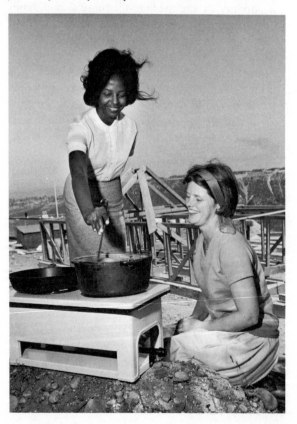

Lifetime rewards of good eating habits

Young people need to know what to eat because they are making the transition from childhood to adulthood and can reap lifetime benefits by establishing sound eating habits early. Girls grow fastest between 13.5 and 14.5 years, boys between 14 and 15.5. Girls usually reach their full height by 15 or 16, boys grow till 19 or the early 20's. Some young people never reach their potential height because of poor eating habits.

*Report: The Wall Street Journal, Feb. 13, 1969, p. 1.

When you attain your full height, you look grown and may feel grown, but studies show that you are neither physically nor emotionally mature until you have time to "firm up" this fast growth. This takes up to eight years. If bones grow so fast that they are weak, they push out of shape. Then your posture is damaged for life. You can pull in your abdominal muscles, but you can't change the bones of stooped shoulders or of a back that has grown into a curve.

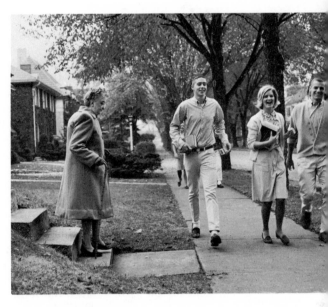

When we are young, we cannot imagine being old. Good eating habits pay off in good posture and a quick, strong step throughout our lives.

Significance of eating habits for teen-age parenthood

At the White House Conference on Children and Youth in 1960, it was reported that 53 percent of all girls between the ages of 15 and 19 were married or had been. One out of every four mothers bearing a first child in the United States in 1964 was a teen-ager. Teen-age fathers increased in our country from 40,000 in 1940 to 106,000 in 1957. Even in this medically-enlightened age, 6 percent of the deaths of 18- and 19-year-old girls were due to the complications of pregnancy and childbirth.*

The 1960 White House Conference brought before us the fact that teen-agers are taking on the responsibility of parenthood, and that they need help. One of the main matters in which the girls need guidance is in nutrition.

Dr. Genevieve Stearns found in studies at the University of Iowa Medical College that poorly-nourished teen-age mothers with a background of poor eating habits had more than three times as many premature infants as mothers whose eating habits were excellent to fair. This group also had more stillbirths and more deaths of the newborn than well-nourished mothers with a good nutritional foundation.

"The girl who marries during her mid-teens," Dr. Stearns concludes, "is apt to be a girl poorly nourished through most of her lifetime, and to be equally ill-equipped to meet the many psychological problems inherent in establishing a successful marriage and the new family. It is not surprising, therefore, that she is the least successful mother in producing a healthy full-term infant." The youth of today will lead the way tomorrow. We make better use—and less abuse—of food as we come to understand how to use it.

*I. G. Macy, *Nutrition and the Teen-Ager*, Reference Papers on Children and Youth, White House Conference on Children and Youth (Washington, D.C.), 1960.

Meaningful words

anthropologist
calcium
convenience foods
cultural interchanges
folklore
food prejudice
lactation
Recommended Daily Dietary
   Allowances
reproduction
riboflavin
status symbol
superstition
thiamine

Thinking and evaluating

1. In what ways has adequate food influenced world history in the past? In the present?

2. What changes in living during your lifetime have directly or indirectly influenced your own state of nutrition? That of others in your family? Your country? The world?

3. In what ways do our eating habits in America reflect the culture of other nations? How have the eating habits of others influenced your family? You?

4. Discuss with your friends good eating habits and poor ones. Do you think they wish to improve their eating habits? How could this be done through snacks? Meals? Which eating habits do you consider to be poor ones?

5. Consider the superstitions, prejudice, advertising, ignorance, indifference, and other factors that influence the eating habits in your family. Your eating habits. Those of your friends. Which do you consider the most significant for you? What foods do you like most? Dislike?

6. What do you understand to be the difference between the terms "poorly fed" and "well-fed"?

7. How do you account for the fact that so many in America fall below the recommended diet when we have such an abundance of food in the variety needed, are the most prosperous nation on earth, and have dependable nutritional information?

8. What does research reveal about the diet of teen-agers? In your judgment, how do the eating habits of young people in your community compare with the studies reported in the nation as a whole?

9. Why do both young women and young men need good eating habits? Why is this so important for the girl? In what ways does the father influence the eating habits of the family? How can the mother affect them?

Applying and sharing

1. Visit your library and look up references relating to the life span of the people in different nations. Do you see a relationship between their diet and their life span? Report what you find to your group and to your family.

2. Talk over with your family what you learned in this chapter. What are the problems, if any, in the eating habits of your family? In your own eating habits?

3. The teacher might divide the class into groups, each making a study of a different way in which our country has contributed and is contributing to the improvement of its people's diets. Those of people in other countries. Each group might then report and discuss what has been learned in the study.

4. Keep a record of the food you eat for one week. Use a notebook so that you can refer to this record throughout this study. Write down everything you eat or drink and the amounts at meals and between meals. Keep this record for future use. See pages 29–30, Chapter 2, for a guide on how to keep such a record.

5. If there is a returned Peace Corps volunteer living in your community, discuss with your teacher the possibility of inviting this person to share with your group his or her experiences in the country where he or she worked, particularly as regards the eating habits of the people.

the meaning of a balanced diet

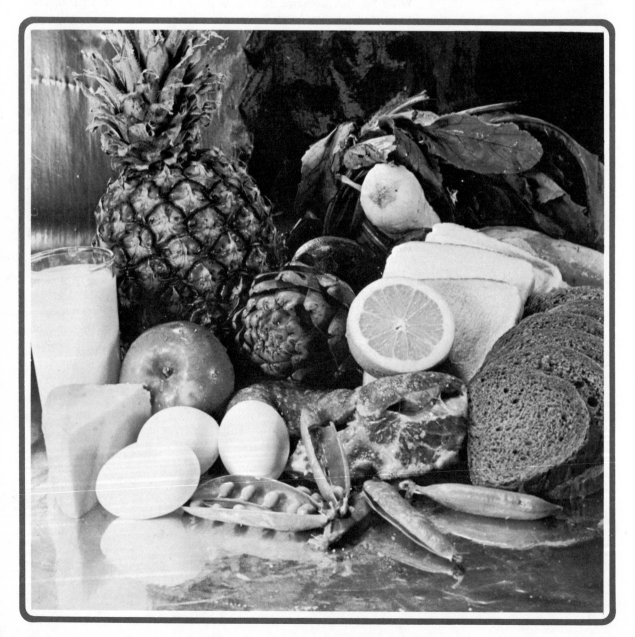

Nutrition and health

A balanced diet is one that provides the variety of foods in sufficient amounts daily to meet the changing needs of the body. It provides a basis for good nutrition and sound health.

Nutrition is the science of food as it relates to health, appearance, physical vitality, mental alertness, and length of life. It has also been defined as the chemistry of life. Today we have a large fund of knowledge, built up by specialists, to guide us in eating a well-balanced diet. But we cannot obtain this knowledge by heeding the advertising about foods, for this is often slanted to sell the food. Dependable knowledge of nutrition is not inherited, nor can we absorb it casually. It must be learned and put into use to help us eat wisely for good health. Before we start our study of the specific foods that make a balanced meal and day's diet, let us discuss a few basic concepts that can help us better understand the role of food.

Food is the material that helps our bodies develop, from tip to toe, according to our hereditary pattern. If we eat wisely, we can reach our full genetic potential. If there are deficiencies in our diet, they will affect our growth and development.

Nutrients are the different tiny parts of a food. These are broken down in digestion. Chemists find that the body is made up of some 50 nutrients. When we eat a balanced diet, this remarkable body of ours can manufacture about 25 of these. Fortunately, we do not have to learn the names of all nutrients in order to include them in the daily diet. They fall into five general classes: carbohydrates, proteins, fats, vitamins, and minerals. With the aid of enzymes, hormones, and water, different tissues select different combinations of nutrients to make and remake us and keep us functioning.

The balanced diet and calories

Many of us confuse a "balanced diet" with counting calories. A calorie is not a food at all, any more than a gallon or a ton is a food. A calorie is a measure of heat—specifically, the amount of heat required to raise the temperature of one gram of water one degree centigrade. A large calorie is the amount of heat required to raise the temperature of one kilogram of water (2.2 pounds) one degree centrigrade. The large calorie is used in the study of food. The body must have fuel for energy. Energy-heat is measured by this unit.

It takes a smaller amount of lead than of oranges to produce a ton, but both have weight. Similarly, it takes a smaller amount of soft drinks, candy, or potato chips to meet the body's energy requirement than oranges, but both have energy-producing substance—and there the comparison ends. The aim of a balanced diet is to keep the supply of food eaten for energy in balance with your needs for good nutrition. "A well-fed horse can pull a heavy load, and a well-fed man has strength of muscle and of brain, while a poorly nourished man has not," observed Dr. W. O. Atwater, a pioneer in nutrition, in 1894.

When we say that a food is fattening, we mean that we eat more of one or all of these three nutrients (shown in Table 2–1) than the body can immediately use. Thus the excess is stored as fatty tissue on the body, technically called adipose tissue.

Recommended daily dietary allowances*

The purpose of the National Research Council is to help the Federal Government in its efforts to

---

Recommended Daily Dietary Allowances, 7th ed., National Academy of Sciences Publication No. 1694 (Washington, D.C., 1968).

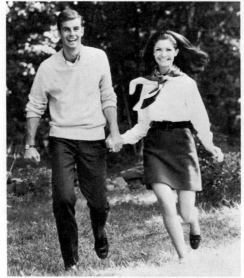

Nonmetallic elements
compose 96% of the body:

OXYGEN	65%
CARBON	18%
HYDROGEN	10%
NITROGEN	3%

Mineral elements compose
about 4% of the body:

CALCIUM	
PHOSPHORUS	2.3% to 3.4%
POTASSIUM	
SULFUR	
CHLORINE	0.95%
SODIUM	
MAGNESIUM	
IRON	0.004%
MANGANESE	0.0003%
COPPER	0.00015%
IODINE	0.00004%

and others in such small
amounts as to be considered
unimportant at present.

give the people the benefits of scientific knowledge. The depression led, in 1936, to the first nation-wide survey of the food eaten by the American people. It was revealed that about one-third of our population had poor diets. The establishment of the Food and Nutrition Board during World War II led to the first published set of recommendations aimed at improving the nation's eating habits.

The members of the Food and Nutrition Board are selected for their ability to interpret nutrition research and for their sound judgment. They are appointed by the National Research Council and meet at least every five years to review (and, when practicable, to improve) their recommendations as our needs change and as research throws new light on these needs.

Seven new nutrients added to recommended diet

The rapid progress of research made it possible for the Board in 1968 to refine its recommendations by adding seven new nutrients to those formerly recommended. These include three B vitamins—B_6, B_{12}, and folacin (folic acid)—one

fat-soluble vitamin—E—and three minerals—phosphorus, iodine, and magnesium. The amounts needed for each age and sex is given in the Appendix, pages 446–447. As we discuss the various food groups, we shall deal with the major food sources of each of these nutrients.

The outstanding difference between the 1968 edition of the Recommended Daily Dietary Allowances and the 1964 edition is the lowering of calorie requirements. This is due to our life of increasing inactivity. Schoolchildren in pioneer America often walked two to five miles a day to school. Their parents burned up energy in other rugged activity. While some of us are still quite active physically, there is a general trend toward inactivity. Some people will not even walk one block to buy a loaf of bread. This decline in physical activity explains why the Board has recommended a reduction in calorie intake for an adult man from 4500 daily (the amount recommended between 1941 and 1948) to 2800. For women in the same age group, the drop is from 3000 daily to 2000.

Technology has contributed to our increasing inactivity. Machines do the heavy work for men. Women have convenience equipment, convenience foods, and little outdoor work around the home,

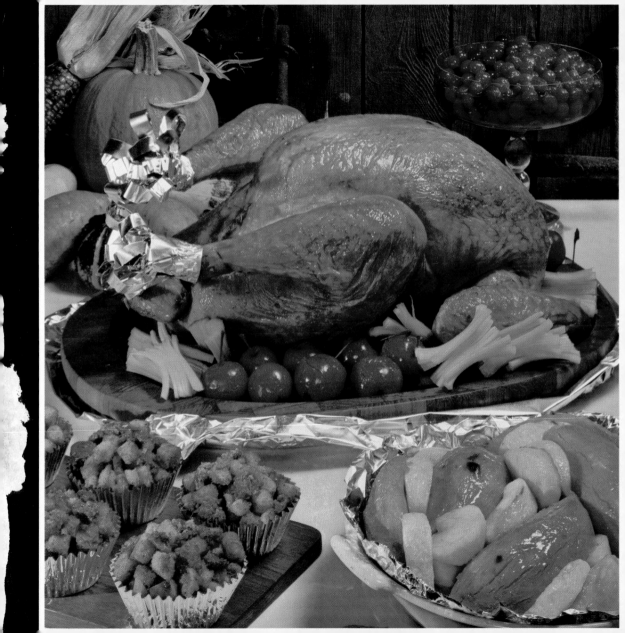

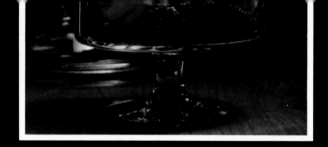

(right) Dried fruits—rich sources of natural sugar—make excellent desserts and snacks.

Ham steak with white grapes, crisp salad, and scalloped rice—a tempting. nourishing meal for any occasion.

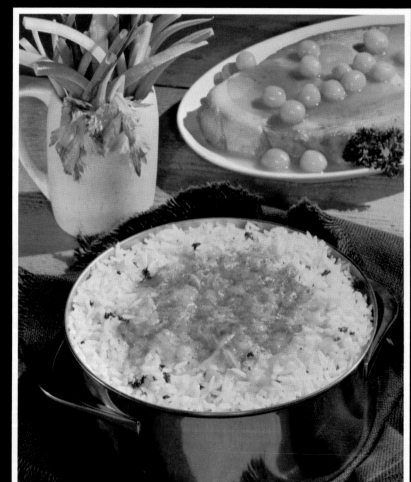

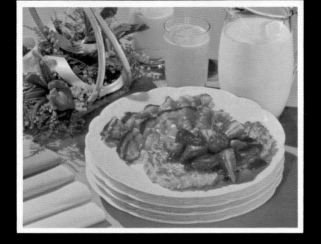

(left) *A breakfast as cheerful and invigorating as a bright spring morning.* (below) *For a "different" roast beef dinner, serve macaroni-bean salad, Swiss chard, herbed bread, and fruit with sharp cheese.*

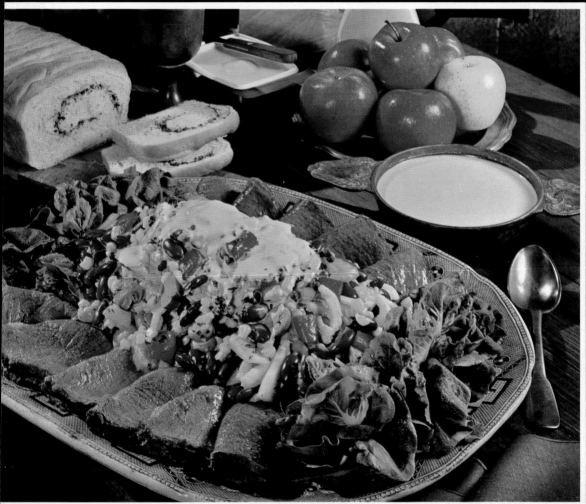

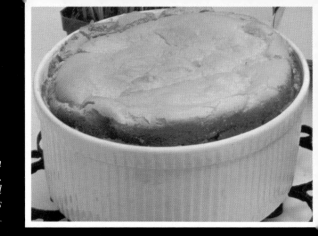

(right) *Cheese soufflé is a light, nutritious dish that is ideal for lunch, brunch, or supper.*
(below) *An American version of a traditional Greek dinner: roast leg of lamb with special spices and side dishes.*

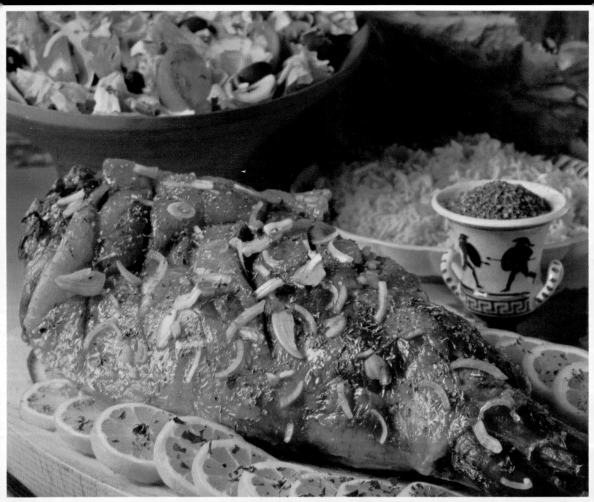

Baked chicken Provençal and salad provide important nutrients recommended for sound health.

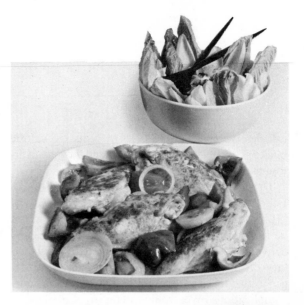

table 2–1 **How the Body Uses the Three Nutrients That Yield Energy-Heat (Calories)**

(1 gm)	CALORIE YIELD	MAIN FUNCTION IN THE BODY	HOW EXCESS AMOUNTS ARE USED
CARBO-HYDRATE	4	Burned to yield energy-heat. Spares the use of protein. Helps use fat.	Stored as glycogen (sugar) in small amounts. Changed to fat and stored as body fat.
FAT	9	Burned to yield energy-heat. Forms tissue fat. Has other necessary functions.	Stored as body fat. Changed back to carbohy-drates to be burned for energy as needed.
PROTEIN	4	Builds and repairs body tissues. Essential for life and growth. Part of team to form hor-mones, enzymes, anti-bodies, and every cell in the body. Small amount burned to yield energy (after elim-inating nitro-gen), if needed.	Changed to carbohydrate to be burned for energy or to be con-verted to fat and stored as fat.

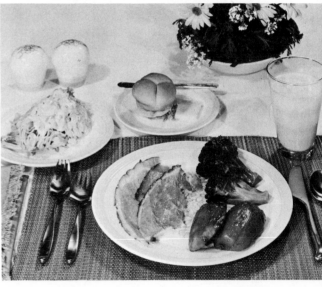

This balanced dinner is both satisfying and nutritious. As it is quite high in calories, the dessert should be fresh fruit.

and are constantly looking for shortcuts to "save energy." Medical authorities advise us to use energy. We simply add pounds of stored fat if we eat like the physically active and act like the phys-ically inactive. Naturally, we don't burn up the calories we eat. The purpose of reducing caloric intake is to help us control the tendency to overweight.

Dr. W. H. Sebrell, the 1968 chairman of the Food and Nutrition Board, sums it up this way: "It is our feeling that a better level of health would be reached if the population were more physically active, and there is growing evidence that a sedentary life is one of the causes contributing to degenerative disease and obesity with their many complications. We would prefer to see physical activity increased, rather than caloric intake further reduced."*

The Board's advice regarding intake of calcium, vitamin A, and vitamin D remains the same. The requirements for the B vitamins are slightly adjusted. The amount of iron is raised, because of the high rate of anemia; that for protein is lowered from 1.0 grams per kilogram of body weight (2.2 pounds) to 0.9 gram per day. The requirement for vitamin C is increased for the very young and slightly decreased for older age groups. Thus, through the services of scientists who serve on this board without pay, we have the benefit of the best advice on what constitutes a good diet.

Water

While water is not a nutrient, it is a part of every cell in the body and constitutes about one-half the body weight. About one and a half cups of water is formed in the end products of oxidizing the food we eat. Figure 2–2 shows the amount of water in different foods we eat.

*W. H. Sebrell, Jr., "Recommended Dietary Allowances, 1968 Revision," *Journal of the American Dietetics Association*, Vol. 54:2, February 1969, pp. 101–108.

fig. 2–2 **AMOUNTS OF WATER IN VARIOUS FOODS***

Food	Percent
VEGETABLES, FRESH	90%
FRUITS, FRESH	85%
MILK, WHOLE	87%
BREAD, ENRICHED	36%
EGGS	74%
BEEF, HAMBURGER	60%
CHICKEN, BREAST	58%
LIVER, BEEF	57%
FISH, HADDOCK	66%

*Source: *Nutritive Value of Foods*, U. S. Department of Agriculture Home and Garden Bulletin No. 72 (Washington, D.C.: U. S. Government Printing Office, 1963).

Regular exercise is important for good health, now and in the future.

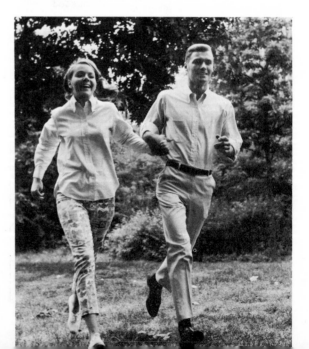

Water is needed for every body function, and therefore for the use of all nutrients and the removal of waste products. It helps regulate body temperature and all mechanical functions of the body, even moving the joints.

The recommendations for good eating (Table 2–2) are meant for normal, healthy persons of all age groups. They are not the minimum needed to prevent nutritional deficiency disease. Nor are they optimal—producing the highest nutrition.

table 2–2   *Recommended Guide to Good Eating—Use Daily*

FOUNDATION FOODS	
MILK GROUP:	3 or more glasses milk—children (1 glass equals 8 oz., or ½ pt.) 4 or more glasses milk—teen-agers 2 or more glasses milk—adults 3 or more glasses milk—expectant mothers 4 or more glasses milk—lactating mothers Cheese, ice cream, and other foods made with milk can supply part of the milk requirement
MEAT GROUP:	2 or more servings (a serving is 3 oz.) cooked lean meat, fish, poultry, glandular meats; 2 eggs; 2¼ oz. cheddar-type cheese Dry beans, peas, nuts as alternates
VEGETABLE-FRUIT GROUP:	4 or more servings (a serving cooked is ½ cup; or 1 whole potato, ear of corn, medium apple, orange, or banana, etc.) A dark green or deep yellow vegetable at least every other day A citrus fruit, tomato, raw cabbage or other vitamin-C-rich foods A potato or equivalent Other vegetables and fruits
BREAD-CEREAL GROUP:	4 or more servings a day according to need (a serving is 1 slice bread, or ⅔ cup cooked cereal, or 1 oz. or 1 cup of ready-to-eat cereal) Whole-grain or enriched or restored
ADDITIONAL FOODS	
FATS:	Some in the form of vegetable oil high in linoleic acid to season food
SWEETS:	To make the diet more palatable and satisfying in proportion to individual need
VITAMIN D:	In the form of fortified milk or vitamin concentrate, under direction of physician during growth, pregnancy, and lactation—400 I.U. daily

table 2–3 *Translating the Pattern for a Balanced Diet into Balanced Daily Meals and Snacks*

PATTERN	BREAKFAST MENU	MENU ALTERNATES
FRUIT OR JUICE (Rich in vitamin C)	Whole orange	½ grapefruit, citrus juices, tomato juice, ½ cantaloupe, berries, other fruits in season
MAIN DISH (Protein)	Scrambled egg with cottage cheese	Whole-grain or enriched cereal cooked with nonfat dry milk; ready-to-eat cereal and milk; French toast; pancakes, waffles, spoon bread; lean ham, broiled chops, liver, kidneys, or fish; cheese, peanut butter, cottage cheese, bean soup, liverwurst sandwich
MILK (Fortified with vitamin D)	1 8-oz. glass, whole or skim	Cheese, yogurt (nonfat, low-fat, or whole), hot chocolate, milk shake
BREAD Whole-grain or enriched	1 slice or more	Toast, plain; hot quick breads; sweet breads (if calories permit)
SOFT MARGARINE, BUTTER, OR VEGE-TABLE OIL	1–2 t.	More or less, according to need
SWEET	1 t.-1 T. jam	More or less, according to need
HOT BEVERAGE	Coffee or tea	Sugar, cream, or lemon added, according to taste and need

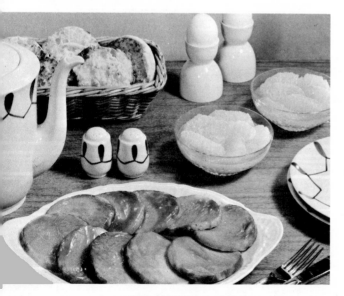

This breakfast supplies a variety of important nutrients to start your day off right.

Principles for planning balanced meals

A good day's diet results from knowing how to plan each meal and snack of the day and how to prepare these foods so that you and your family enjoy eating them. In the next 10 chapters, we will come to understand better why we need some foods from each group in each meal, and how to prepare them. The following is the pattern for a balanced meal.

1/Include in each meal approximately a third of the protein needed during the day, some of this coming from animal foods, such as milk, red meat, poultry, fish, organs, and eggs.

2/Include in each meal a variety of foods to provide essential minerals and vitamins, as listed

PATTERN	LUNCH OR SUPPER MENU	MENU ALTERNATES
MAIN DISH (Protein)	Tuna fish salad	Other fish salads, chicken or turkey salad, bean or fruit salad; chef's salad, egg salad; cottage cheese; hot casserole dish using cheese, baked beans, meat, fish, or poultry with any combination of vegetables and/or rice, noodles, bulgur, or macaroni products; omelet; soups, such as bean, meat-vegetable, fish or poultry chowder, pea, lentil, or minestrone; sandwiches, such as meat, fish, poultry, cheese, eggs, peanut butter, baked beans, hamburgers, frankfurters, or liverwurst; enchiladas with cheese filling; tacos with beans, meat, or cheese filling
BREAD Whole-grain or enriched	Hot corn muffin	Other hot muffins, popovers (plain), toasted English muffins, crackers, fresh yeast bread, any quick bread
MILK	1 8-oz. glass	Cottage cheese; other foods as suggested for breakfast
BUTTER, SOFT MARGARINE, OR VEGETABLE OIL	1 t.	More or less, according to need
DESSERT	1 banana	Fresh fruit in season, canned, or frozen; ice cream, ice milk, pudding; cookie, gingerbread, deep-dish fruit pie

PATTERN	SNACK MENU	MENU ALTERNATES
FRUIT	1 apple	See Table 2–5 for alternates

PATTERN	DINNER OR SUPPER MENU	MENU ALTERNATES
MEAT, FISH, POULTRY, ORGAN MEAT, OR ALTERNATE	Baked fresh ham	Lean pork (fresh or cured), lean beef, lamb, chicken, turkey; fish, shellfish; liver; beans, peas, lentils (dried); cheese
STARCHY VEGETABLE	1 med. baked potato	White or sweet potatoes, parsnips; hot breads; rice, macaroni products, bulgur; dumplings
GREEN OR YELLOW VEGETABLE	½ c. collards (cooked)	Turnip greens, spinach, dandelion greens, kale, broccoli, Swiss chard, lettuce; summer squash, corn, carrots; cauliflower, string beans, zucchini squash; others
RAW VEGETABLE SALAD OR FRESH FRUIT	½ cantaloupe	Other fresh, canned, frozen, or dried fruit; raw finger vegetables or salad
BREAD Whole-grain or enriched	1 slice or more	Toast, hot quick breads, sweet breads (if calories permit)
SOFT MARGARINE, BUTTER, OR VEGETABLE OIL	1–2 t.	More or less, according to need
BEVERAGE	Coffee or tea	Sugar, cream, or lemon added, according to taste

PATTERN	SNACK MENU	MENU ALTERNATES
MILK AND COOKIE	Milk and cookie	Fresh fruit, before bed, if desired and needed

in Table 2–2. Well-selected food from each food group will do this.

3/A vitamin C-rich food is desirable in one meal, and helpful in each. Use a raw fruit or vegetable at least once during the day.

4/Use liver and seafood at least once during the week.

5/Combine foods for variety in nutrients and flavor—bland with sharp; in texture—crisp with soft; and in color—contrast.

6/Serve no large meals or small meals, but divide the amount of food about equally, with breakfast slightly smaller and dinner not too large.

7/If you or any other member of the family has an overweight problem, plan meals high in roughage—rich in vegetables and fruits, low in fats and sweets (see Chapters 11, 12, and 20).

8/When snacks are eaten, select them to fit into the total food need for the day, lest you gain weight.

Fish should be served at least once a week. This provides generous protein with low calories and low fat.

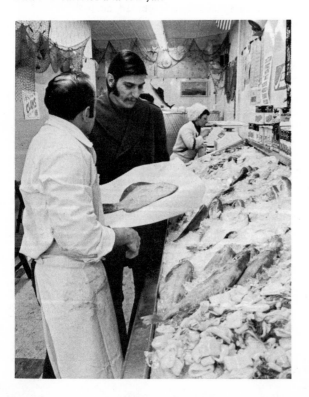

table 2–4 Nutritious Low-Calorie Snacks for Any Age

MILK AND MILK PRODUCTS	Plain milk, nonfat milk shake, nonfat malted milk, spiced milk, ice milk; low-fat cheese; pizza made with cheese; low-fat yogurt
FRUITS	Fruit drinks; fresh raw fruit; dried fruit; canned or frozen fruit
VEGETABLES	Finger vegetables—raw celery, lettuce, cucumbers, tomatoes, radishes, carrots, green or red peppers, broccoli, cauliflower, peas, etc.
MEAT	Meat, poultry, fish, or other protein foods, such as eggs, peanut butter, or baked beans, in sandwiches with whole-grain or enriched bread
OTHERS	Home-popped corn with 1 T. vegetable oil per ⅓ c. corn added; dry-roasted peanuts (without added fat); angel food cake, sponge cake

As we proceed in our study, you will learn how to control weight by careful selection of each food in the diet. Consider the nutrients in each meal and each day as a unit. Such an understanding will protect you from fad diets.

Before a doctor can prescribe a cure, he must diagnose the disease. Similarly, you can diagnose how good your present eating habits are. One way to do this is by a dietary study of yourself. Keep a record of the food you eat for one week—everything you eat and drink at meals, and everything between meals. Then analyze it and compare the results to RDA, pages 446–447.

7/Take one typical day's diet at each season and calculate the amount of each nutrient it contains. Use the table on pages 448–455 (in the Appendix).

To calculate the calories derived from each nutrient in the food, follow a simple formula. Using milk as an example: in one glass of milk there are 9 grams each of protein and fat (3.5 percent fat) and 12 grams of carbohydrate. Each gram of fat yields 9 calories and each gram of protein or carbohydrate yields 4. Multiply the number of grams by the number of calories that each of the nutrients yields, to learn the number of calories from that nutrient.

How to keep a dietary record for one day or more

1/Have a separate notebook for this purpose and keep it for future reference.

2/List the date, day of the week, meal, and snacks as: September 25, Monday, Breakfast, Lunch, Dinner, Snack (if any).

3/Write down everything you consume at each meal or between meals (every food or beverage).

4/State the measure of what you eat. For example, for dinner: ½ cup of carrots, 1 baked potato, ¾ cup tossed green salad, 1 glass of milk, 2 slices of roast beef, 1 roll, 1 pat of butter (½ tablespoon), gingerbread (1½-inch square), plus 2 tablespoons of applesauce, black coffee.

5/Estimate the amount of fat and sugar used in seasoning foods and include it in your listing.

6/Keep your first record for seven consecutive days, if possible. Repeat this procedure at each season of the year.

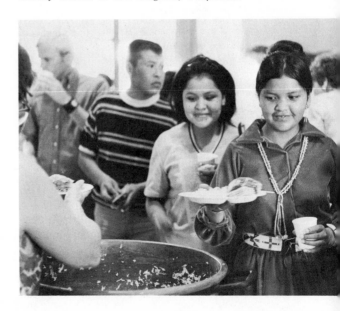

These American Indian teen-agers are learning the principles of good nutrition at the Signal Hill Community Center in Los Angeles, California.

This is a hearty, well-balanced breakfast. How would you cut down on calories to meet modern dietary recommendations?

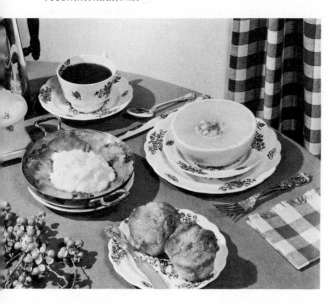

Protein:	9 x 4 = 36	(calories)
Fat:	9 x 9 = 81	
Carbohydrate:	12 x 4 = 48	
	———	
Total calories	165*	

It is of value to you to keep a complete record of all that you eat and drink, so that you may have an idea of your eating habits. Select typical meals and snacks you regularly eat. If you wish to keep this in chart form, follow the plan in the table of Nutritive Values of Foods in the Appendix. Then total the amounts per meal and per day, including the snacks.

---

*In round numbers, the total calories in 1 glass of milk is usually listed as 160, owing to variation in fat content.

Meaning of metabolism

Some people think a balanced diet doesn't matter. This mistake is often due to lack of familiarity with that important word *metabolism*. Almost four centuries ago, Sanctorius, an Italian with a fine mind and strong curiosity, first looked into the question of metabolism. Every day he weighed himself, weighed all of the food and drink he took, and then weighed himself again. The discrepancy puzzled him. Although he didn't know enough chemistry or have the right equipment to find out what becomes of the food that is eaten, he has been called the father of experiments in metabolism.

Not to be confused with digestion, **metabolism is the term used to describe all the chemical changes that take place in the tissues of the body.** Metabolism consists of two processes, anabolism and catabolism. During anabolism, food is chemically changed so as to build cells in body tissue, to maintain the healthy cells we have and to repair those that are deteriorated. Catabolism is that part of the process that destroys old, useless tissues. It also breaks down waste products into simple substances—oxygen, hydrogen, carbon, and nitrogen products—which are eliminated in excretions. Thus, through metabolism, the foods we eat are chemically taken apart and nutrients are released for their work. New tissues are formed. Food is oxidized for immediate use as energy-heat. If there is a surplus, it is stored as fat.

We read much about basal metabolism and often physicians advise that it be measured. What is it? **Basal metabolism is the very least amount of energy required to keep the internal life processes going.**

To be accurately measured, basal metabolism must be tested 12 to 15 hours after the last food

Workers in the Head Start program take turns cooking special dishes representing their different backgrounds.

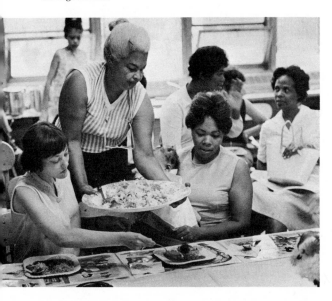

was eaten, and when the person is lying at complete and comfortable rest. Basal metabolism shows how much energy, or how many calories, the body at rest uses for its internal workings—how much is needed to keep the heart beating, the blood circulating, the lungs breathing, and the temperature controlled, and for its other involuntary functioning.

How food is transformed into the person you are

Digestion

Digestion is the process of breaking down food, both mechanically and chemically, so that it can be absorbed and distributed for use. Table 2–5 is a simplification of this process. It begins in the mouth while the food is being chewed. Chewing

grinds food into small particles, moistens it with saliva, and releases nutrients. Ptyalin (ti′ ə lən), an enzyme in the salivary juice, starts sugar and starch digestion. Simple sugars are split, ready for absorption, and cooked starch is broken into smaller molecules (dextrin). The food is swallowed.

Now an amazing kind of involuntary automation occurs. In the stomach, the food pulp is churned about by strong muscular contractions. It mixes with swallowed saliva and the digestion of carbohydrates continues in the upper part of the stomach. Gastric juice flows in and protein and fat begin to be digested, but digestion of starch and sugar halts. This is due to the acid in the gastric juice, which stops the action of the ptyalin. The food is slowly pushed out of the stomach into the approximately 24-foot length of the small intestine, where the major part of digestion takes place. The liver produces bile. The gall bladder, which stores bile, now gradually releases it. Bile produces a fine emulsion of fats, and enzymes can now split the complex fat molecules into smaller and separate parts (fatty acids and glycerol). The pancreas adds its enzymes to those of the intestinal juice. The digestion of protein, carbohydrate, and fat is completed in the small intestines.

Recent research indicates that digestion is aided by certain vitamins in the B-complex group, including folic acid (folacin). Vitamin K seems to play a role in aiding the process, and there are "friendly" bacteria that are useful, too.

Absorption

Digestion completed, the small intestine becomes the arena in which absorption also takes place. The undigestible cellulose from fruits, vegetables, and whole-grain cereal-bread forms bulk. The

fig. 2–3 **THE COURSE FOOD TRAVELS TO BECOME PART OF YOU***

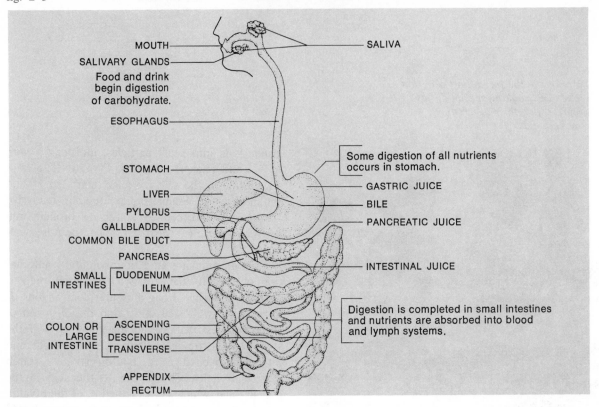

MOUTH — — SALIVA

SALIVARY GLANDS

Food and drink
begin digestion
of carbohydrate.

ESOPHAGUS

Some digestion of all nutrients
occurs in stomach.

STOMACH

LIVER — GASTRIC JUICE

PYLORUS — BILE

GALLBLADDER — PANCREATIC JUICE

COMMON BILE DUCT

PANCREAS

SMALL
INTESTINES { DUODENUM
ILEUM — INTESTINAL JUICE

COLON OR
LARGE { ASCENDING
INTESTINE { DESCENDING
TRANSVERSE

Digestion is completed in small intestines
and nutrients are absorbed into blood
and lymph systems.

APPENDIX

RECTUM

table 2–5   *Process of Digestion*

NUTRIENT	FOOD	SPLIT BY DIGESTIVE JUICES DURING DIGESTION*	FUNCTIONS IN BODY
PROTEIN	Meat, poultry, fish, organs, milk, cheese, eggs, legumes, nuts, cereal grains, others	Broken into amino acids; absorbed into bloodstream	Build tissues in all parts of body for growth and repair. On a team to build hormones, enzymes, antibodies, and some vitamins. Help regulate body functioning. Used as energy, if needed. Excess stored as fat.
FATS	Oils; hard, soft, and semi-soft fats; fats in foods, visible and invisible	Fatty acids and glycerols absorbed by blood and lymph after being finely emulsified in small intestines	Concentrated energy-heat. Provide essential fatty acids. Help in absorption and use of fat-soluble vitamins. Give flavor and satiety to diet. Perform other functions.
CARBOHYDRATES	Starch and sugars	Glucose—absorbed by blood Fructose Galactose	Low-cost energy. Simple sugar gives only energy-heat, flavor. "Complex" starch carries other nutrients.

*By splitting apart proteins, fats, and carbohydrates, digestion makes available to the blood all the vitamins, minerals, and other nutrients the body needs. The way to acquire good nutrition is from well-balanced meals.

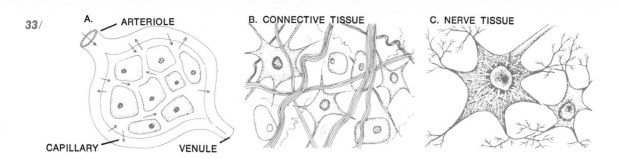

A. ARTERIOLE — CAPILLARY — VENULE

B. CONNECTIVE TISSUE

C. NERVE TISSUE

muscular contractions known as peristaltic (**per ə stol′ tik**) waves, which have mixed and pushed the food during digestion, also force the bulk against the more than five million *villi* lining the wall of the small intestine. (See Figure 2–4). These villi are made up of many folds of fingerlike tissue. It is estimated that if the villi could be spread out they would have an absorptive surface of about 45 square feet or more. This would cover the floor of a room nine feet by five feet. The villi close around the nutrients pressed against them and absorb them into the bloodstream.

The importance of balanced meals

The importance of a balance of food in a meal is brought home to us more vividly the more we understand how it is absorbed. Calcium cannot be absorbed from the digestive tract without vita-

fig. 2–4: *(X) Wall of the small intestine; (Y) Lining of intestinal wall, composed of tiny villi; (Z) Structure of a villus.*

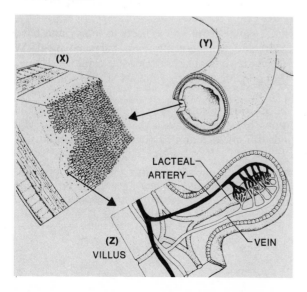

(X)

(Y)

LACTEAL
ARTERY

(Z)
VILLUS

VEIN

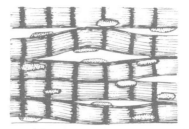

D. MUSCLE TISSUE

fig. 2–5: *Different cells make different types of body tissues from the nutrients supplied by the blood.*

min D. Vitamin B_{12}, which is highly important in blood formation, goes to waste unless a substance called the intrinsic factor is present in the gastric juice. The fat-soluble vitamins—A, D, E, and K—require the presence of fat for absorption. Water-soluble vitamins, minerals, and simple sugars are absorbed directly from the small intestine, as are the amino acids that result from the splitting of proteins, carbohydrates, and fats. Other fats, as well as the fat-soluble vitamins, may pass through the villi into the lymph system, where they undergo change before entering the bloodstream.

The process of digestion and absorption is an indication of how wonderfully we are made, as well as how important our food choices can be. We determine what we shall eat, but after that the process is beyond the control of our will. Absorption is selective; the body takes control. The following drawings help us understand how body cells work with no assistance on our part except to provide them with proper food.

Figure 2–5a shows how close the blood supply is to each cell. The arrows indicate how nutrients from the food you eat and waste from the cells diffuse back and forth. The tiny, porous capillaries are the final means of transportation for this exchange. It is not an orderly procession like an assembly line belt, but a constant motion of "moving and bouncing in all directions," as the physiologist A. C. Guyton* states it.

Utilization

After the food is digested, absorbed, and carried finally to each cell in the body, the cells perform their functions for us in building and rebuilding specific types of body tissues. Though cells differ, they have much in common. Each is an independent automaton that lives and grows. When body tissue is injured or wears out, the cells divide and make new cells, provided they have the combination of nutrients to do the job. They use the different nutrients from the food you eat to make and remake you.

Meaningful words

anabolism
balanced diet
basal metabolism
calorie
carbohydrate
catabolism
fat
food absorption villi
food digestion
food utilization
metabolism
minerals
nutrients
nutrition
protein
ptyalin

Thinking and evaluating

1. What is a balanced diet? Does a daily food guide assure one? Explain.

2. What does the RDA table in the Appendix mean to you now? Do you think more knowledge of different foods could give it even deeper meaning? How might this help your life now? Later?

3. Using a seven-day record of the food you ate, and Table 2–1 and those in the Appendix, calculate the total calories you had in your diet from carbohydrates, from protein, and from fat. Save the calculations for future reference.

4. On the basis of your seven-day record, how would you rate your own diet? What are its weaknesses? Its strengths? Can you improve it? How?

5. Do you think that a young man who expects to marry and have a family needs to understand what constitutes a balanced meal? A balanced day's diet? Explain your answers. Do you think he should assist in doing the shopping or preparing meals if his wife works outside the home?

6. What are the basic food groups? How might one follow the general recommendations but fail to have a balanced diet? Do you think you need a guide for meal planning, or an understanding of foods, or both? Why?

7. Explain the principles for planning a day's balanced diet, including meals and snacks. Why should snacks be considered as part of the daily food plan?

---

*A. C. Guyton, *Textbook of Medical Physiology* (Philadelphia: W. B. Saunders Company, 1966), p. 4.

8. Explain how food is changed from the time it is eaten until it becomes part of your body through digestion, absorption, and utilization by body tissues. How would you explain this to a person who lacks understanding of why we need a balanced meal and a balanced diet?

Applying and sharing

1. Using the sample outline on pages 29–30, make a record of the food and beverages you consumed yesterday. For values refer to the table of Nutritive Values in the Appendix. Analyze each meal and each snack separately. Then add up the calories, protein, fat, calcium, iron, and vitamins listed. Look up the recommended allowances for your age group in the RDA table in the Appendix and compare the totals for the day under each heading. How do you rate? Is this day's diet typical?

2. Using Table 2–2 and also the principles for planning balanced meals (pages 26 and 28), plan menus on a low-cost budget that you would enjoy eating and preparing if you were a young bride. Plan menus for a guest dinner eaten at the table; on the patio; at a picnic; for a special family occasion.

3. Of the meals you planned, prepare at home those for one day. Serve, eat, and analyze them. How can you improve on your food selections or their method of preparation?

4. Try to communicate to your family what you have learned in this chapter and how it can help you. Discuss why we need balanced meals and how to plan them.

meat for
enjoyment and stamina

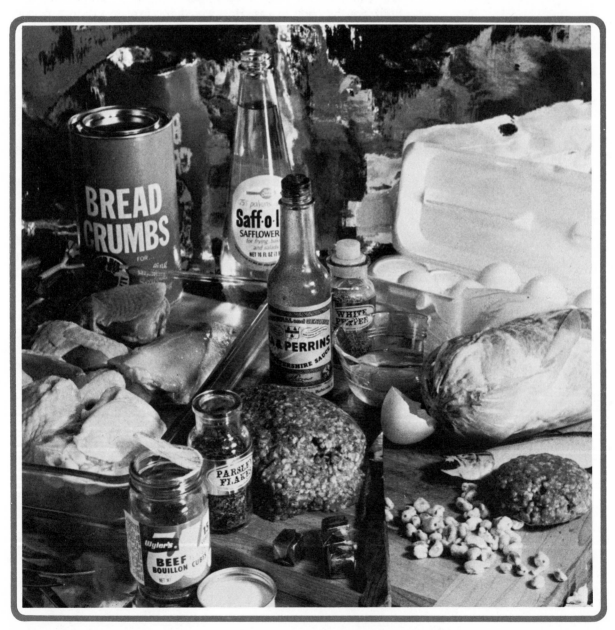

Meat for enjoyment

The juicy flavor and mouth-watering aroma of meat form the center of interest in a meal, whether it is in a public place or in a private home. Our forefathers required a sturdy diet. Meat became a symbol of plenty to them, after the hunger and poverty so many had known in the lands from which they came. We still relish meat as a favorite dish.

As Figure 3–1 shows, we ate more meat and paid more for it in 1965 than we did in 1955, and more beef and poultry than any other meats. Today we are spending more for meat than for any other food group.

Meat for stamina

The high-quality protein in meat gives us strength to do our work, helps make children grow, and enables older people to maintain their vigor. The B vitamins, unknown until 1926 and even later, nevertheless helped our forefathers. These vitamins are found in meat, especially liver and organ meats. The minerals—iron, iodine (in sea fish), phosphorus, magnesium, and traces of many others—add zest to life and full growth for children. The fat in meat was much more important to our forefathers, who performed hard physical labor, than it is for us today, since we live such inactive lives physically.

Another point in its favor is that meat is almost completely digested, and is for that reason a desirable food for all ages, from infants of a few months to the elderly.

Can a food with so many attributes have any weaknesses? How do its advantages measure up against its disadvantages?

Some disadvantages of too much meat in the diet

1/The chief disadvantage is the cost. All of us like the taste, and some people believe that a meal is not a meal without a large serving of meat. But its high cost makes meat absorb an excessive proportion of the food budget. Does the price you pay for your meat take money from other required foods—milk, vegetables, and fruits? Unless you are on a quite liberal food budget, you cannot afford to have meat in every meal and still buy the other foods necessary to keep the diet well-balanced. There are other, less expensive sources of good protein that can help you keep your diet and your budget in good balance.

2/Meat has some nutritional weaknesses. All meats are low in calcium and vitamin C, and most (except liver) are low in vitamin A—chief nutrients that are too low in our diets. In this chapter and Chapter 11, you will see that highly-saturated fat is one problem in meat for most of us today.

3/The bacterial flora of meat is putrefactive, but this is of no significance when you have some fruits, vegetables, and milk in the meal.

4/The mineral ash of meat is acid when oxidized (burned) in the body, but this is of no consequence on a balanced diet.

Since a good protein dish is the first thing we think of in planning a meal, let us look into the nature and sources of protein.

Protein and you

Protein forms the nucleus (center) of all cells, and is therefore essential for all growth and repair of each tissue. It is the essence of life. A Dutch

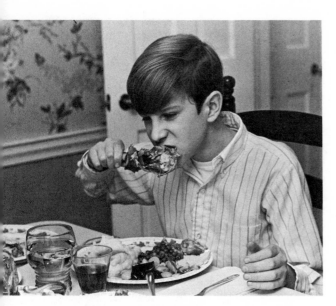

Meat lends zest and enjoyment to a meal. A turkey leg is a great treat on festive occasions.

physician-chemist, G. J. Mulder, in his studies found a "life substance" in plants and animals that was essential for life. While he did not isolate it, he named it protein, which means in Greek "of first importance." It is the only nutrient that contains nitrogen and is the largest and most complex molecule found in food. It consists of a complex group of amino acids and also contains carbon, hydrogen, oxygen, frequently sulfur, and sometimes phosphorus, iron, iodine, and other elements.

Protein in the body

It is not surprising that there is more protein in your body than any other nutrient—half the dry weight. A tenth is in your skin, a fifth in your bones, and a third in your muscles. The thick part of the blood is 95 percent protein, and protein serves important purposes in the fluid, too.

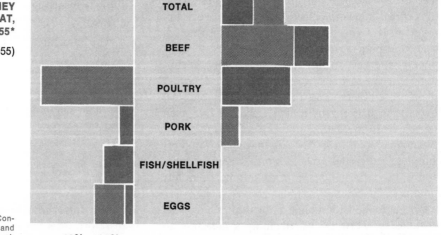

fig. 3–1   **USE AND MONEY VALUE OF MEAT, 1965 AND 1955***

(Percent change 1965 and 1955)

Quantity   Price

TOTAL

BEEF

POULTRY

PORK

FISH/SHELLFISH

EGGS

−20% −10%   0   +10% +20% +30% +40% +50% +60%

*Nationwide Household Food Consumption Surveys, Spring 1965 and Spring 1955, Agricultural Research Service, USDA.

table 3–1 *Meat Consumed Per Person in the U. S. in 1965**

MEAT NAME	AMOUNT PER PERSON (Pounds)
FISH	10.6
CHICKEN AND TURKEY	40.8
OTHER MEATS	166.6
Total	218.0

*National Food Situation, National Science Foundation Publication No. 115 (Washington, D.C., 1966).

Protein in plants and animals

Plants synthesize (produce) protein right out of the energy of the sun, the oxygen in the air, and the water and nitrogen in the soil. One group, legumes, can take nitrogen from the air, as well as from the soil. Animals can make protein from plants. Since we eat both plant and animal foods, we are able to use both to advantage. But the proteins in plants lack some essential amino acids that man must have; therefore, we must supplement plants with animal proteins that contain all the amino acids.

Nature of the protein molecule

Amino acids

A protein molecule has been compared to the letters of the alphabet. There are some 22 amino acids in protein, each with its own name and function. When the body has the other nutrients it needs, it can make about 14 of these. Eight must be supplied in food; these are called essential, for without them we cannot live.

Complete protein

A food that contains all the essential amino acids in the required amounts is said to be a complete protein. Meat, poultry, all kinds of fish, organ meats, milk and milk products, and eggs are our complete protein foods. Every meal should contain some quantity of one or more of these animal foods to meet the body's need for essential amino acids.

Partially complete protein

The protein in vegetables, cereal grains, and fruits lacks one or more of the essential amino acids or does not contain large enough amounts of all of them. Plant foods are spoken of as containing partially complete protein—or limiting protein, to use the newer term. The best plant foods for protein content are soybeans, peanuts, and chick peas.

An incomplete protein cannot promote growth, reproduction, or lactation, nor can it sustain life. Gelatin has been advertised as a protein for building fingernails. Although this food is 100 percent protein, it is an incomplete protein lacking some of the essential amino acids. Unless these essential amino acids are supplied by other foods in the diet, the gelatin alone cannot promote growth. The gelatin advertising shows how people can be led to the wrong conclusions by citing percentages without clearly stating their meaning. To illustrate, one foundation work in experimental nutrition by Amy

Meat is one of our richest sources of protein.

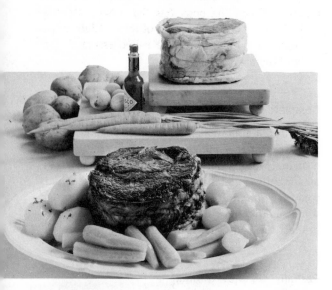

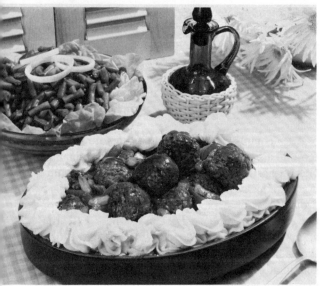

Meat contains all the essential amino acids and is thus valuable at all stages of life.

L. Daniels and Ruth Bennett White* at the University of Iowa reveals that, when healthy young white rats were fed gelatin as the only protein in an otherwise adequate diet, they failed to grow and became weak and feeble, developed unattractive skin, fur, and posture, then had convulsions and died.

Modern science has found a sound basis for the historic custom of eating some bread with meat, milk, or eggs and having some vegetables and fruits in a meal. You can have high-quality protein at less cost when you eat animal foods with plant foods, for then the partially complete protein of the latter is used well.

How protein helps our lives now and later

Protein for normal growth

When infants, growing children, and young people have some, but not enough, high-quality protein in the diet, they do not grow normally, but are stunted. Protein deficiency is also noticeable in adults. Older people are weak and feeble when protein is deficient, a weakness that may occur in younger people, too. The muscle tissue is soft and flabby and lacks strength for normal work and play, and poor posture results. Protein is required for the formation of the genes that carry our hereditary traits, the enzymes that spark

*Amy L. Daniels and Ruth Bennett White, "Vitamin B_1 in Relation to the Development of the Thyroid and Thymus Glands of Suckling Young," and "Influence on the Development of Suckling Young of the Addition of Certain Amino Acids in the Diets of the Mothers," *Society for the Proceedings of Experimental Biology and Medicine*, Vol. 27, June 1930.

chemical reactions within cells, the hormones that regulate body processes, and the gamma globulin and antibodies that fight bacteria and viruses and give us immunity to some diseases. It forms a large part of the blood and is quite important in the use of nutrients inside cells, in the spaces between cells, and in the lymph.

Protein for resistance to disease

Sufficient high-quality protein gives us resistance to disease and viruses and also provides mental alertness and helps our personality. With it, we are more sociable and relaxed, can concentrate, are interested in our work, and have a healthy mental outlook. These are all characteristics of good nutrition.

DEFICIENCY DISEASES. American babies do not get the protein-deficiency disease kwashiorkor (kwä′ shē ör kər)—also called red boy, because the hair turns a red-orange color—but many young children have it in developing nations after they are weaned and placed on the adult diet. This disease does respond to treatment. A virtual miracle takes place when a better diet is instituted, especially with the addition of dry milk. But this food must be imported.

Because of our new knowledge of the chemistry of food and nutrition, great strides are being made to help people meet their protein need with foods they can grow. One agency working to develop such foods is the Institute of Nutrition for Central America and Panama. This institute has produced a food called incaparina, which is a mixture of corn, cottonseed meal, sorghum, and yeast. Children who eat this food don't get kwashiorkor, and those who have it can be cured with incaparina, because the amino acids it contains are sufficiently

well-balanced. Usually, when a person lacks sufficient good protein, he is also deficient in important vitamins and minerals.

PROTEIN SOURCES. Most Americans today are getting enough protein and about two-thirds of it comes from animal sources. Some people on reducing diets, expectant and lactating mothers, some teen-agers, some vegetarians, and some who eat excessive amounts of sweets and fats are not getting enough good-grade protein.

How the body adapts

What happens when the body does not have enough good-grade protein in the diet? First, it

A high-protein diet promotes mental and physical alertness and energy.

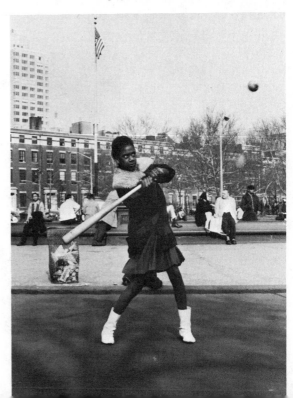

takes amino acids from the liver, then from the muscles or other tissues. The liver is a depot for most nutrients, but the protein reserve there is low. When the body begins to take protein from our tissues to maintain the processes of life, we are destroying ourselves. This makes us look old and tired prematurely and develop other symptoms of aging or ill health.

How protein works best

Protein is better used by the body when it is about equally divided among the three meals of the day than when it is slighted at breakfast or lunch and overeaten at dinner. This was demonstrated in an experiment with college girls at the University of Nebraska. They were placed on a controlled diet that was adequate for the day as a whole. But when two glasses of milk were taken with dinner

and no milk at breakfast, the protein was not retained as well as when one glass was taken with each meal.

If you have one slice of toast, butter, jam, orange juice, and coffee for breakfast, you have only 3 grams of protein. If, for lunch, you have a bag of 10 potato chips, a soft drink, and a candy bar, you have another inadequate snack-type lunch yielding only 1 gram of protein. Then, if at dinner you eat a 6-ounce steak, you get 40 grams of protein. A glass of milk adds 9 grams of protein; a baked potato, 3 grams; a half-cup of green peas, 4½ grams; lettuce salad, 2 grams; and a half-cup of applesauce, ½ gram. Dinner adds up to 59 grams of protein—enough to meet your need for the day. But it will not be as well used as it would be had you taken 27 of the grams of protein in the form of one glass of milk at each meal and had an egg or cereal plus milk at break-

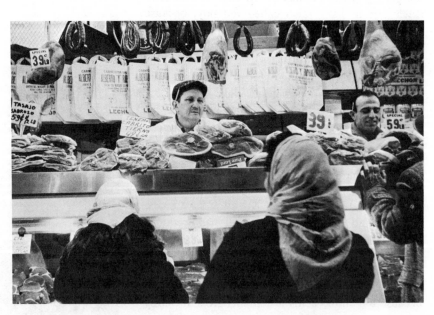

Most Americans get enough protein. It is largely from animal sources.

fast, with part of the day's meat in a sandwich at lunch.

Understanding these principles helps us realize the importance of eating a well-balanced meal at regular intervals.

The pathway of protein in the body

When we eat protein from plants or animal foods, during the digestive process the protein is broken apart by enzymes into amino acids. These fragments of proteins of all kinds are absorbed and travel in the bloodstream. Each tissue needs a specific combination. The hair, skin, and nails need amino acids that contain sulfur, for example. As the amino acids circulate through the microscopic capillaries, each cell traps the combination it needs. It must have all present at one time or none. It is unfortunate for us that it cannot take what is there and wait until the others it requires come along. This makes it imperative that we have the balance we need in every meal.

What, then, determines our need of protein? And how much should we eat each day?

Translating our daily need of protein into meals

The need of protein relates to:

1/Growth. The faster the growth, the greater the need of protein.

2/Size. The larger a person is, the more body tissues he has to maintain.

3/Special conditions. Pregnancy, lactation, and disease require more protein.

When one does not eat enough protein food to maintain life processes, repair tissues, and grow, it is growth that suffers the first loss in children, and repair of worn tissues in adults.

Exercise and protein

Research has disproved an old belief that the more a person exercises, the more protein he needs. Exercise requires more calories to burn as energy, but not more protein, unless muscle growth takes place during the exercise. Athletes need a balanced diet like the rest of us.

Recommended allowance

The recommendations for the amount of protein for each age group each day are given in Table

For a newborn infant, milk supplies all the necessary protein. As he grows older, he requires more from meat and other foods.

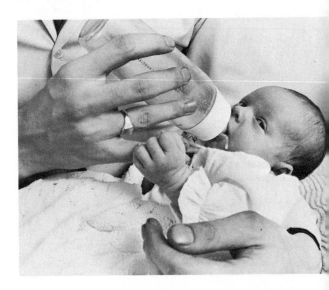

fig. 3–2   **DISTRIBUTION OF AMERICAN DOLLARS IN TERMS OF NUTRIENTS***

NIACIN	41%
PROTEIN	36%
FAT	34%
THIAMINE	29%
IRON	28%
RIBOFLAVIN	22%
VITAMIN A**	22%
CALORIES	19%

Figures based on the use in the daily diet of beef, veal, lamb sheep, hogs, and poultry, but do not include fish.

*R. J. Lee and H. W. Harper, "Meat and Poultry Inspection," *Protecting Our Food: The Yearbook of Agriculture 1966* (Washington, D.C.: USDA), p. 281.

**Most of the vitamin A found in meat is in liver.

3–2. This amounts to 0.9 grams per kilogram of body weight for the "reference" man—age 22, weight 70 kilograms (154 pounds). In the daily food guide, it is recommended that we include at least two servings daily from the meat-egg group, with an occasional alternate from the legume group. About one-half to two-thirds of the daily protein should come from animal foods—meat, eggs, milk, and cheese—and about one-third to one-half from cereal-breads and vegetables, especially dried beans, dried peas, and nuts.

Comparison of a dietary survey made by the USDA Research Service in 1965 with a similar study made in 1955 reveals that the only two nutrients that were improved in the diets were protein (by 3 percent per person per day) and

table 3–2   *How to Meet the Daily Recommended Protein on a Balanced Diet*

PERSONS	AGE	RECOMMENDED PROTEIN DAILY (Grams)	PROTEIN PROVIDED BY RECOMMENDED FOOD GROUPS Measure of Food	Grams (approx.)
CHILDREN	1–3	25	1 quart milk	36
	3–6	30	1 egg	6
	6–8	35		
	8–10	40	3 ounces cooked lean meat, poultry, fish	17–23
Girls	10–12	50		
Boys	10–12	45	Total animal protein	59–65
GIRLS & WOMEN	12–14	50	4 slices bread, or	
	14–75 +	55	3 slices + 1 serving cereal	8
Pregnancy	3rd–9th month	65	4 servings vegetables and fruits,	
Lactation		75	including potato, but not dry beans	4
			½-cup serving dry beans or peas	7
BOYS & MEN	12–14	50	Total plant protein	19
	14–22	60		
	22–75 +	65	Total protein for day	78–84

*Computed from *Nutritive Value of Foods*, Home and Garden Bulletin No. 72, USDA, and *Recommended Daily Dietary Allowances*, Food and Nutrition Board, National Research Council, National Academy of Sciences, 1968 (see pages 446–447).

Dried beans and other legumes should be substituted for meat occasionally. They are good protein foods and are high in iron.

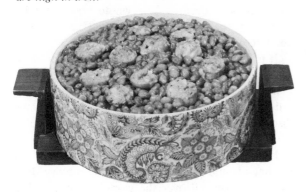

Fish is an excellent source of protein and is low in fat and calories.

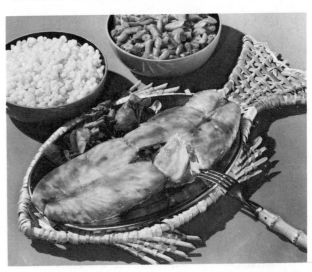

iron. This is attributed to an increase in the amount of meat eaten daily. Even so, there are some children, teen-age girls, and older women whose diets are too low in protein. It would seem that this lack is in the intake of milk, rather than meat, for their diets are also too low in calcium.

When the body has met its need for building and maintaining cells, it then promptly removes the nitrogen from the amino acids and eliminates it as waste products. What remains beyond this need is either burned as energy or stored as body fat.

Meat helps build red blood

The blood is a swift-moving lifeline for the body. We depend on it to carry oxygen from the lungs and the nutrients absorbed from food to the remotest parts of the body, and also to remove waste.

The meat group of foods provides important nutrients to build red blood. But before we consider what these are and how they help us, let us first discuss the blood itself.

Nature of blood

The blood is composed of hemoglobin, plasma, and red and white cells. It is the red cells that concern us here.

Red blood cells

The red blood cell is known technically as erythrocyte (**i rith′ rə sīt**) and is commonly called the red corpuscle. It is shaped like a biconcave disc and is flexible like a bag. It can squeeze through narrow capillaries that have a diameter as small as a hair. This enables us to receive nourishment and oxygen in every cell, from the bones to the retina of the eye. Thus growth and tissue repair proceed normally when the blood is normal.

The normal blood of an adult man contains over five million red blood cells per cubic millimeter of blood, and that of a woman averages about four and one-half million. It is estimated

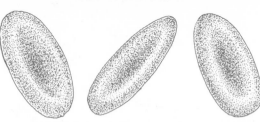

fig. 3–3 **RED BLOOD CELLS**

that an adult's body contains 25 to 35 trillion red blood cells.

Hemoglobin (hē′ mə glō bən) is the thick part of the blood and plasma is the fluid part. The normal hemoglobin content of the red cell is 16 grams per 100 milliliters of blood for an adult man and 14 grams for a woman. If the hemoglobin falls far below normal or if it has too few red cells (usually both occur at the same time), anemia develops.

Red cells are made in the bone marrow. This takes place in all bones up to age 20. At that time, the long bones become too fat in marrow, and the cells are made in the bones of the vertebrae, the sternum, and the ribs.

Red cells are not made for a lifetime, as are arms and legs. Each lives only about four months. The membrane gets old and falls apart. The spleen is the chief organ that destroys the cells. About 80 percent of the iron in the hemoglobin of the cells is salvaged and stored in the liver, the spleen, and the bone marrow for future use in constructing cells.

The amount of blood in the body is four to five quarts in an adult, or about 7 percent of the total weight. Let us consider the nutrients needed to make it.

Functions of iron

Iron is essential for building red blood cells. It combines with protein and vitamins, especially B vitamins, to make hemoglobin. Myoglobin (mī ə glō bən), which is found in muscle tissue, works with oxygen to help regulate tissue oxidation, or the burning of nutrients to release energy.

Iron is required for the formation of enzymes and has been found in minute amounts in all cells.

Its value in the diet is far out of proportion to the small amount needed. The whole body contains only four to five grams of iron. That is about enough to make one stout pin.

It is iron that is responsible for the red color of the blood. When iron is too low, the body cannot make the quality of hemoglobin or the number of red cells required. The blood is pale and the disease referred to as hypochromic anemia results. There are other types of anemia as well.

Reports of the World Health Organization tell us that anemia is one of the major dietary deficiency diseases all over the world. Teen-age girls and women are especially affected. It is also found among older people, infants, and children.

Causes of anemia

Anemia may result from (1) a deficiency of iron in the diet, (2) acute or chronic hemorrhage, (3) disease and other factors, such as atomic explosions, excessive exposure to X ray, and radiation affecting the formation of red blood cells, and (4) a deficiency of folacin or of vitamin C.

Effects of anemia

Anemia increases the work load of the heart. The body is synchronized to the point that, when there are too few red cells with too little hemoglobin, the heart increases its rate of beating. It is thrilling to realize how the body tries to help us. It tries to compensate by speeding up and sending more oxygen through the body in a given amount of time.

You may recognize this by palpitation of the heart or breathlessness, both characteristics of anemia. Other symptoms are the feeling of being constantly tired or tiring easily from slight exertion. Resistance to infection and disease is lowered. Often the color is pale, especially that of the eyelids, earlobes, and lining of the alimentary canal. In long-term anemia, the skin becomes dry and wrinkled and the nails flatten and lose lustre.

Types of anemia that relate to diet

Hemorrhagic anemia

Hemorrhagic (**hem ə raj′ ik**) anemia occurs acutely when there is an accident that causes severe bleeding, bleeding ulcers, frequent nosebleed, or severe loss of blood at childbirth. This type is treated by blood transfusions, which help maintain the normal value and volume of the blood. The blood usually comes from blood banks. It is important that both patient and donor eat an iron-rich diet, for the donor may develop nutritional anemia himself if he gives as many as five blood donations a year.

Iron-deficiency anemia

Iron-deficiency or nutritional anemia is the result of a poorly balanced diet, or one that lacks sufficient iron to make up for losses. Common causes of this disease are (1) a long-term diet too low in iron, (2) the regular loss of blood in menstruation, (3) occasional long or excessively heavy menstrual periods, or (4) excessive loss of blood at childbirth. Anemic mothers usually produce babies that have too low an iron reserve. The infants exhaust this reserve quickly and become anemic, unless the diet is intelligently managed. This is extremely important and is discussed in detail in Chapter 14.

Girls and women who follow fad diets to reduce or control weight usually have a diet deficient in iron and often become anemic. You will not make that mistake.

Pernicious anemia and vitamin B_{12}

Pernicious anemia is a disease, once fatal, in which red blood cells are too few in number and far too large. It is now controlled by vitamin B_{12}. A Nobel prize was shared in 1934 by Doctors G. H. Whipple of the University of Rochester and G. R. Minot and W. P. Murphy of Boston for finding the cause of this disease and how to control it.

Whipple discovered the intrinsic factor in 1920. Normally, this can be made within the body as part of the gastric juice that flows into the stomach. But in pernicious anemia this process does not occur.

Six years later, after many experiments, Minot and Murphy found that patients with pernicious anemia, when fed one-quarter to one-half pound of liver daily, could produce red blood cells again.

These findings touched off extensive research in the United States and England. And in 1948, within the same month, universities in both countries announced that they had discovered a red crystalline substance that was identified as vitamin B_{12}. It was also called the extrinsic factor—that is, coming from food or from outside the body. Further experiments disclosed that the intrinsic factor must combine with the extrinsic factor (vitamin B_{12}) before it can be absorbed from the digestive tract.

In 1955 the chemical formula of vitamin B_{12} was announced. It is the largest, most complex molecule known, with the exception of protein. Now, when one five-millionth to five five-millionths of one gram of B_{12} is injected into the muscle, it can restore normal blood. It makes the person comfortable, since it eliminates the nervousness associated with this disease. It also promotes growth and helps the body use amino acids.

table 3–3 Iron Content in Various Foods*

FOOD GROUP	KIND OF FOOD	WEIGHT OR MEASURE	APPROXIMATE AMOUNT OF IRON (Milligrams)	FOOD GROUP	KIND OF FOOD	WEIGHT OR MEASURE	APPROXIMATE AMOUNT OF IRON (Milligrams)
MEAT, FISH, POULTRY, EGGS	Pork liver, raw	3½ oz.	19.2		Blueberries	1 c.	1.4
	Lamb liver, raw	3½ oz.	10.9		Cantaloupe	½	0.8
	Calf liver, raw	3½ oz.	8.8		Banana	1	0.8
	Beef liver, raw	3½ oz.	6.5		Avocado	½	0.7
	Chicken liver, raw	3½ oz.	7.9		Grapefruit	½	0.5
	Liverwurst	3½ oz.	5.9		Orange, navel	1	0.5
	Lamb kidney	3 oz.	7.6		Apple	1	0.4
	Beef heart	3 oz.	5.0		Endive, green, raw	2 oz.	1.0
	Oysters, raw	½ c.	6.6		Spinach, cooked	½ c.	2.0
	Clams, raw	3 oz.	5.2		Turnip greens, cooked	½ c.	0.8
	Shrimp, canned	3 oz.	2.6		Collards, cooked	½ c.	0.6
	Beef, loin, broiled	3 oz.	3.0		Broccoli, cooked	½ c.	0.6
	Hamburger, lean	3 oz.	3.0		Brussels sprouts, cooked	½ c.	0.9
	regular	3 oz.	2.7		Sauerkraut	½ c.	0.7
	Pork roast	3 oz.	2.7		Coleslaw	1 c.	0.4
	Ham, cured	3 oz.	2.2		Carrots	½ c.	0.5
	Lamb roast	3 oz.	1.4		Pepper	1	0.5
	Chicken, ½ breast and bone	3.3 oz.	1.3		Potato, peeled, boiled white	1	0.8
	Chicken drumstick, fried	2.1 oz.	0.9		sweet	1	1.0
	Eggs	1	1.1	CEREAL-BREAD	Oatmeal, cooked	1 c.	1.4
VEGETABLES, FRUITS	Beans, dried, cooked	1 c.	4.9		Bread, white, enriched	1 slice	0.6
	Peanuts	½ c.	1.5	MILK, MILK PRODUCTS	Milk	1 c.	0.1
	Peanut butter	2 T.	0.6		Cheese, American cheddar	1-in. cube	0.2
	Peas, green	½ c.	1.5	SWEETS	Sugar, white	1 T.	trace
	Figs, dried	2 whole	1.2		Molasses, light	1 T.	0.9
	Apricots, cooked	½ c.	2.6		blackstrap	1 T.	3.2
	Prunes, cooked	½ c.	2.3				
	Tomato juice, canned	1 c.	2.2				

*Adapted from *Composition of Foods,* Agriculture Handbook No. 8 (Washington, D.C.: USDA, 1964) and *Nutritive Value of Foods,* Home and Garden Bulletin No. 72 (Washington, D.C.: USDA, 1970).

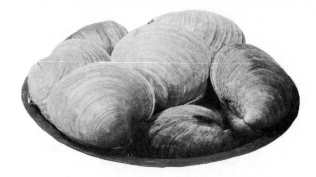

Liver is the richest source of vitamin B_{12}, which is also found in organ meats, muscle meats, shellfish, eggs, and milk. Those who eat a balanced diet have all that is needed for normal health.

Macrocytic anemia

Macrocytic anemia (also called megablastic anemia), found chiefly in women during pregnancy and lactation, and in infants, is discussed in Chapter 7. It is caused by a deficiency in folic acid (folacin), a B vitamin.

Daily need of iron

To build basic stamina, males from 10 to 14 and females from 10 to 35 need 18 milligrams of iron in the daily diet. After age 14, the daily requirement for males drops to 10 milligrams daily.

Girls need more iron in their daily food and they can avoid anemia if they learn to like iron-rich foods early in life. Girls lose blood, and iron with it, regularly through menstruation. The loss of iron during menstruation has been found in studies to be about 1 milligram per day.

Foods rich in iron

Unfortunately, iron is quite low or completely lacking in many foods that people enjoy eating. And of that which occurs in food, only about 10 percent is absorbed. It is not equally well absorbed from all foods.

Like other nutrients, it is dependent on teamwork. To be effective in its absorption and use, it needs copper, vitamin C, protein, the intrinsic factor in hydrochloric acid in the stomach, a large number of B vitamins, and other nutrients, known

and perhaps still unknown. Table 3–3 lists foods rich in iron.

Liver of all types is a rich source of iron. Pork liver ranks at the top. It carries a generous amount of copper, too. Kidney, heart, and spleen are rich sources. Among fish and shellfish, clams and oysters are quite high in iron. The lean muscle of meat, eggs, dried beans, dried peas, nuts, raisins, dried apricots, prunes, and the green leaves of vegetables are good sources. Plan your menus for a week at a time and balance them for each day, to be sure you have some liver or other iron-rich meat in your meals.

Importance of iodine

Iodine is needed to make thyroxin, a hormone secreted from the thyroid gland, that regulates the cells' use of energy. When a person does not have sufficient iodine in the diet to enable the thyroid gland to make the necessary thyroxin, the gland strains to meet the body's need. It becomes over-stimulated and enlarged, resulting in simple goiter.

Iodine and seafood

Observant people noted that those who ate seafood and the plants growing near the sea did not have goiter. Through research in nutrition, we have learned why. Seawater, seaweed, and salt-water fish contain iodine.

Inland Switzerland and some parts of inland France had high rates of goiter. In our country, the goiter belt stretches from the inland East to the inland West. In Akron, Ohio in 1920, nearly 2500 girls took part in a classic experiment that is helping us today. About 2000 girls had slightly enlarged thyroid glands; 246, moderately enlarged

Iodine deficiency still appears among the Swiss, as seen in the "simple" goiter of this young woman.

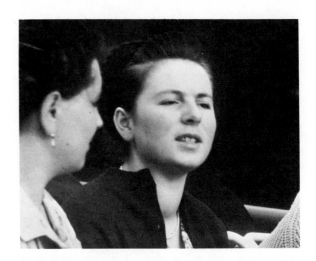

glands; and 39, toxic goiters. Out of the 2000 treated with a small amount of sodium iodide in the drinking water, only 5 developed thyroid enlargement, as compared with 500 in the control group who did not take the iodine-water.

Frequently, a condition that causes a disease in man will also affect the animals that live in the same area. Cows, sheep, mares, dogs, chickens, and pigs in the goiter belt developed enlarged thyroids. In 1916, Wisconsin reported millions of pigs born hairless and defective to mothers with deficient thyroxin in the blood.

Iodized salt

Iodized salt has proven effective in preventing simple goiter. Nevertheless, studies show that goiter increased in the United States from 1955 to 1970, and that the use of iodized salt dropped from 80 to 40 percent. Iodized salt is available in food markets throughout the country. Through the use of iodized salt and seafood, simple goiter can be prevented.

Role of niacin

Niacin, along with vitamin B_{12}, is an outstanding vitamin found in meats. No other food contributes so much B_{12} to the diet. When people have too little of this vitamin, they develop pellagra, a disease that haunted our own South until cereal-breads were enriched (see Chapter 9).

You may have read the exciting true story of how Dr. Joseph Goldberger proved that pellagra is caused by a poor diet, specifically by insufficient niacin. He fed prisoners the very diet eaten by those afflicted by the disease and produced pellagra in them. He then cured it with a good balanced diet.

Importance of tryptophane

Research has revealed why pellagra has been associated in people's minds with corn. This grain contains only a small amount of the amino acid tryptophane (**trip′ tə fān**), which is essential for life. With the aid of suitable bacteria and vitamin B_6, tryptophane is chemically changed into niacin right in the digestive tract. It was not "bad" corn that was causing pellagra, as believed, but a diet deficient in good-quality protein and niacin.

Today we know that when the diet contains sufficient good-grade protein, as in meat, eggs, and milk, **the body can increase the amount of niacin by one third.** This is why milk, for example, can prevent pellagra—its niacin content is low, but the tryptophane is high.

Other foods rich in tryptophane, besides meat, poultry, fish, eggs, liver and other organs, include peanuts, peanut butter, and brewer's yeast. Fair sources are milk, whole grains, enriched cereals, legumes, potatoes, and some green leafy vegetables. Gelatin lacks tryptophane, and therefore its 100-percent protein is incomplete.

Functions of Niacin

Like other B vitamins, niacin is soluble in water. It is not easily destroyed by cooking, acid, or alkali. Like riboflavin and thiamine, it serves as a

table 3–4 *Niacin Content in Common Portions of Food**

FOOD APPROXIMATE MEASURE (Per 100 gm—3½ oz.)**	NIACIN mg
Peanut butter	14.7
Liver, beef, raw	13.6
calf, raw	11.4
Tuna fish, canned, solids	11.9
Heart, beef, raw	7.5
Salmon, canned, red	7.3
Meats, lean muscle, avg., raw	4.6
Peas, dried	2.2
fresh	3.7
Bread, whole wheat	2.8
enriched white	2.4
unenriched white	1.1
Beans, dried, cooked, 1 cup	1.3
Nuts (not peanuts), avg., 1 cup	1.7
Fruits, dried (except raisins), avg., cooked, unsweetened	2.3
Cornmeal, whole, dry, 1 cup	2.3
degerminated, enriched, 1 cup	4.8
Corn, sweet, fresh, cooked, 1 ear	1.0
Rice, white, enriched, cooked, 1 cup	2.1
Lima beans, fresh, cooked, 1 cup	2.2
Oatmeal, cooked, 1 cup	0.2
Broccoli, cooked, 1 cup	1.4
Leafy vegetables, avg.	1.1
Fresh fruits, avg.	0.3
Cheeses	0.1–0.2
Eggs, whole, fresh	0.1
Milk, whole, fresh, 1 cup	0.2
Potato, 1 med., white	1.7
Sweet potatoes	0.7
Oil and fats	0.0
Sugar	0.0
Carbonated beverages	0.0

*Adapted from *Composition of Foods*, Agriculture Handbook No. 8 (Washington, D.C.: USDA, 1963) and *Nutritive Value of Foods*, Home and Garden Bulletin No. 72 (Washington, D.C.: USDA, 1970).

**Amount, except where otherwise stated.

coenzyme in the exchange of oxygen within cells and the release of energy in the body.

Niacin makes many contributions to our physical, mental, and emotional health. We know this because, when people have too little of it, they become emotionally distressed and suffer anxieties, depression, confusion, and hallucinations. Mentally, they are in a stupor. Physically, they develop a bright red dermatitis on the hands and all parts of the body exposed to light, and often have diarrhea as well. All these symptoms are relieved by a diet containing adequate meat, milk, eggs, fruits, and vegetables.

Niacin and blood cholesterol

Recent studies indicate that blood-serum cholesterol can be lowered when niacin is taken in large amounts. More work is needed before definitive conclusions are drawn. Niacin is now being used by some physicians in the treatment of cardiovascular disease.

It is well to remember that when we eat the variety of foods we have been discussing, the diet will include a sufficient amount of niacin.

Other B vitamins

Riboflavin, thiamine, and some quantity of most other B vitamins are found in meat, poultry, fish, and eggs. Liver is our richest food source of B vitamins. Pork has been elevated to a position of distinction by the research on thiamine in meats. A serving of roast pork contains seven times as much thiamine as roast veal and over 15 times as much as a serving of roast beef. This is shown in the table of Nutritive Value of Foods, page 454.

Role of fat

Most red meat is high in fat content. The amount of fat, which ranges from 10 to 40 percent, depends on the animal and the cut and grade of meat. Fish, chicken, and turkey contain less fat than goose, duck, and red meats. Young animals and poultry contain more lean and less fat per pound than older ones. Experiments are under way to produce pork with less fat and more lean, for it is the lean that we value most.

The trend is to lower the fat content of our diet for weight control and for other health reasons.

French country inns usually roast meat before an open grate. This method eliminates part of the fat and retains the tenderness of the meat.

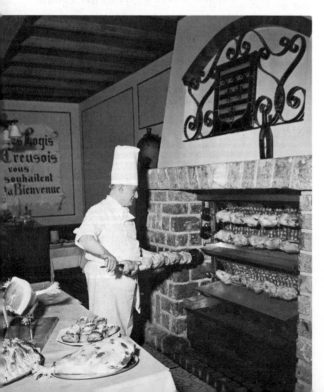

The fat in meat is saturated; that in fish is not. (Fats are discussed in detail in Chapter 11.) Research shows that the kind and amount of fat in the diet are associated with some types of heart and circulatory disease.

There are more calories from fat in meat than from protein. It is well to learn to calculate caloric content in planning meals and selecting food. For instance, using the table of Nutritive Values in the Appendix, you will find that there are 306 calories from fat and 68 from protein in a 3-ounce serving of roast beef. We arrive at these figures by multiplying the number of grams of fat (34) by 9 (the number of calories in 1 gram of fat) and the number of grams of protein (17) by 4 (the number in one gram of protein). In the roast beef, fat yields over four times as many calories as does protein. Eggs contain more calories from fat (54) than from protein (24). If you wish, you can work out the calories from each food you eat, using the table in the Appendix. This record can help you now and later.

The "hidden" fat

Commercial cold cuts are a good example of how fat creeps into the diet. A frankfurter, which appears to be solid lean meat, actually contains 7 grams of protein and 15 grams of fat, yielding 28 calories from protein and 135 from fat. Four slices of bologna yield 24 calories from protein and 126 from fat. Two ounces of dry-type salami yield 56 calories from protein and 198 from fat. The same amount of boiled ham has 44 calories from protein and 90 from fat. The fat in this can be seen and most of it cut off. One and three-fourths ounces of liverwurst (not smoked) yields 32.4 calories from protein and 109 from fat, but more iron in proportion than any fresh meat, except liver itself, and more vitamin A and riboflavin.

The "magic" of liver

Anthropologists found in some primitive societies that liver was believed to have "magic" properties. It was given to young children, pregnant and lactating women, the sick, and the aged. It was also used for special conditions, such as sore eyes and night blindness. It was considered the most desirable part of any animal. It is reported that head-hunters actually were primarily after the livers.

Modern nutrition explains the "magic" of liver. This organ is a depot for some quantity of almost every nutrient in the body, except calcium. Liver is richer than any other food in iron, vitamin A and D, and the B vitamins, including B_{12}. A 4-ounce serving of liver has as much vitamin A as 3 pounds of butter or fortified margarine.

The heart, kidney, and spleen, while not so rich in nutrients as liver, contain more than other meats. The stomach, called tripe, is valuable for some known, and possibly many unknown nutrients it provides.

Thus we see why it is important to include one serving of liver in the weekly menu. It helps fill in gaps in a fair diet and enriches a good one. It is especially useful for girls and women from the time the menstrual cycle begins until it ends, for those on reducing and low-fat diets, for pregnant and lactating mothers, for growing children, for anyone during or following an illness (unless prohibited by the physician), and for those who tend to be anemic.

Vitamin D and rickets

In 1909, a Russian physician prescribed cod-liver oil for a four-year-old child who had never walked because of rickets. After taking the cod-liver oil for two months, the child had absorbed and laid down enough calcium and phosphorus in the bones to start walking. Vitamin D, a fat-soluble vitamin that the cod liver contains in large amounts, is often called calciferol (kal sif' ə rol), the bone-hardening vitamin, the sunshine vitamin, and the antirachitic (ant i rə kit' ik) or rickets-preventing vitamin. It is essential in the team of nutrients that build and maintain hard bone structure.

You may never have seen a case of rickets. But if you have seen a person with bowlegs, knock-knees, enlarged wrists or ankles, or ribs with little bumps on them, you have seen mild manifestations of this disease. Children are most affected in infancy and early growth. The vitamin D in a mother's diet greatly affects the normal development of the expected baby, and she needs more during pregnancy and lactation.

Rickets occurred in our country and in northern Europe, where there were long periods with little sunshine, and in large industrial cities where there was heavy smog of much cloudiness. It was noticed that, where mountains shut out the sunshine (as in the valleys of Switzerland), the children had rickets; but on the sunny heights of mountains or in tropical areas this disease was not present.

The cause of this crippling disease remained a mystery until the twentieth century. Now we know that, unless enough vitamin D is present, calcium and phosphorus—even in abundant amounts—cannot produce strong bones and teeth. Ribs may become deformed, causing a pinched chest with crowded internal organs. When a young child with rickets stands, its leg bones bend, producing bowlegs or knock-knees.

A form of this disease called osteomalacia (ä stē ō mə lāsh'ē ə) causes the wrists and ankle bones to soften at any age. The skulls of growing children may become misshapen. The teeth are thinner, and the enamel may have pits and fissures similar to those resulting from vitamin-A deficiency.

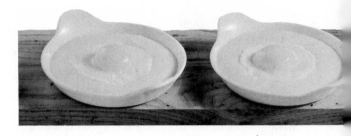

Benefits of sunshine

When the sun shines directly on the skin, the ultraviolet rays activate a form of cholesterol, a fatty substance that lies beneath the skin, and it can produce vitamin D. This explains why rickets is seldom found in sunny, tropical countries. But clouds, clothing, dust, fog, smog, windowpanes, and even dark pigment in the skin cut out the ultraviolet rays, preventing the formation of vitamin D by the body.

Dietary needs

In the RDA Table on pages 446–447 you will note that 400 International Units of vitamin D are recommended daily for infants and all children until growth is completed. This does not mean that we stop needing it when we are grown, for calcium and phosphorus cannot do their repair work without it. However, once the structure of bones and teeth is formed, most adults get sufficient vitamin D in the diet and sunshine to maintain bony structures in the body.

Sources of vitamin D

Liver and fish-liver oils are the best sources of vitamin D in our diets, and egg yolk also contains

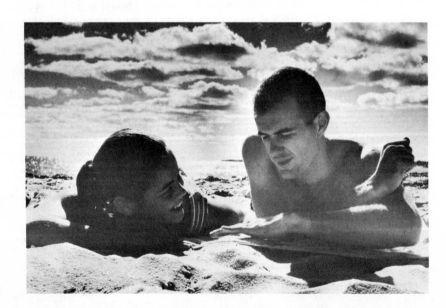

The sun's rays falling directly on the skin help the body produce vitamin D.

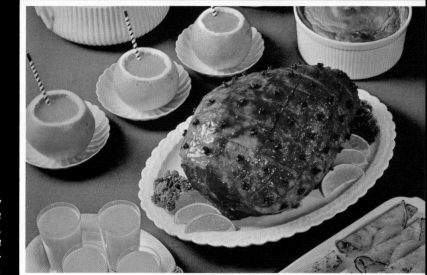

(right) *Be prepared for hearty appetites—and compliments—when you serve this zesty brunch.* (below) *Crown roast of pork is a masterpiece that gets a royal welcome on any dinner table.*

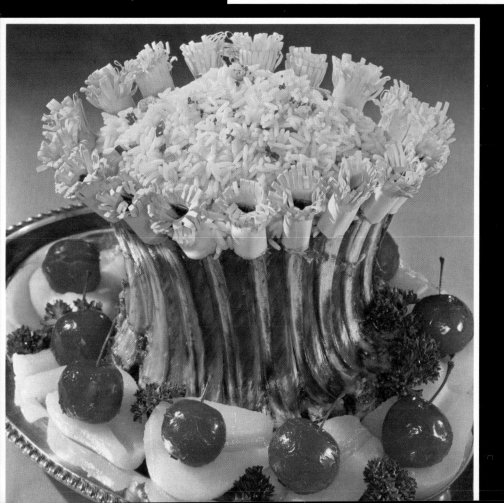

(top left) *A tempting—and balanced—meal can be easily prepared in the broiler.* (top right) *For contrast in flavor, color, and texture, serve stuffed veal roast with red cabbage and applesauce.* (bottom) *Steak, marinated in wine with herbs, is a gourmet dish for any occasion.*

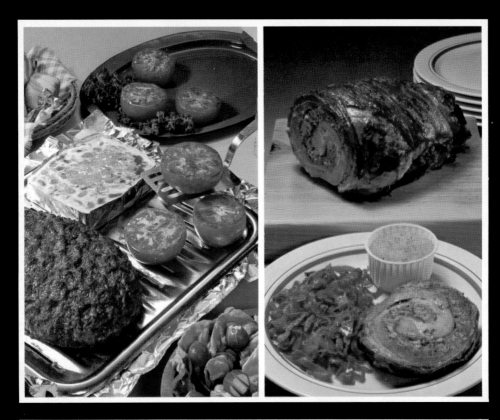

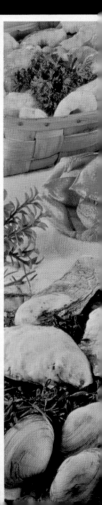

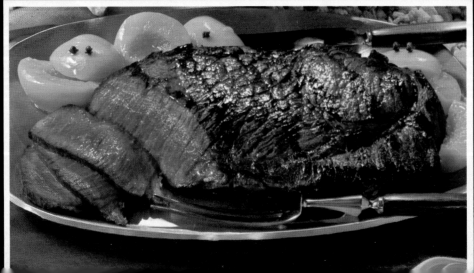

Can anyone resist a hearty beef stew?

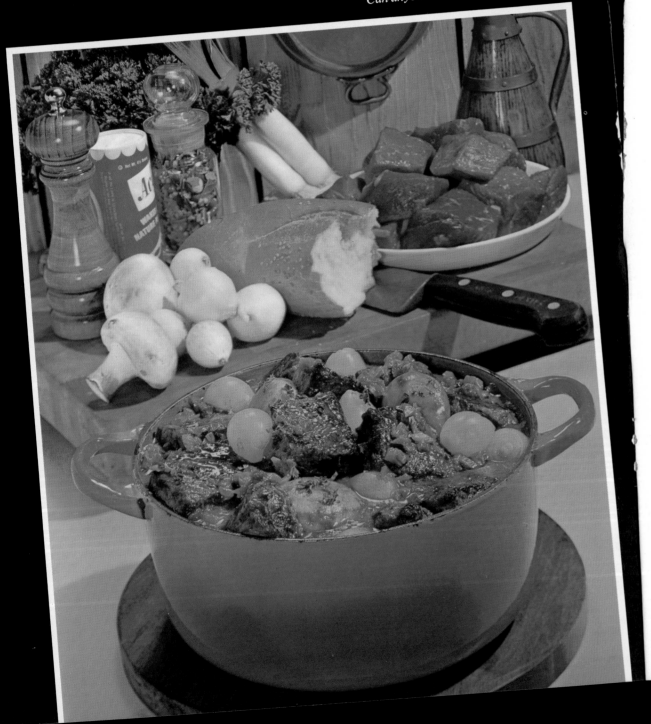

fig. 3—4 THE PARTS OF AN EGG

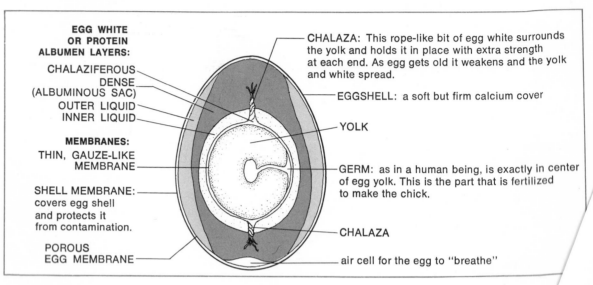

EGG WHITE OR PROTEIN ALBUMEN LAYERS:
CHALAZIFEROUS
DENSE (ALBUMINOUS SAC)
OUTER LIQUID
INNER LIQUID

MEMBRANES:
THIN, GAUZE-LIKE MEMBRANE

SHELL MEMBRANE: covers egg shell and protects it from contamination.

POROUS EGG MEMBRANE

CHALAZA: This rope-like bit of egg white surrounds the yolk and holds it in place with extra strength at each end. As egg gets old it weakens and the yolk and white spread.

EGGSHELL: a soft but firm calcium cover

YOLK

GERM: as in a human being, is exactly in center of egg yolk. This is the part that is fertilized to make the chick.

CHALAZA

air cell for the egg to "breathe"

this vitamin. Today, milk is "fortified" with 400 I.U. per quart. This practice has virtually eliminated rickets in our country. When certain oils are exposed to ultraviolet light, vitamin D can be inexpensively produced synthetically.

Can one get too much vitamin D?

You can get too much vitamin D if you overdose with concentrated vitamins. Some nutritionists think that vitamin D should be added only to milk and that irradiation should be controlled. An excess of this vitamin produces a toxic effect— loss of appetite, vomiting, diarrhea, and calcification of the walls of the blood vessels, the heart, and the soft tissues. This is not caused by natural food or by milk fortified with vitamin D. However, the toxic effect can follow self-medication. A mother applying the concept that, if a little is good, more is better, can give too much to an infant or young child. Even in an older person,

toxicity has been noted when overdose taken, as for arthritis.

Man may not live by meat alone, bu with a higher degree of stamina and his more delectable when meat, fish, po organ meats, and eggs are part of his d

Why egg with meats in

The hen packs into an egg 6 which is so perfectly balanced i the egg is used as the stand other foods. The white is 10 rich in riboflavin, and con cholesterol. This makes it diets for some types of weight control.

The egg yolk contai every nutrient, except ment for the beginnin well-balanced food. of the neatest calor

ance found in foods. If her diet is poor, she lays fewer eggs, but she tends to produce each uniform in nutrients.

Farmers realized this fact and fed their poultry and livestock well-balanced diets long before the homemaker fed her family well-balanced diets. Studies show that, when the hen's diet is high in vitamin A, and when vitamin D is added to the food (or she gets sunshine), more of these vitamins are found in the egg yolk and in the fat of the hen's body.

The amino acids in the egg, especially in the yolk, are the kind required by the cells to build good skin and hair. You won't get this benefit by simply rubbing an "egg shampoo" on your scalp, but you will derive it from the eggs in your meals.

An egg might well be called a little bomb of nourishment. It can make up for the protein deficiency of vegetables, fruits, and cereal-bread, and balances milk in iron. Within the small shell is such a variety of nutrients that the whole body of a chick is made from one egg.

Meaningful words

amino acids
anemia
antibodies
antirachitic vitamin
calciferol
complete protein
enzymes
erythrocyte
essential amino acids
intrinsic factor
gamma globulin

globin
hemorrhagic anemia
—
—omic anemia
—ete protein
—factor
—iency anemia
—rotein
—c anemia

Thinking and evaluating

1. On the basis of the seven-day food record you kept of your own eating habits, did you have a "complete" protein food in each meal? How much did you have in each meal? Compare this record with what you ate yesterday and evaluate whether you are improving or not.

2. What is meant by complete protein, partially complete or limiting protein, and incomplete protein? Give examples of each. What is meant by essential amino acids?

3. In what ways does an adequate amount of protein with all the essential amino acids in your daily diet help your life now? How will it help you in the future?

4. Why is iron so important? What types of anemia can be controlled with food and which nutrients are especially helpful? Why should girls and women learn to include iron-rich foods in the diet every day?

5. In what ways has the discovery of vitamin B_{12} been important for mankind? What other B vitamins are found in meat, poultry, fish, liver, organ meats, and eggs? Which of these foods are most important for niacin content? How does niacin help you?

6. Is it usually the lack of one nutrient in the diet that causes people to get diseases such as pellagra? Rickets? Explain.

7. Why can eggs be used as a meat alternate? In what ways are they superior to legumes? In what ways are legumes a good alternate for the "meat-egg" group in supplying important nutrients?

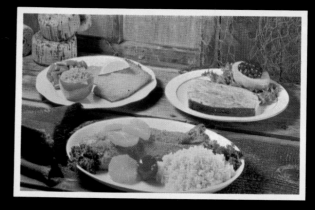

(left) *Fish may be prepared in many delicious ways, and adds low-calorie variety to the week's menus.*
(below) *Fruits of the sea—a treasure in eating for sailors and landlubbers alike.*

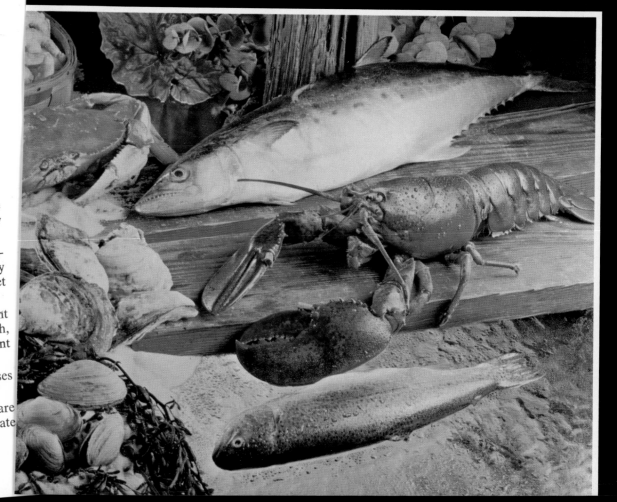

Meaningful words

molecule
niacin
osteomalacia
pernicious anemia
rickets
synthesize
thyroid
thyroxin

8. Do you consider it important to include liver in the diet at least once a week? Explain. In what nutrient is seafood more important than freshwater fish? What kinds do you like best? How many different kinds have you eaten? Why are fish, liver, and eggs so important on a weight-control or low-fat diet? In a normal diet?

Applying and sharing

1. Compare your seven-day food record with the food you ate yesterday. Use the table of Nutritive Value of Foods in the Appendix and figure out the following problems:
   a. How many grams of protein did you eat in each meal? In each day?
   b. What percent of the day's calories was derived from protein? From fat?
   c. How many milligrams of iron were there? Of niacin?
   d. How do you rate your intake, as compared with the recommended quantities for each nutrient?

2. On the basis of this comparison, which foods helped most in meeting your recommended daily allowance of each nutrient? Where were there any weaknesses? Make a plan showing how you can improve.

3. Plan daily menus for the meals and snacks in one week, showing how you would use the variety of meats listed in the table of Nutritive Value of Foods on page 454, to make a balanced meal each time and stay within the budget of your family at present. How would you change the plan to meet the needs of a lower-cost budget?

4. Write to the Department of the Interior for information on fish as a food and for recipes using various kinds.

5. Look up ways to prepare liver in a variety of cookbooks and try four different recipes at school and at home. Do the same for sea fish.

6. Share with your family what you have learned in this chapter.

7. In studying the table of Nutritive Value of Foods in the Appendix, can you understand why eggs have had an important place in the diet of mankind throughout history? How would you evaluate the importance of an egg in the daily diet? Recheck the menus you planned and underscore the places where you use eggs in meals. Prepare eggs four different ways for breakfast and lunch as part of a balanced meal.

meat in meals

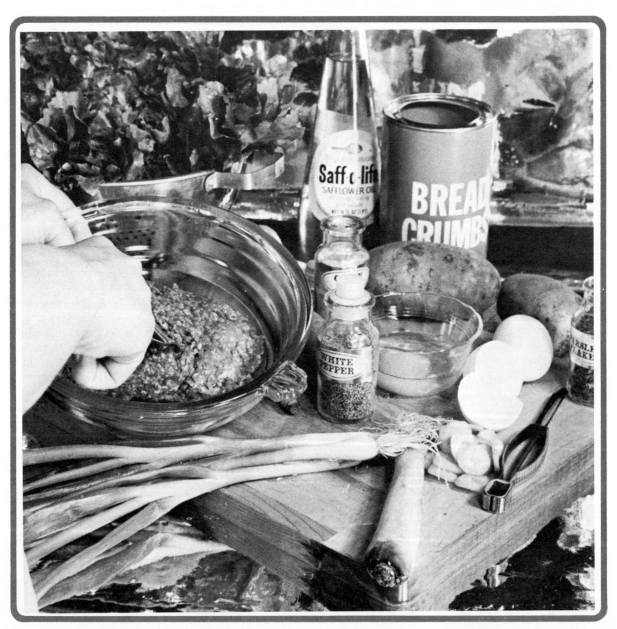

In 1844 Nathaniel Hawthorne, the American author, did his own cooking for a short time while his wife was away. He took especial delight in preparing a corn beef, following a recipe in the currently popular *Sarah Hale's Cook Book*, and wrote that the result was "exquisitely done" and "such a masterpiece in its way that it seems irreverential to eat it. Things on which so much thought and labor are bestowed should surely be immortal."

Hawthorne's happiness is the crowning triumph of all food management—the joy of seeing well-selected food so exquisitely prepared that it is a "masterpiece." No food provides more day-to-day mealtime pleasure than meat. No food takes more of the food dollar. This amounted to 36 to 40 percent of the total spent on food in 1965.

This poses a dilemma for young people establishing their own homes. Many are accustomed to eating higher-quality, more expensive meat than they can afford on a low food budget, which many have in the first years of marriage. A wife wishes to please her husband in the meals she prepares, and the kind of meat he likes is a key food in the meal. You will be able to resolve this conflict—and provide delicious meats in your meals, yet stay within your food budget—when you have completed this study.

Types of meat

There are many kinds of meat on the market (see Table 4–1), and many things to learn about managing it. Let us learn how to select meat wisely and prepare it "exquisitely." Then we can have in our meals the meat we enjoy, and at the same time include the amount of vegetables, fruits, milk, and other foods we need.

Composition of meats

Meat is the flesh of animals, poultry, and fish. It is composed of lean muscle fiber, connective tissues, fat, and bone. Lean muscles carry the vitamins, minerals, and protein. This is the part we count as a serving of meat. It is the main flavor and texture in meat.

Connective tissues

Connective tissues are creamy-white, threadlike strands that bind the muscle fibers in little bundles, and the muscle to the bones. These are quite tender in fish, young poultry, lamb, pork, and some cuts and grades of beef. They are tough in older poultry, beef, and skinny or poorly nourished animals. The connective tissue must be tender to begin with, or become tender during cooking, if meat is to be tender and enjoyable to eat. Old animals and exercised parts of an animal produce tougher connective tissue. (See the chart on meat cuts.) This is quite an important point to remember in selecting meat and cooking it. The connective tissue yields gelatin when slowly cooked in moist heat.

Bone

Bone is a part of meat that we do not usually eat, except in canned salmon and sardines and the gristle of pigs' feet. (Gristle is the connective tissue around joints.) Bone in meat, fish, and poultry is quite an important part of the meat for Eskimos and others who have little or no milk and cheese in the diet. Among many primitive peoples, the bones are cooked until soft and the gristle, which is rich in calcium, is eaten. Bones are discarded by most Americans. Thus the more bone in a cut of meat, the less lean and the higher the cost of lean per pound.

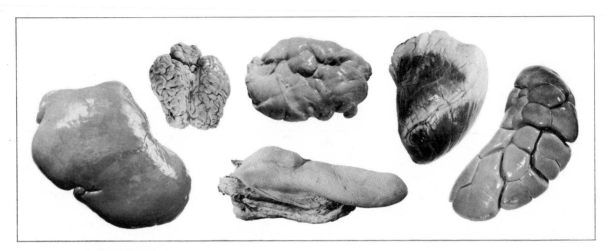

Which is the most nourishing of all the organ meats?

Buying a large roast is good economy. It supplies planned leftovers that will mean ready meals for the future.

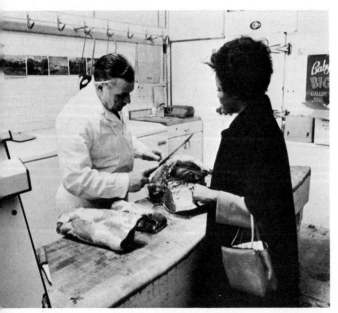

Fat

Fat relates directly to the quality of the meat, the kind and breed of the animal, its diet, and the care it has had. Well-nourished animals produce meat that is tender, juicy, and interlaid with fat. Poorly fed ones lack fat and the meat is tough. The highest quality of meat (Prime Grade) has the most fat interlaid with the lean. Each succeeding lower grade has less fat streaked through the lean and is less tender. When an animal runs on the range, it has less fat and tougher meat than animals restricted to close quarters.

Fat surrounds the carcass of animals and poultry just beneath the skin. Veal, which is beef three months old or younger, has so little fat that the meat is tough unless properly cooked. Broilers have little fat, but their meat is tender.

Lamb and pork usually contain a thick layer of fat around the carcass, as do most other meats. Fish is lowest in fat, but it is tender when properly cooked, for it has very little connective tissue. The fat of poultry is yellow-tinged and contains some vitamin A and carotenes. Animal fat is white, with the exception of older beef, which has a creamy tinge and contains a small amount of vitamin A.

Understanding the way meat is made enables us to make wiser decisions in selecting and cooking it. It also helps us save money when we buy it.

table 4–1   *Kinds of Red Meat, Organs, Fish, and Poultry*

RED MEAT	ORGANS (Variety Meats)	FISH	POULTRY
Beef	Liver	Salt water	Chicken
Veal	Heart	Fresh water	Turkey
Pork, lean	Kidneys	Shellfish:	Duck
(not	Sweetbreads	Oysters	Goose
bacon or	Brains	Shrimp	Squab
fatback)	Lungs	Crab	Cornish
Lamb	Tripe	Clams	hen
Mutton	Tongue	Lobster	Pheasant
Goat		Scallops	Wild
			birds

Analysis of meat by R. M. Leverton and G. V. Odell revealed that cooked pork has slightly less fat than similar portions of beef or lamb. From the standpoint of meal planning, the summary of their research (Table 4–2) is valuable.

Selecting meat: grades

Quality of meat depends on (1) grade, (2) cut, (3) age of the animal, (4) nutrition of the animal, (5) methods of processing, and (6) cleanliness and wholesomeness.

Grade of meat indicates the quality of the whole carcass, the tenderness of the lean and the connective tissue, and the juiciness. It also indicates how the meat should be cooked to develop its best texture and flavor. Table 4–3 is designed to help you see at a glance the different grades of beef, beginning with prime, which is top grade. Each succeeding grade is slightly lower in quality than the grade above it.

If you familiarize yourself with the different grades and their characteristics, it can help you learn the grades quickly by looking at the meat in the store. Beef is used as the example, for it is the most graded meat. There is more tough meat in beef than in any other kind.

Prime grade

Prime grade meat is the élite. The lean is fine-grained and smooth as velvet. Tiny streaks of fat are intermingled with the lean. This is called marbling. Well-marbled meat has exceptional tenderness and juiciness, and "melts in the mouth." Most prime-grade meat goes to the better restaurant trade. It can be ordered from your butcher.

table 4–2   *Comparison of Protein and Fat with Calories in Cooked Meat**

KIND OF MEAT	CALORIES Per 100 gm	PROTEIN Per 100 gm or 3½ oz.	FAT Cooked
BEEF			
Lean	209	32.5	7.8
Lean plus marble	266	29.6	15.4
VEAL			
Lean	192	33.6	5.3
Lean plus marble	213	32.7	8.1
PORK			
Lean	194	30.7	7.0
Lean plus marble	240	28.5	13.1
LAMB			
Lean	188	28.6	7.3
Lean plus marble	258	26.6	16.1

*SOURCE: R. M. Leverton and G. V. Odell, *The Nutritive Value of Cooked Meat*, Miscellaneous Publication MP-49, Oklahoma Experimental Station, Oklahoma State University, 1958.

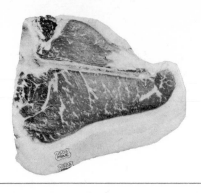 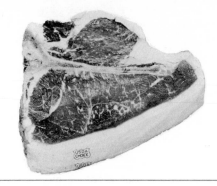

Grades of steaks

table 4–3   USDA Grades of Meat in Order of Quality

BEEF GRADE	CHARACTERISTICS
U. S. PRIME	Cherry-red color in fresh beef, darker in "ripened" meat. Fine-grained; firm; lean, with white connective tissue, much marbling of fat in lean portion.
U. S. CHOICE	Firm-grained; firm; lean, with white connective tissue, less marbling of fat.
U. S. GOOD	Coarser-grained; lean, with creamy-white connective tissue, less fat in lean and around it.
U. S. STANDARD OR U. S. COMMERCIAL	Darker red color; coarser lean, with darker connective tissue, less fat.
U. S. UTILITY	Lowest grade on the market, and usually not seen on meat counters.
CANNER AND CUTTER	Not seen on the market; used for processed meat products.

Choice grade

Choice grade is the one most used in the home. It is tender, but has less fat, with less marbling, and costs less than prime grade.

All pork is tender. Research shows it is not fatter in the lean parts than either beef or lamb. This dispels an old-fashioned belief about it.

Grade stamps

The grade of meat is stamped on the outside of the carcass in rows, with a purple harmless vegetable dye. Look for the grade. Meat is graded by trained specialists, according to standards set by the federal government. Grading is voluntary and some meat companies train their own graders according to established standards.

Brand names

Meat companies also use brand names for different grades. This can be quite confusing to the homemaker. There are some 21 different brand names used for different grades of ham, for instance, by six different meat companies. Which would you rate as a higher grade, Select or Arrow? Star, Banquet, or Quality? Fancy, Rex, or Puritan? These brand names range from top grade to fourth grade.

The homemaker is better served by a system of numbers (with 1 as top and the rest in descending order) or letters of the alphabet, beginning with A as the top grade and working downward for lower grades. When brand names are used, grade identification should also be present. The consumer may have to work to get this accomplished.

Poultry grading

Poultry is graded by federal government standards as A, B, and C, as shown in the photograph of grade stamps, and by characteristics, as in Table 4–4. A is the top grade.

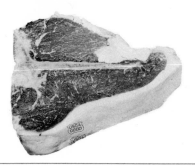
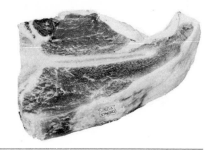

Fish ungraded

Fish is not graded. This is because all of it is tender. The degree of freshness depends on the individual market, and should be carefully checked by the purchaser.

Grading of other meats

Veal is graded from Prime to Commercial. Pork is graded U.S. Choice, Medium, and Cull. Lamb is graded U.S. Prime, Choice, Good, Utility, and Cull.

All grades that bear the mark come from animals that were wholesome and clean at the time of grading. The characteristics of beef are typical of meats of other animals in the same grade. See Chapter 17, pages 316–317 for the federal safeguards taken for inspection of meat and poultry.

The highest grades are cooked by dry heat (broiling and roasting), as indicated in Table 4–8. In Prime Grade, such cuts as round and chuck are tender and juicy when roasted or broiled.

Remember that the protein, vitamins, and minerals in meat are more concentrated in the lower grades that have more lean and less fat. The homemaker can choose lower grades of meat and feed her family better at less cost. She needs to learn how to prepare lower grades so that they are tender. Good grade and Standard grade are excellent choices for one who wishes to get the most meat and nutrients for her food dollar and also to enjoy a full-flavored meat.

Cuts of meat

Cuts of meat must be learned, as the name of the cut is not stamped on meat as the grade is. The charts (pages 64–67) can help familiarize you with cuts, but the meat markets are a far better place to test what you know. The cut of meat indicates tenderness or toughness, the price to pay, and how to cook it. The lower the grade, the bonier or fatter the cut, the lower the cost should be.

How to select cuts of meat

An easy way to remember cuts is that the least exercised portions are the most tender in the animal. There are fewer tender cuts, for they lie along

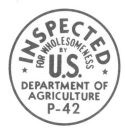

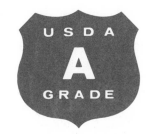

Poultry grade stamps

fig. 4–1 **BEEF CHART** Retail cuts of beef and where they come from

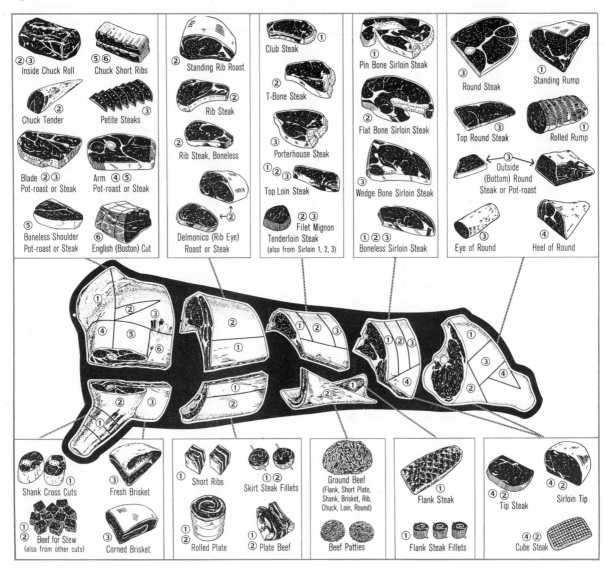

Inside Chuck Roll ② ③
Chuck Short Ribs ⑤ ⑥
Chuck Tender ②
Petite Steaks ③
Blade ② ③ Pot-roast or Steak
Arm ④ ⑤ Pot-roast or Steak
Boneless Shoulder ⑤ Pot-roast or Steak
English (Boston) Cut ⑥

Standing Rib Roast ②
Rib Steak ②
Rib Steak, Boneless ②
Delmonico (Rib Eye) Roast or Steak

Club Steak ①
T-Bone Steak ②
Porterhouse Steak ③
Top Loin Steak ① ② ③
Filet Mignon Tenderloin Steak ② ③
(also from Sirloin 1, 2, 3)

Pin Bone Sirloin Steak ①
Flat Bone Sirloin Steak ②
Wedge Bone Sirloin Steak ③
Boneless Sirloin Steak ① ② ③

Round Steak ③
Standing Rump ①
Top Round Steak ③
Rolled Rump ①
Outside (Bottom) Round ③ Steak or Pot-roast
Eye of Round ③
Heel of Round ④

Shank Cross Cuts ①
Fresh Brisket ③
Beef for Stew ① ② (also from other cuts)
Corned Brisket ③
Short Ribs ①
Skirt Steak Fillets ① ②
Rolled Plate ① ②
Plate Beef ① ②
Ground Beef (Flank, Short Plate, Shank, Brisket, Rib, Chuck, Loin, Round)
Beef Patties
Flank Steak ①
Flank Steak Fillets ①
Tip Steak ④ ②
Sirloin Tip ④ ②
Cube Steak ④ ②

the backbone and upper ribs—and they cost the most per pound. Table 4–8 shows that tender cuts are cooked by dry heat. A skinny old animal of low grade would take longer to cook than a well-fed young animal, by any method. The tougher cuts require moist heat in cooking. The method most favored today is to take a choice or prime grade and roast it at a low temperature for a longer period of time until it is tender.

Ripened meat

Ripening or "aging" of beef adds to the cost but improves the flavor. Ripened meat has hung in a refrigerated warehouse for two to three weeks. This process allows the enzymes to act on the lean and connective tissues and make the meat more tender, juicy, and delicate in flavor. The hindquarters, ribs, and loins of beef are ripened, and lamb may also be ripened. Those who know the

fig. 4–2 **VEAL CHART** Retail cuts of veal and where they come from

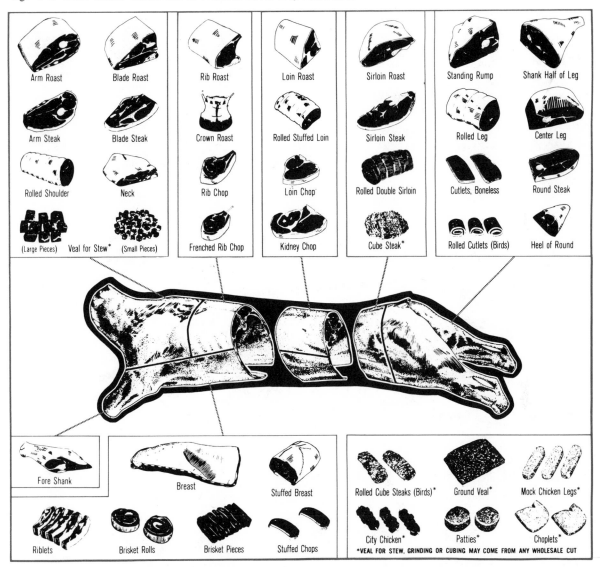

Arm Roast	Blade Roast	Rib Roast	Loin Roast	Sirloin Roast	Standing Rump	Shank Half of Leg

flavor of ripened beef prefer it above all others, even though it is slightly higher in price. It is darker in color than unripened beef.

Cured meat

Cured meat is made by heavily salting fresh meat and letting it stand in the brine. The meat most commonly cured is pork. The hind legs are hams; the forelegs, Boston butt and picnic ham; the side, bacon. Bacon is not considered meat, but fat. We buy it and enjoy it for flavor. It is expensive. Canadian bacon comes from the loin and is lean, but expensive.

Some cuts of beef, such as the rump, plate, round, and brisket are cured. This is called corned beef. So much cured ham is used that the price is about the same as that of fresh ham.

fig. 4–3 **PORK CHART** Retail cuts of pork and where they come from

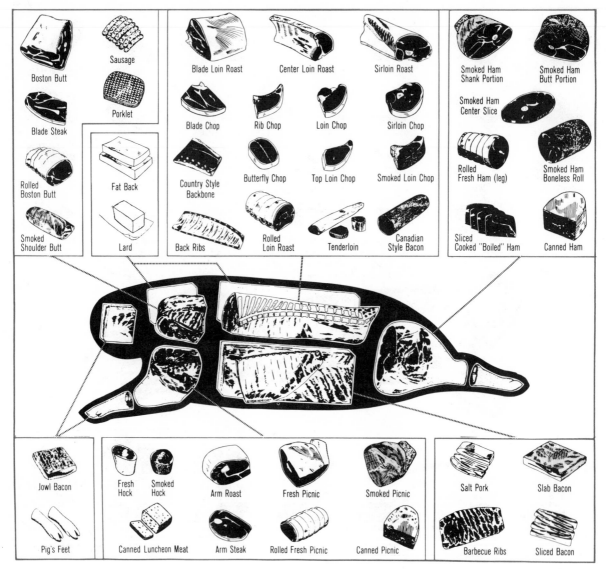

Boston Butt · Sausage · Porklet · Blade Steak · Rolled Boston Butt · Smoked Shoulder Butt · Fat Back · Lard · Blade Loin Roast · Center Loin Roast · Sirloin Roast · Blade Chop · Rib Chop · Loin Chop · Sirloin Chop · Country Style Backbone · Butterfly Chop · Top Loin Chop · Smoked Loin Chop · Back Ribs · Rolled Loin Roast · Tenderloin · Canadian Style Bacon · Smoked Ham Shank Portion · Smoked Ham Butt Portion · Smoked Ham Center Slice · Rolled Fresh Ham (leg) · Smoked Ham Boneless Roll · Sliced Cooked "Boiled" Ham · Canned Ham · Jowl Bacon · Pig's Feet · Fresh Hock · Smoked Hock · Canned Luncheon Meat · Arm Roast · Arm Steak · Fresh Picnic · Rolled Fresh Picnic · Smoked Picnic · Canned Picnic · Salt Pork · Slab Bacon · Barbecue Ribs · Sliced Bacon

Processed meats

Processed meats cost more per pound than many fresh meats, though canned ones are made from the lowest grades and toughest cuts. Meats are processed by canning, drying, freezing, freeze-drying, and pickling.

The nutrients and flavor of frozen meats, poultry, and fish are equal to those of the fresh unfrozen variety. Some harmful bacteria are de-stroyed by freezing, but meat spoils quickly once it is thawed. Any processed meat, once opened, should be stored in the refrigerator. Canned and frozen fish enables inlanders to have this food whenever they want it, and thus enjoy a better diet. Some frozen and canned meats compare favorably in price with fresh varieties. It is good management to keep a supply of processed meats, poultry, and fish on hand for convenience and for emergencies.

67/

fig. 4-4 **LAMB CHART** Retail cuts of lamb and where they come from

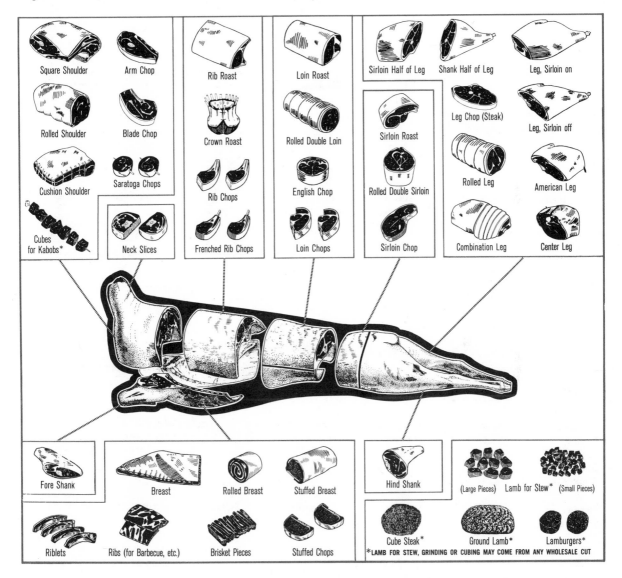

Dried beef

Dried (or chipped) beef is an example of low-grade meat or tough cuts that can be processed (in this case cured in brine, dried, and thinly sliced) into an epicure's choice and sold at a fancy price. This meat illustrates the price we pay for the labor, time, and equipment used in processing some foods. For instance, in 1969 one brand of sliced dried beef sold at 50 cents a 2-ounce jar. This is at the rate of $4.00 per pound! A bride who is accustomed to eating chipped beef on hot biscuits, waffles, or toast at her mother's home may reach for a small jar of this beef for a **Sunday** breakfast and not realize the actual cost per pound.

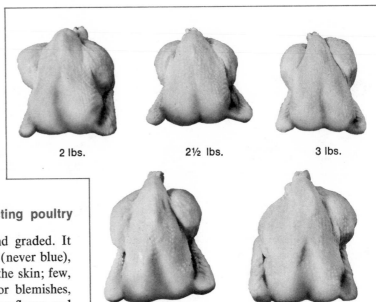

2 lbs.   2½ lbs.   3 lbs.

3½ lbs.   4 lbs.

How would you grade these chickens?
How would you cook each?

Selecting poultry

High-quality poultry is inspected and graded. It
has firm, thick flesh of a yellow tinge (never blue),
with a layer of yellowish fat beneath the skin; few,
if any, pinfeathers; and no bruises or blemishes,
though these do not affect nutrients or flavor and
make the poultry cost less. The grading indicates
that it is clean and wholesome.

table 4–4   A Guide for Selection and Use of Poultry

KIND	WEIGHT Lbs.	CHARACTERISTICS High-quality	HOW TO USE
ROASTING		Firm breastbone; fleshed breasts; pliable, smooth skin; yellowish and evenly distributed fat	Roasted whole in oven (stuffed, if desired, with bread, cornbread, rice, bulgur); barbecued on spit; roasted in parts
Chicken	3–6		
Turkey	5–26		
Capon	3–6		
Goose	4–10		
Duck	1½–4		
FRYER Whole or parts	2–3	Has less fat; breastbone flexible cartilage; short legs; well-fleshed	Broiled; fried disjointed; baked
BROILER	¾–2	Same as fryers. More pinfeathers on young birds	Split in halves down back and breast; broiled in stove on grill
CORNISH HEN	¾–1	Breast broad; well-fleshed; flexible breastbone; wings flexible when pulled	Roasted, stuffed as above
FOWL	3–6	Same as roasting chickens (older birds, tougher)	Stewed; chicken and dumplings; casseroles; salad; sandwiches; fricassee; soup; croquettes; pies; hash

Selecting fish

High quality in fish is best judged if it is bought whole. Odor is the most important indication of freshness. A fresh fish has little odor, and each has the natural odor for its kind. Once the fish begins to deteriorate, the odor becomes strong and offensive.

In a fresh fish, the eyes should bulge as in a live fish and be bright and shining, not dull or slimy. The gills should be firm, red-pink in color, and free from mucus. The scales should have a bright sheen, as if the fish were just caught, and should not stick together. The flesh should be firm and should spring back when touched.

Most fish is frozen as soon as it is caught. Some is canned immediately. This fish is of high quality, if it bears the marks of federal inspection on the cans.

Determining cost of meat

Cost in meat is related to (1) grade, (2) cut, (3) age, (4) method of processing, (5) amount of fat and bone, and (6) kind of meat, fish, or poultry. Usually red meats and shellfish cost more per pound than other kinds. Hidden costs of meat include fuel and preparation time, the way it is cooked, and the way it is served.

Calculate the cost of meat on the basis of how many four-ounce servings of raw, lean meat a pound yields. It takes half a broiler or a plateful of tiny riblets from a young lamb to make a serving. Yet a pound of ground lean beef will yield four good servings and a pound of flesh-fish, such as fillet, yields three to four servings. (See Table 4–7 for the recommended amount to buy per serving.)

Most fish is frozen as soon as it is caught.

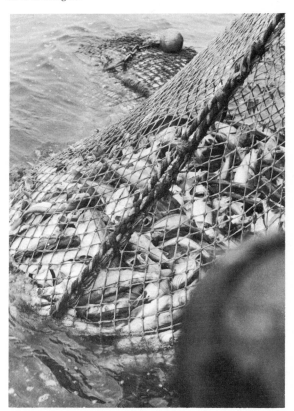

Tenderizing meat

Tenderizing meat improves its tenderness and quality. Hams are an example of the quick "tenderized-cured" process which takes two weeks, as compared with the old-time brine method, which required six weeks. Enzymes are injected into the meat, carrying other curing agents as well. These circulate through the tissues, making them more tender and moist and softer in texture. Many people prefer this. Others like the dry hard cure, like the Virginia hams.

table 4–5   *A Guide for Selection and Use of Fish*

KIND	CHARACTERISTICS (High-quality)	HOW TO USE
FISH:		
Mackerel	Flesh firm, colored, highest in fat	Broiled, baked, fried (Add lime or
Sardines	Odor: clean, mild, fresh	lemon.)
Shad		
Eel		
Herring		
Halibut	Fresh or frozen	Thaw frozen
Haddock	Low fat; firm flesh—no fingerprint	Broiled, baked, fried, or poached
Swordfish	when pressed; white or pink flesh for	Add seasonings with oil and rub in
Snapper	its kind	to improve flavor. Add lime or lemon.
Flounder	Odor: for its kind, not strong or	Cook at low temperature to destroy
Black bass	offensive	odor.
Trout		
Cod		
Salmon		
Pickerel		
SHELLFISH:		
Oysters	Fresh, canned, and frozen	Stewed, creamed, scalloped, fried
	Firm, plump, little odor	Raw as first course (on half-shell)
	Season: September to April	Serve with lemon, lime, or sauce.
Scallops	Firm; almost odorless	Deep-fried, pan-fried, fritters, chowder
	Season: September to March	
Clams	Buy only unbroken shells.	Chowder; raw, on half-shell; steamed;
	Quahogs, little neck—both round	broiled; boiled; juice; in appetizers
	shape	
	Season: All year	
	Soft-shell—long shape	
	Season: May to October	
Crab	Fresh, frozen, canned	Cocktail, salad, deviled, casserole,
	High-quality—back fin, white claw	scalloped
	Season: Hard-shell, all year; soft-shell	
	summer	
Shrimp	Flesh firm, color pink	Cocktail, salad, boiled, fried, curried,
	Season: All year	casseroles, appetizers
Lobsters	Select only live or boiled. If alive,	Broiled, boiled, cocktail, salad
	should be very active to touch.	
	Season: fresh—summer; frozen,	
	canned—all year	
Fish roe	Shad, sturgeon (caviar)	Appetizer, sandwich
(eggs)	Fresh or canned	Shad roe—broiled, poached, casserole

Meat may also be tenderized by breaking or softening the fibers—the muscle and connective tissues. In the markets, a machine is used for this purpose. At home, use a hammer or a spiked hammer. Grinding the meat or using a tenderizing powder over it are other ways to tenderize low grades and tough cuts so that they may be broiled. Low-temperature moist heat is a sure way to soften tough fibers.

Storing meat, poultry, or fish

Refrigerating fresh food

Fresh meat, poultry, fish, and cold cuts, as well as frozen foods, should be purchased last in shopping. These should be stored in the coldest part of the refrigerator. Fresh, unfrozen meat should be loosely wrapped if it is not to be cooked on the day it is purchased. Tight packaging increases the growth of microorganisms and hastens spoilage. The outside of packaged meat should be wiped with a paper towel before it is placed in the refrigerator. Fish should be wrapped so that no odor escapes into the refrigerator or freezer. It should be washed just before cooking, and all excess water absorbed on paper towels.

Storing leftover cooked meat

Leftover cooked meat should be cooled quickly and placed in the coldest part of the refrigerator. It should be used within a day or two. For freezing, it should be tightly sealed and placed immediately in the freezer, for best flavor. Stuffing should be removed from poultry and frozen in a separate container.

table 4–6 *Meat Storage Time Chart**
Maximum Storage Time

MEAT	REFRIGERATOR**	FREEZER
FRESH		
Beef	2–4 days	6–12 months
Veal	2–4 days	6–9 months
Pork	2–4 days	3–6 months
Lamb	2–4 days	6–9 months
Ground beef, veal, lamb	1–2 days	3–4 months
Ground pork	1–2 days	1–3 months
Variety meats	1–2 days	3–4 months
PROCESSED		
Luncheon meats	1 week	Not recommended
Sausage, fresh pork	2–3 days	Not recommended
Sausage, smoked	3–7 days	Not recommended
Sausage, dry and semidry (unsliced)	2–3 weeks	Not recommended
Frankfurters	4–5 days	2 weeks
Bacon	5–7 days	2 weeks
Smoked ham, whole	——	60 days
Beef, corned	1 week	2 weeks
COOKED		
Leftover meat	4–5 days	2–3 months
FROZEN COOKED FOODS		
Meat pies	——	3 months
Swiss steak	——	3 months
Stews	——	3–4 months
Prepared meat dinners	——	2–6 months

*SOURCE: *Lessons on Meat* (Washington, D.C.: National Live Stock and Meat Board).
**The range in time reflects recommendations for maximum storage time from several authorities. For top quality, fresh meats should be used in 2 or 3 days, ground meat and variety meats should be used in 24 hours.

Using frozen meat, fish, and poultry

Frozen precooked meat should be used within the time schedule in Table 4–6. Frozen oysters should be used within a month and frozen cured pork or sausage within two months. The date should be marked on the food when it is put in the freezer. To save money and time and make a convenient meal easily and quickly, precooked meats should be used on the days when it will help most—when the homemaker is busy or ill, or a family emergency arises.

Frozen meat, whether cooked raw, should be thawed gradually in the refrigerator, if space and time permit. Some juice and nutrients escape in thawing. These should be saved and added back at the end, or, if the meat is cooked, replaced as the food is reheated.

How much to buy?

If your budget permits, plan to have a good animal protein food in each meal. For each person, allow at least three ounces of lean meat, fish, or poultry when cooked, not counting fat or bone. This applies to older children, teen-agers, and adults. Allow about two ounces of lean meat for children under six.

The cost of meat varies with the economic condition of our country, the locality, the season, and the store in which it is purchased. But the relation of nutrients in each kind of meat is stable. Hence three ounces of rib roast of beef or pork chop costs more and yields less protein than the same amount of lean round roast of beef, halibut, or beef liver any year.

Table 4–7 illustrates how a young couple, or anyone on a low food budget, can have a good

table 4–7   Nutrient Comparison of Meats and Alternates*

ITEM	SIZE OF SERVING**	PERCENT OF DAILY ALLOWANCE PER SERVING**				
		Protein	Iron	Thiamine	Riboflavin	Niacin
Ham	3 oz.	29	21	38	11	29
Beef rib roast	3 oz.	29	22	4	9	30
Pork chops	3 oz.	29	22	59	12	36
Beef chuck roast	3 oz.	32	22	3	10	29
Halibut	3 oz.	33	6	4	4	74
Beef liver	3 oz.	30	55	18	198	105
Eggs, large	2 eggs	19	22	7	16	1
Peanut butter	2 T.	12	5	3	2	43
Dry beans	¾ cup cooked	16	30	8	6	12

*Adapted from Louise Page and Eloise Cofer, "Your Money's Worth," *Food: The Yearbook of Agriculture* 1959 (Washington, D.C.: USDA), p. 570.
**For an average adult. Meat servings are cooked meat without fat, gristle, and bone:

protein food in each meal at the price they can afford to pay. In 1968, for instance, beef rib roast was 25 percent higher in some sections of the country than in others, while eggs were lower per dozen. Prices change, but the percent of nutrients yielded by one pound remains stable.

Principles for cooking meats and eggs

Cooking meats

The aim in cooking meat is to produce the most delectable dish possible from the kind chosen. It should be tender in texture, juicy, of fine aroma, of good color, and, best of all, flavorsome when ready to eat.

When meat is cooked, there is a loss of moisture and a change in color, the fat melts, the proteins coagulate, and when moist heat is used the collagen (gristle) softens and releases gelatin. These changes improve the flavor of meat and also make it more digestible. Cooking also destroys harmful bacteria.

The proteins in lean meat and egg white coagulate at a much lower temperature than boiling water (at about 140°F). At a high temperature, protein hardens in both the muscle fibers (albumin and globulin) and the connective tissue (collagen and elastin). This makes meat and eggs tough, rubbery, and dry, regardless of the grade or cut. Understanding this is one basis for successful meat cookery.

LOW-TEMPERATURE COOKING. Low temperature is the key to cooking meat to make it tender, juicy, and mellow in flavor. This is preferred for the highest grades and tenderest cuts, as well as the lower grades and tough cuts. There is less loss of moisture at low temperature, and less shrinkage. Generally, it is recommended that red meat be roasted at a temperature of 300°F, and poultry and pork at 325°F. However, a 1970 study comparing beef roasted at 200°F and 300°F confirmed earlier findings that the lower temperature yielded more servings per pound, thus costing less; that the meat was juicier, more tender, and more flavorsome; and that fewer nutrients were lost in drippings. It must be remembered, however, that low-temperature cooking requires a much longer period of time.

COOKING TIME. The time required depends on the kind of meat, grade, cut, method of cooking, thickness, and size of meat. Time is approximate when given in minutes per pound. A meat thermometer is a sure way of knowing that you allow the right amount of time. It will tell you when the pork is at 185°F, the temperature at which you can be sure that all harmful bacteria are destroyed. It can enable you to serve the roast rare or medium rare without guessing.

Methods of cooking meat

The methods recommended for cooking various meats are illustrated in Table 4–8.

DRY HEAT. This is used in broiling and roasting, for prime and choice grade meat and tender cuts, or tenderized lower grades and tougher cuts. The tender cuts of meat suited to cooking by dry heat are listed in Table 4–8. Broiling and roasting provide maximum flavor and nutrients in red meats, poultry, fish, and organ meats.

Panbroiling. Panbroiling is cooking without fat. This method is used for any cut or kind of meat that may be broiled. The technique differs in that the meat is browned and turned, then cooked

Chicken is one of our most popular meats for roasting, broiling, or barbecuing.

The moist heat method of cooking produces tender, juicy meat and flavorsome vegetables.

to the desired doneness, using a thick, firm-bottomed skillet or grill.

Microwave. This is a form of dry heat that is used by restaurants, institutions, and airplanes, and in a few homes. It is becoming less expensive and saves much time. The microwave oven creates heat by ultrahigh frequency, causing molecule agitation and energy-heat release. It holds promise for wider use. One drawback has been poor browning. This is corrected by conventional oven browning. Micro-cooking is now available in lower-price ovens for the home.

table 4–8 **Basic Methods of Cooking Meat, Poultry, Fish, and Organ Meats**

| KIND | DRY HEAT | | MOIST HEAT | | |
	Broiling	Roasting*	Frying (pan)	Braising	In Liquid
BEEF*	Steaks:	Rib	Round steak	Pot roast	Soups and stews
	Porterhouse	Standing	Ground steak	Steaks	Brisket
	T-bone	Rolled	T-bone steak	Lower round	Short ribs
	Sirloin	Rump	Rib steak	Arm	Shank
	Tenderloin	Sirloin	Club steak	Blade	Plate
	(Filet	Loaf	Filet mignon	Flank	Neck
	mignon)		Sirloin steak		Flank
	Club				Heel of round
	Rib				Corned beef
	Top round				Cross-cut shank
	Loin tip				
	Ground				
VEAL	None—	Loin	Cutlet	Breast	Neck
	too lean	Leg	Chops	Steak	Riblets
		Rack	Steak	Loin	Breast
		Shoulder	Cube steak	Chops	Flank
		(Rub roasts	Ground	Kidney	Shank
		with oil.)		Cubes	Heel of round
				Ribs	
PORK**	Canadian bacon	Loin	Ham, fresh or	Chops	Ham
	Bacon	Sirloin	cured	Spareribs	Picnic ham
	Ham slice	Ham, fresh or	Bacon	Shoulder steaks	Shoulder butt
	Smoked shoulder	cured	Canadian bacon	Tenderloin	Shank
	(No fresh pork	Spareribs			Hocks
	should be	Ham loaf			Tenderloin
	broiled.)	Picnic ham,			
		fresh or			
		cured			

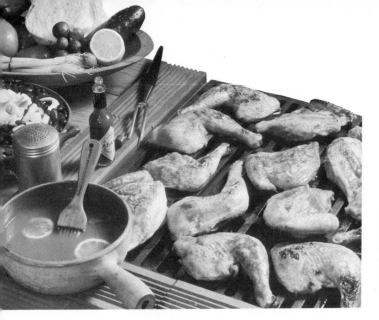
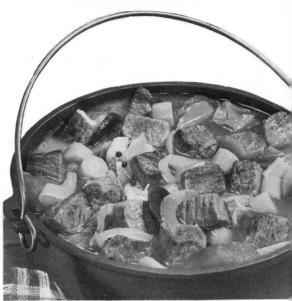

| KIND | DRY HEAT | | MOIST HEAT | | |
	Broiling	Roasting*	Frying (pan)	Braising	In Liquid
LAMB	Chops Loin Rib Sirloin Shoulder Steaks Ground	Leg Shoulder Loaf	Chops Loin Shoulder steak Ground	Chops Shoulder Breast Neck Shank	Neck Flank Shank Riblets Breast
VARIETY ORGANS	Liver, (lamb, veal, or chicken) Kidneys Sweetbreads		Liver (lamb, veal, chicken, pork, or beef) Brains	Liver Kidneys Heart Sweetbreads Brains	Brains Kidney Tongue Sweetbreads
POULTRY	Broilers	Broilers Young hens Hen turkeys Young tom turkeys Ducks Geese	Fryers Broilers	Hens Fowls	Hens Fowls Old roosters Old tom turkeys
FISH	Fish is so tender that any kind may be cooked in any fashion that you like.				

*Latest research shows that 200°F is the most desirable temperature for roasting beef, for economy, juiciness, tenderness, and flavor. A meat thermometer should be used.

  Rare beef—Internal temperature 140°F; Color: red to pink inside

  Medium—Internal temperature 160°F; Color: pink

  Well done—Internal temperature 170°F; Color: brown

  Pork, lamb, and poultry are roasted and cooked well done.

**Pork—Fresh: The aim in roasting fresh pork is to reach an internal temperature of 185°F, which can be achieved by cooking for a longer period at a lower temperature (225°F). The time to allow will depend on the size and shape of the roast. The same advantages of low-temperature roasting for beef hold also for pork and lamb.

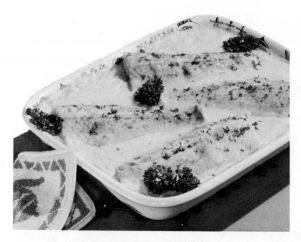

Poached fish, using herbs and spices, is a delightful taste treat.

MOIST HEAT. This method is used for cooking lower grades and less tender cuts of meat. Table 4–8 shows the cuts most suited to moist heat. The purpose of cooking meat with moist heat is to soften the connective tissue and release the collagen from the gristle.

Braising. Braising differs from stewing or cooking in liquid in that the meat is first seasoned. It may or may not be dredged in flour, but it is always browned on both sides. A small amount of water or other liquid is added. It is covered and cooked at a low temperature until done.

Cooking in Liquid. This includes soupmaking, stewing, and simmering meat for slicing, such as pot roasts. The meat may be browned first or not, according to your preference. Liquid and seasonings are added and the mixture is simmered in a heavy covered kettle. The meat and liquid should occupy no more than one-half the capacity of the pot. Cooking in a pressure saucepan until tender saves two hours or more in time. Vegetables are added when the meat is tender, and are cooked crisp-tender. The fat is skimmed off and most of the vitamins, minerals, and amino acids remain in the meat, vegetables, and liquid, since the latter is part of the soup or stew.

Deep-frying. This is a very quick method of cooking. Fat, preferably vegetable oil high in linoleic acid, is heated to 350° to 400°F. The food is lowered into it in a basket. Because of the high temperature and the danger of splashing, extreme care should be exercised when cooking. Water should never be used to put out a fire caused by fat.

Flavor

Each method of cooking meat produces an entirely different and distinctive flavor. Dry heat gives a

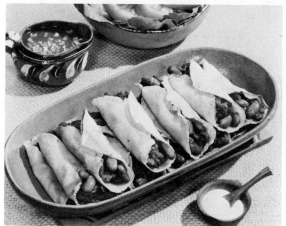

Enchiladas, made with tangy spiced beans, are a favorite alternate for meat.

flavor most people like best. However, we know that a properly cooked pot roast, chicken and noodles, or poached salmon is a delightful eating experience. Using variety in methods of cooking the same meat sparks the imagination and the appetite.

Loss of nutrients

Experimental studies show that much thiamine is lost in cooking meats. Thiamine loss ranged from 60 percent in roast meat to 70 percent in broiled meat. Stewed meat lost 75 percent, but much of this was retained in the liquid. About 90 percent

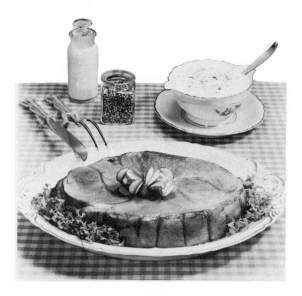

Ham steak, garnished with parsley and radish roses and served with horseradish sauce, is an attractive and nutritious dish.

of the thiamine was retained in pan-fried meat, as the fat seals in nutrients from oxygen. There was little loss of riboflavin and niacin, which drip with the juice into the brown drippings, where they can be used in gravy or juice.

Gourmet variations with herbs and spices

Creative use of seasonings

The homemaker who can make a delicious dish out of an unattractive piece of meat, as the British do with kidney pie, is in a distinguished class. Part of this skill lies in using garlic, onion, pepper, and other herbs and spices to bring out a subtle flavor. However, herbs and spices are used so delicately in the hands of a culinary artist that you cannot guess what is in a dish, but you know it is delicious. Table 22–1, page 396, gives gourmet variations for seasoning meats, poultry, fish, and eggs with herbs and spices.

Your creativeness is developed by experimenting with a variety of herbs and spices when you cook. When you create a tasty dish, you add enjoyment to the family's diet. But a word of warning: As with fine perfume, a small amount of herbs and spices enhances the meat, while a large amount drowns out its natural flavor. Measure what you add. Record it. Vary the amount, until you hit the one that you and your family likes best. For instance, a small amount of curry powder (a mixture of spices) can enliven a dish, but twice the amount may destroy the good flavor. Tarragon chicken is quite different from thyme chicken, and chicken with chili peppers differs from both of them. See the Cookbook for gourmet variations in cooking red meats, poultry, fish, and eggs.

Garnishes for eye and taste appeal

Garnishes add a delightful color and flavor to different kinds of meats. Table 22–1 shows a number of garnishes to spark your imagination and creative skill. Place garnishes carefully on the meat or around it, and use only enough to enhance the meat itself, but not so much that the meat is hidden.

Planned leftovers

For economy and convenience, it is wise to prepare larger quantities of meats and save some for future use. This extra food is called planned leftovers. By taking advantage of lower prices for "specials," and by larger quantity buying, you save shopping time, energy, fuel, and cooking time.

You can make your own convenience meat, ready to serve, with a minimum of preparation

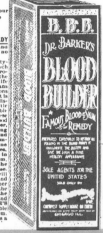
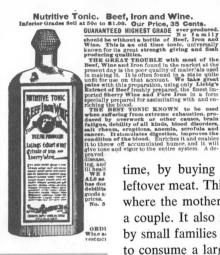
A turn-of-the-century catalogue ad

time, by buying a large roast that will provide leftover meat. This is especially helpful in a family where the mother works outside the home, or for a couple. It also makes possible the use of roasts by small families that could otherwise not be able to consume a large roast at one time. It comes in handy for the young mother who is going to the hospital or returning with a new baby. How can it be done?

Cook a boned roast of beef, ham, or turkey. Buy a large one when there is a special price, if your freezer space permits. Roast the beef rare. Then cut it in meal-size sections, seal it airtight, and freeze it immediately after the first meal. When you are ready to use the beef for the next meal, remove it from the freezer in the morning (when you plan to use it for dinner) and place it on the refrigerator shelf. It should be just thawed, or almost so, when you place it in a pan in a low oven. You will have to experiment to find the proper time allowance. Get the meat hot, like freshly-cooked meat—and no more. Even beef can taste as juicy and good as when fresh-roasted, if you reheat it just enough, but not too much, and serve it at once.

A large roasted turkey or chicken, ham, fresh pork, lamb, or veal may be treated similarly. Pork, however, must be cooked well-done to begin with. Flavor is better if the meat is not sliced until it is ready to serve.

Buying eggs to save money

Make the best use of your food dollar by selecting eggs according to the use you wish to make of them, the grade of fresh ones, and the size or weight. Fresh eggs cost the most, and the higher the grade the higher the cost.

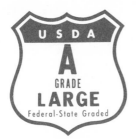 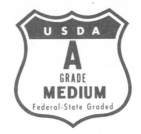

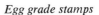

Egg grade stamps

Grades of eggs

The grade is indicated by AA, A, and B. The highest grade is AA. Each grade has a high, firm yolk and a thick, firm white, but AA is the firmest. Use top grades for poaching, boiling, and frying and lower grades for various cooked dishes, including scrambled eggs and omelets.

Size and weight

The size and weight of eggs are other keys to selection. Figure 4–0 shows the names of the various types of eggs, by size and weight. Generally, if there is less than a 7-cent price spread per dozen eggs between one size and the next smaller size in the same grade, buy the larger size. To illustrate, if extra large eggs cost 65 cents a dozen and large ones cost 60, the extra large size is the best use of your money.

Also consider the needs of your family. An adult may prefer an extra large egg, but if there is a small child a small egg may help him eat it all and enjoy it. It is a psychological victory for him to "eat it all." Keep two sizes on hand when children are small.

Standards for fresh eggs are set by federal and state authorities. The shield is on the carton to guide you. It means the grade on the box was correct at the time it was placed there.

Candling is a mass way of determining freshness. It determines grade by the thickness of the white and the yolk. During inspection and grading, eggs are weighed for size.

Color

The color of the shell depends on the breed of chicken. The color of the egg yolk depends on the kind of feed. Deep yellow color indicates that the hen has had carotene-rich food. Hens eat green grass and can convert carotene from it into vitamin A. Since vitamin A is colorless, a light yolk may have even more vitamin A than a darker-yellow one which has more carotene (see Chapter 5).

Storing eggs

Eggs should be stored in the refrigerator in a covered container, with the large end up, so that the air sac is at the top. Research shows that eggs stored in the refrigerator for three weeks deteriorate less than eggs stored at room temperature for three days. As eggs get older, chemical changes take place that Americans don't like. In countries where people are accustomed to eating unrefrigerated eggs, the people enjoy the flavor of old but sound eggs.

Leftover yolks should be stored in the refrigerator in a covered jar, and should be covered with water. Yolks should be used within one or two days, but egg whites will keep in the refrigerator for a week. Yolks or whites may be stored frozen at 0°F or lower. The frozen eggs should be thawed and used in the same way as fresh ones.

Dried eggs

The drying of eggs in flat dishes in the sun has been practiced in the Orient for centuries. Dried egg solids are on our markets whole, or as yolks or whites, and provide the nutrients of fresh eggs at lower cost. Read the label to see if it bears the U.S. inspection mark, which indicates that the product was prepared from wholesome eggs under sanitary conditions. Use dried eggs as an alternate for fresh eggs, as shown in Table 4–9. Store dried eggs, before and after opening, in a tightly closed container in the refrigerator.

How to use dried eggs

Use dried eggs only in recipes that require thorough cooking, as in baked foods. When you use them in other foods, boil the food which contains the dried egg for 12 minutes. This applies particularly to casserole dishes after they reach the boiling point. This precaution is to ensure a safe product.

Without knowing it, each of us has eaten dried eggs many times in bakery foods, in restaurants, in institutional meals, in many kinds of mixes, and in precooked convenience foods. The flavor is pleasant, and they are a good alternate for fresh eggs. Dried eggs are used by commercial companies because they cost less. We can use them for the same reason in cooking, if we care to do so.

Uses of eggs

Eggs are used (1) to thicken a mixture, (2) to leaven, (3) to bind or emulsify, (4) to make a foam, and (5) to improve the flavor and nutrients in beverages and in many dishes.

Thickening foods

Eggs thicken soups, sauces, soufflés, custards, floating island, puddings, cream-type pie fillings, and ice cream. In thickening power, one whole egg is equal to two yolks or two whites. To help prevent curdling, stir the hot liquid into the egg mixture, and not the other way round. Research at Cornell University has resulted in the recommendation that the egg be cooked with sauces for puddings using tapioca, flour, and the like, rather than the old way of adding eggs at the last on top of the stove and cooking until the mixture is thickened.

Cooking in a double boiler helps control the temperature after eggs are added and prevents curdling. Heating milk before adding it to a custard mixture hastens the baking. Custards bake more evenly if they are set in a pan of hot water. Use the same technique for corn puddings, other puddings, and soufflés. Do not cover custards or egg mixtures in the oven, as browning is a desirable part of the flavor. If an egg sauce curdles, beat out the lumps with a blender or an egg beater.

Leavening

Eggs leaven mixtures. This lightens and increases the volume of cakes and breads. Angel food, sponge, and chiffon cakes are completely dependent on eggs to lighten them. Soufflés, leavened with eggs and combined with cheese, chicken, fish, ham, or vegetable, or made as desserts, give an elegant touch to a meal. Learning to make one soufflé enables you to make many, to delight your family or guests—a mark of a creative and artistic hostess.

table 4–9 *How to Convert Dried Egg Powder to the Equal of Fresh Eggs*

FRESH EGG	DRIED EGG	WATER (Lukewarm—118°F)
1 whole egg	2½ T.	2½ T.
1 egg white	2 t.	2 T.
1 egg yolk	2 T.	2 t.

Emulsifying

Eggs emulsify, that is, bind together two or more ingredients that separate naturally, such as oil and vinegar. Thus they help make different mayonnaise types of salad dressing or hollandaise sauce smooth.

Making foams

Eggs used to make a foam, as in meringues, angel food cakes, sponge cakes, chiffon cakes, or soufflés, produce larger volume and blend with other ingredients better when at room temperature. Often the recipe calls for salt or acid (cream of tartar is acid) to be added when the foam begins to form. This is to lower the temperature (and thus coagulate more quickly) and to give a firmer texture to the egg white, enabling it to hold more air and thus increase lightness. When sugar is added during the beating of egg whites, it takes longer to reach the desired peak of stiffness. This is because sugar raises the coagulation temperature. It also takes longer, therefore, to bake a very sweet custard than an unsweetened egg-milk mixture.

Eggs also glaze baked foods and are used to give firm structure to croquettes and meat loaf, and for batter in frying.

Raw egg white: to be avoided

When the egg white is raw, the protein avidin combines with biotin in the egg and can prevent its absorption by the body. Biotin, an essential member of the B vitamin family, is needed as a co-enzyme for a larger team of nutrients in using starch, sugar, and fat, and may perform still-unknown services for us.

At the University of Georgia, interesting studies by Virgil Sydenstricker and his associates showed what happened when large amounts of raw egg white were fed in an otherwise balanced diet. A rash developed on skin, which became dry and scaly, and there were changes in skin color. The tongue became sore, nervous symptoms developed, and abnormal electrocardiograms were recorded. Loss of hair, anemia, skin hemorrhages, scaly and greasy skins, and nervousness were also noted in animals that ate raw egg white. The interesting thing in the studies was that when the subjects were fed egg that was cooked until the white was firm, all unfavorable symptoms disappeared.

It is not likely that you will eat so much raw egg white as to deprive your body of the amount of biotin it needs. But there is no reason to eat raw eggs and take chances of developing an allergy to them, when there are so many delicious ways

table 4–10   Temperatures and Time for Baking Representative Egg, Meat, Milk, and Cheese Dishes

TYPE OF PRODUCT	OVEN TEMPERATURE Degrees F	APPROXIMATE BAKING TIME Minutes
Cheese soufflé (Baked in pan of hot water)	350	30–60
Custard (Baked in pan of hot water)	350	30–60
Macaroni and cheese	350	25–30
Meat loaf	300	60–90
Meat pie	400	25–30
Rice pudding (raw rice)	300	120–180
Scalloped potatoes	350	60

table 4–11   *How to Use Eggs, Red Meats, Organ Meats, Poultry, and Fish for Breakfast**

EGGS	RED MEATS	ORGANS	POULTRY	FISH
Boiled	Canadian bacon	Sautéed chicken	Fried chicken	Broiled fish
Poached	Ham, cured	livers	Broiled chicken	in season
Blindfolded	Lamb chop	Broiled kidney	Turkey hash	Creamed fish on
Fried	Texas steak	Broiled liver	Turkey croquettes	corn muffins
Shirred	Creamed chipped	and bacon	Creamed chicken	Smoked fish
Scrambled	beef	Broiled	on hot biscuits	
Scrambled with	Ham and eggs	sweetbreads		
cheese				
Omelet				
Creamed				
French toast				
Popovers				
Spoon bread				
Pancakes				

*For a balanced breakfast, add a citrus fruit or juice or other fruit in season, bread, a spread, milk, and coffee (if desired). For a hearty breakfast, add a dish of cereal, jam, or preserves, if the diet permits the added calories.

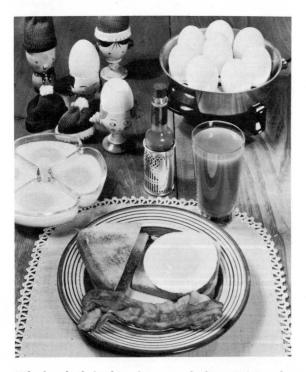

Whether boiled, shirred, or poached, eggs form the core of a good breakfast. Why should egg white always be cooked?

to eat them cooked. Besides, raw eggs may contain the harmful salmonella microorganism (discussed in Chapter 17). None of these disadvantages are present in cooked eggs. Adding raw eggs, therefore, to any beverages, salad (as in Caesar), desserts (as in gelatin ones), or sherbets is not a desirable practice.

How many eggs?

How many eggs do we need in a week? Unless there are specific medical reasons for you to limit egg intake, it is considered that one daily is valuable, not only for the protein, but also for the variety of other nutrients it brings, and at least four to five should be eaten per week.

Use of meats and eggs in meals

Divide your money for meat and eggs so that each meal has a fair serving of one of these foods or has an alternate in the form of cheese, dry legumes, or nuts.

table 4-12   **How to Use Eggs, Red Meats, Organ Meats, Poultry, and Fish for Lunch****

EGGS	RED MEATS	ORGANS	POULTRY	FISH
Quiche Lorraine	Meat sandwich	Liverwurst	Chicken or	Tuna fish salad
Salad	beef, veal,	sandwich	turkey salad	Crab, shrimp, or
Sandwich	pork, lamb	Brain salad	Sandwich	lobster salad
Popovers	Soup	Kidney pie	Soufflé	Sandwiches
Stuffed	Stew	Any used for	Creamed	Poached
Cheese soufflé	Casserole	breakfast	Curried	Chowder
Meat or vegetable	Hamburger	Liver casserole	Any used for	Broiled
soufflé	Frankfurter		breakfast	Casserole
Welsh rarebit	Salad			
Eggs à la	Chili			
goldenrod	Meat loaf			
Spoon bread	Ham bits with			
Omelet	lentils or beans			
Deviled				
In casseroles				

**For a balanced lunch, add to one of these main dishes a raw or cooked vegetable or both; milk, tea, or coffee; bread and butter, and a simple dessert or fresh fruit. Eggs may be used at dinner in any of the ways suggested for lunch or breakfast.

table 4-13   **How to Use Eggs, Red Meats, Organ Meats, Poultry, and Fish for Dinner*****

EGGS	RED MEATS	ORGANS	POULTRY	FISH
Creole eggs	Roast meat:	Broiled liver	Roast	Chowder
Egg and vege-	Beef, Veal,	Liver pâté	Oven-fried	Baked
table casserole	Fresh Pork	Liver loaf	Southern fried	Roast, stuffed
Egg and seafood	Ham, Lamb	Pan-fried liver	chicken	Broiled
casserole	Broiled meat:	Liver sausage	A la king	Fried
Ham-and-egg	Chops	Liverburgers	Casserole	Casserole
shortcake on	Steaks	Liver-vegetable	Stew	Fish cakes
corn bread	Pot roast	casserole	With dumplings	Canapes
Grits soufflé	Braised stew	Liver pilaf	With noodles	Fish sticks
Egg and seafood	meat	Stuffed heart	Turkey steaks	Salad
salad	Barbecued beef	Braised heart	Turkey loaf	Appetizer
Turkey soufflé	Barbecued pork	Heart-vegetable	Turkey chowder	
Chicken soufflé	Shish kabob	soup	Pie	
Enchiladas	Meat loaf	Broiled kidneys	Loaf	
	Meat patties	Beef-kidney pie	Fricassee	
	Chili con carne	Sautéed chicken	Hash	
		livers		

***For a balanced dinner, serve at least 3 ounces per serving of cooked lean meat, organ meat, poultry, or fish without fat or bone. When eggs are the main protein dish, serve 2 eggs or the equivalent per serving. Add a cooked green or yellow vegetable (or another succulent one), a medium-sized potato or alternate (corn, macaroni, rice, bulgur, kasha, noodles), a raw vegetable salad or fresh fruit, milk, bread and butter if needed, dessert of choice if fruit is not used, and coffee or tea for adults.

Think in terms of a week and plan your menus so that you will have variety in your meals each day. For instance, during the week you will wish to serve liver and seafood or fish once or more. There are hundreds of different ways to serve these foods. One restaurant in Los Angeles, for example, serves omelets in 36 different ways, ranging in cost from $1.75 to $9.00 per omelet.

Tables 4–11, 4–12, and 4–13 give a few examples of how eggs, red meats, organs, poultry, and fish may be used in different ways at breakfast, lunch, and dinner.

The choice of meat at dinner is the focal point in planning the meal. It also is the major source of enjoyment. Most of us prefer the best serving of the day at dinner. This is fine, so long as we keep our choices in balance for the whole day's diet, and for the dinner itself. We should not concentrate on meat to the exclusion of the milk, vegetables, and fruits that we need. The plan of a balanced dinner given in Chapter 2 is an excellent guide.

By good management, we can have a food from the meat group in each meal at any budget level, and at the same time not neglect the other foods we need. Indeed, you can share with Hawthorne the delight that such an achievement in the meal as a whole "should surely be immortal."

Meaningful words

"aging" meat
albumin
avidin
bacteria
biotin
braising
broiling
candling
canner and cutter grade
carotene
choice grade
coagulation
collagen
commercial grade
cull grade
"cured" meat
elastin
gelatin
globulin
good grade
"marbling"

Thinking and evaluating

1. What foods from the meat group did you include in each meal and snack yesterday and today? What other foods did you eat that included animal protein? How does this add up for each meal? How can you improve it for economy and nutrients?

2. Explain what is meant by grades of meat. Which costs the most? Which contains the most fat? The most lean? The most nutrients? How does an understanding of grades of meat help you save money in buying it? In controlling weight? In planning meals?

3. Why does an understanding of the different cuts of meat in our modern supermarkets (where most meat is cut and prepackaged) help you save money in cooking it?

4. What different factors affect the cost of meat per pound? Do any of these relate to the nutrients it contains? How can you save money by taking these factors into account when you shop for meat?

5. If you were a bride on a low food budget, how would you decide whether to buy beef, pork, lamb, veal, poultry, fish, or cold cuts? Fresh, frozen, dried, or canned meats? Explain your reasons. How would you store each kind? Why would you serve liver during the week? Seafood?

6. Explain why it is important to have variety in the meat, fish, poultry, organ meats, and eggs and in the way you use each of them in meals. When would you use dried beans, peas, nuts, or cheese as

Meaningful words

medium grade
microwave
pan broiling
prime grade
processed meat
ripening meat
salmonella
standard grade
tenderizing
utility grade

meat alternates? Show how to balance the meal when a meat alternate is used.

7. Give examples of the use of eggs to (a) thicken, (b) leaven, (c) emulsify, (d) glaze, (e) give firm structure, (f) coat, (g) foam, and (h) use in a balanced breakfast seven days a week.

8. How many different kinds of meat, fish, and poultry have you eaten? Which do you like best? Which would you like to learn to include in more menus? Which method of cooking each type of meat or eggs do you like best? Which methods have you not tried?

Applying and sharing

1. (a) Visit a large meat department in a supermarket and note the grades, cuts, and prices of beef, veal, pork, lamb, different kinds of liver, poultry, fish, shellfish, and cold cuts. This may be done more efficiently by dividing the class into groups, and pooling your information, but there is no substitute for seeing each kind for yourself.

(b) Do the same for eggs, comparing size and cost.

2. On the basis of what you learned in your visit, and in this and the preceding chapters, plan balanced menus for a young couple for one week and include a good source of protein that gives variety in each meal on (a) a low food budget, (b) a moderate budget, (c) one meal for guests. How did you use seafood? Liver? What was the cost per day of each meat? Eggs?

3. Evaluate the commercials you hear on television and radio concerning taking any products for iron deficiency. How would you use meat to help meet this need?

4. Practice cooking meat at school and at home by the (1) dry heat methods of cooking; (2) moist heat methods of cooking. (Select recipes for ways to prepare each of these: red meats, fish, poultry, and organ meats on a low budget; a moderate one, and a liberal one. Try one in each category.)

5. What conclusions do you draw from your experience in cooking different kinds, cuts, and grades of meat? Poultry? Fish? Organ meats?

6. Select recipes and prepare eggs using four different ways to enliven breakfast and lunch. What did you learn by this experience that can improve your diet now?

7. Make a plan to put into practice at home what you have learned about meat, poultry, fish, organ meats, and eggs.

the lifelong benefits of milk

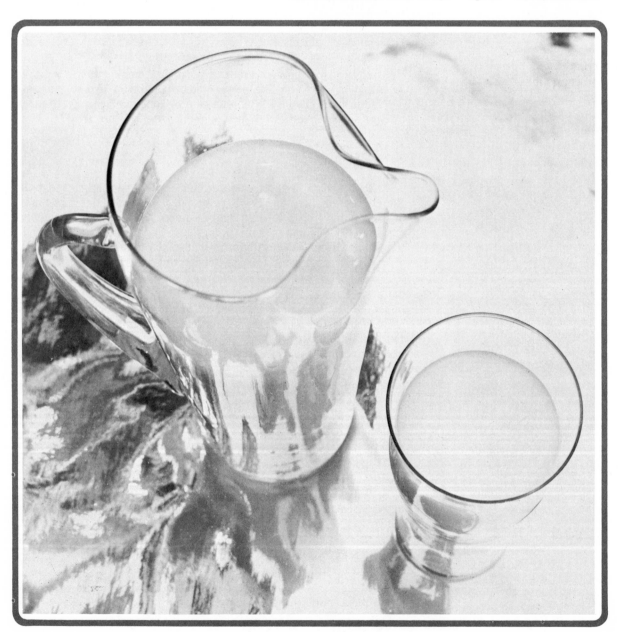

The first food

Milk is the only food nature provides to nourish us when we are born. It is the first food for lower animals, too, from a 1-ounce kitten to a 400-pound baby elephant. This is due to the wide variety and generous amount of nutrients milk contains. These nutrients maintain life, promote growth, and help give resistance to disease. Hence it is surprising that such an important food is also associated with false notions.

In this chapter we shall turn to scientific research to explode some of these mistaken beliefs. Then, on the basis of facts, you can make up your mind as to how much and what kind of milk or milk products you wish to include in your daily diet.

Are allergies to milk genuine?

Some are. These can be determined only by a trained professional (a physician), not by a layman. Studies show that only about 10 percent of all allergies are caused by food, and few of these are caused by milk. A few babies are temporarily allergic to some forms of cow's milk. Tests show that when it is boiled, evaporated, dried, or acidulated and used in a formula, most babies are not allergic to it. Those who are usually outgrow the allergy.

Studies show that many who claim to be allergic to milk or other food may dislike the flavor, odor, or texture or may have some emotional antipathy to it, which can cause an effect similar to that of a real allergy. Milk helps us in many ways.

Milk helps the complexion

A clear, smooth, pretty complexion is one of the evidences of good nutrition that we can see, and we prize it. People of all ages have serious skin diseases in countries where the milk content in the diet is inadequate.

Acne and diet

In our country, acne is probably the most common skin disease. It is found among some young people as they change from adolescence to adulthood.

Acne is not caused primarily by a poor diet, though it can be helped by a good one. According to the American Medical Association's Committee on Cutaneous Health and Cosmetics, acne is caused primarily by hyperactive oil glands in the skin. They retain secretions and become inflamed. This occurs most frequently on the face and neck and across the shoulders in the back. At this period of life, there is an increase in the amount and variety of hormones secreted into the bloodstream, which is thought to contribute to the problem. Physicians usually recommend that those with skin problems avoid eating fatty or fried foods, chocolates, candy, cola-type drinks, nuts, pastries, and excess sweets—good advice for most of us for other reasons, as well.

The most important aspect in the dietary prevention and treatment of skin problems, many nutritionists and dermatologists agree, is that the diet of young people should be highly nutritious and adequate to meet their needs during the period of rapid physical development.

Combatting misinformation on milk

A false notion on milk in relation to skin problems is held by some. Here are two examples.

In San Diego, California, Mrs. Audrey Hallett of Hoover High School was teaching this sec-

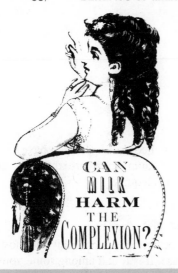

CAN MILK HARM THE COMPLEXION?

Folklore and superstition

Have you heard that . . .

Milk causes a bad complexion?

Milk is fattening?

Only babies need milk?

Once we are grown we no longer need milk?

Milk causes cancer?

Milk causes sour stomach?

Milk should not be eaten in the same meal with acid foods?

Milk should not be eaten in the same meal with fish?

Milk causes constipation?

Milk causes allergy?

Don't you believe it!

proof to substantiate the advice given his daughter. There was none!

A similar question came to Dr. Philip White, secretary of the Foods and Nutrition Council of the American Medical Association. "Teen-agers in my county are being encouraged to eliminate all dairy products from their diet. The reason given is that a hormone in milk causes acne," wrote a reader of his column in *Today's Health*. The reader wanted to know whether this recommendation was reasonable. Dr. White replied that the recommendation was not, that "dairy products. . . make very significant contributions of calcium, phosphorus, protein, vitamins A and D, as well as riboflavin and other B vitamins. . . . Whoever made the recommendation that teen-agers eliminate dairy foods is going to be hard-pressed to come up with as good sources of the important nutrients, especially for calcium, vitamin D, and riboflavin. . . . To deviate from an adequate diet in an attempt to clear up acne is not only foolish— it is very hazardous." He compared such advice to keeping the top of a convertible down during a rainstorm because of a tiny leak in the roof.

The nutrients that nourish the body as a whole are the ones that give the basis for a beautiful skin at all ages.

Is milk fattening?

Have you ever heard someone say, "Oh, I don't drink milk, because it is so fattening"? What are the facts? A chemical analysis of milk shows it contains 87 percent water, 3.5 percent fat, 3.5 percent protein, 5 percent milk sugar, 0.7 percent minerals, and a wide variety of vitamins.

Table 5–1 is designed to help you see at a glance how milk compares in calories per serving with many other foods you regularly eat. For in-

tion of this book, when she paused to ask how many were drinking milk. Only 50 percent of the class were. What was the reason? Discussion brought out the fact that one girl in the class had been told by her physician to stop drinking milk, because "it was bad for her complexion." She told her friends. Many of them also went to this physician and received the same advice, though most had good complexions. The father of the first girl fortunately knew the facts about milk and confronted the physician, asking for scientific

stance, one 8-ounce glass of whole milk contains 165 calories, while skim milk and plain cultured buttermilk contain only 90 calories. Compare these with a piece of chocolate cake (420 calories), an ounce of potato chips (280 calories), or a piece of apple pie (330 calories).

You intelligently ask, "What am I getting in addition to my calories in a glass of milk?" That is what the remainder of this chapter is about. The answer can help you understand why nonfat milk is recommended for all well-balanced weight-control diets, including reducing diets, and for young people with acne.

Milk: our calcium-rich food

Milk is our most important food for calcium, the most abundant mineral in the body. It composes 1.5 to 2.0 percent of an adult's body weight. Table 5–2 shows how difficult it is to plan meals containing enough calcium without using milk.

Daily requirement

One quart of milk daily meets the recommended amount of calcium for most young people, as do two glasses for most adults. (See the RDA table on pages 446–447.) Table 5–2 shows how much of other common foods it would take to equal the amount of calcium in a quart of milk. Imagine trying to eat 115 hamburgers to get the calcium you need in one day, or 115 boiled potatoes, or 24 cups of cooked carrots, or 144 medium-sized apples!

In making cheese, the calcium stays mainly with the whey, which is drained off. Thus it is difficult to eat more than five cups of either cottage or cheddar cheese to get the needed amount. This points up the significance of using some fluid or concentrated milk in some form.

table 5–1 *Comparison of Calories in Milk with Those in Other Foods**

NAME OF FOOD	NUMBER OF CALORIES PER SERVING
Milk—Whole fluid, 1 8-oz. glass (3.5% fat)	160
Low-fat, 1 8-oz. glass (calories according to percent of fat)	120–150
Nonfat-buttermilk, skim, reconstituted dry or evaporated, 1 8-oz. glass.	90
1 8-oz. glass chocolate-flavored milk	190
1 8-oz. glass malted milk	245
1 piece lemon meringue pie, 4-in. section	305
1 piece apple pie	350
1 piece cherry pie	350
1 piece mince pie	365
1 doughnut, cake type	125
1 plain cup cake, made from mix, without icing	90
with icing	130
1 piece plain cake, 1/9 of 9″ square cake, without icing	315
with icing	400
1 piece chocolate cake with chocolate frosting	445
⅛ of a pizza pie, 14-in. diameter	185
1 plain cookie, 3-in. diameter	50
1 3-oz. hamburger, market ground (not counting roll)	245
1 12-oz. glass beer	150
1 8-oz. glass cola-type drink	95
10 potato chips, 2-in. diameter	115
2 T. peanut butter	190
1 oz. fudge or caramel candy (no nuts)	115
1 cup plain gelatin dessert	140

*Adapted from *Nutritive Value of Foods*, Home and Garden Bulletin No. 72. (Washington, D.C.: USDA, revised 1970).

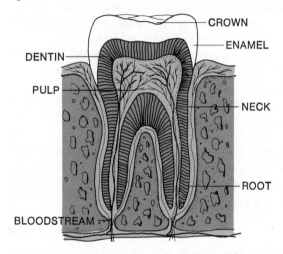

fig. 5–1 **THE PARTS OF A TOOTH**

How bones and teeth are made

The bones and teeth contain about 99 percent of the calcium in the body and 80 to 90 percent of the phosphorus. Milk contains these two minerals in the exact proportions needed to form tiny, needlelike crystals, called trabeculae (**trə bek′ yə lē**). They are set in a honeycomblike framework to make bones and teeth. In the center of the bone are the marrow, the nerve tissue, and a network of tiny blood and lymph vessels. The crystals are surrounded by fluid which traps needed nutrients such as protein, magnesium, vitamins D, C, and A, hormones, and enzymes from the blood as it circulates. By this means growth takes place and tissue is repaired and maintained.

As bones grow, nutrients are laid down on the outside of the long bones, such as the legs. At the

table 5–2 *Amount of Other Foods Required to Equal Calcium Content in 1 Quart of Milk*

1 quart of whole milk provides 1.15 grams of calcium.	
115	hamburgers
115	3-ounce servings of lean roast beef
115	potatoes, boiled in jackets
24	cups cooked diced carrots
31	cups cooked green peas
4	cups cooked turnip greens
576	cooked ears of corn
18	cups cooked green beans
12½	cups cooked dried beans
115	medium-sized bananas
144	medium-sized apples
21	oranges
3	3-ounce servings sardines, with bones
300	1½-ounce servings tuna

same time, absorption of material from the inside of the bone cavity provides a wider hole for the bone marrow. This makes the bone lighter, and enables us to move more easily. A boy may not reach his full height until he is about 21 years of age, but girls usually attain their maximum height by age 18. Teeth are formed in the same way as bone, except that the crystals are larger on tooth enamel and these are the hardest tissue in the body.

Why we need a constant level of calcium in the blood

The blood maintains a constant level of calcium to keep you alive and functioning. This process, which goes on without our being aware of it, is another example of how the human body tries to adapt to its individual circumstances. It must have a constant level of calcium for the following reasons:

1/It helps control the heartbeat. Calcium triggers the contraction that sends the blood pulsing through every tissue.

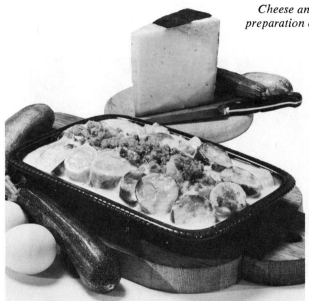

Cheese and milk are used in the preparation of many delicious and nourishing dishes.

2/It serves as a comember of a team to clot the blood. When the blood does not clot, even a small cut can be serious.

3/It promotes the passage of fluid between cells, enabling them to absorb nutrients and oxygen and give off waste, and to make the fluid firmer.

4/It, with phosphorus, is required for normal functioning of nerves and muscles. For instance, when the calcium level in the blood drops, nerves are more irritable. Leg cramps in pregnant women and others have been relieved when milk was increased in the diet. Muscle spasms occur when calcium drops far below the normal level in the blood.

5/It, with phosphorus, helps maintain the acid-base balance, keeping the chemistry of the body automatically functioning properly.

Thus we see that the body has a constant and genuine need for calcium to keep us alive. When we don't provide it with our meals in the amount needed, the body adapts to this lack and takes the calcium it requires from our reserve in the bones. If that "cupboard" is "bare," like the one in the nursery rhyme, our body then takes calcium from living bone structure. Thus we are destroyed in one place to keep us functioning as a whole. This eventually catches up with us.

Calcium and growth

Growth is stunted when there is not enough calcium to meet the needs for body functioning and for laying down the amount required in the bones and teeth. In nations where little or no milk is used, people's bodies adapt to low calcium in the diet by remaining short in stature.

No one knows what a good diet can do for him until he eats it regularly. Diet is important even to attaining potential height.

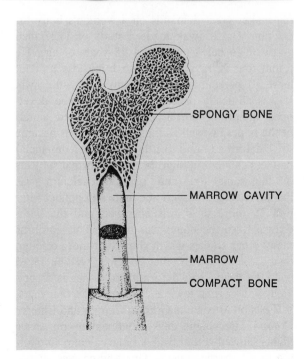

fig. 5–2 **THE STRUCTURE OF BONES** (Human Femur)

SPONGY BONE

MARROW CAVITY

MARROW

COMPACT BONE

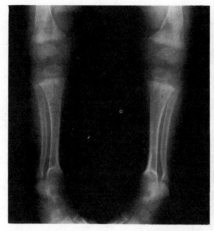 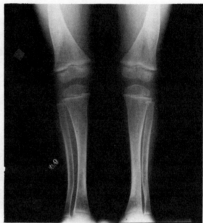

Effects of calcium deficiency: rickets (left) *before treatment,* (right) *after treatment.*

Effects of calcium deficiency

When there is a deficiency in calcium, a person's posture is poor and his jawbones and teeth may be poorly formed. This affects appearance and personality. Curvature of the spine occurs even in young people, and often it affects the middle-aged and elderly.

Osteoporosis (ä stē ō pə rō′ səs) is a crippling bone disease of the middle-aged and older person. While it is associated with such conditions as rheumatoid arthritis, hyperthyroidism, cancer, and scurvy, and with overuse of certain drugs that are demineralizing (cortisone, for example), it is also associated with diet, studies show. It is a condition in which the calcium is withdrawn from the bones, leaving them calcium-poor, with a fragile, porous form.

Dr. Lee Lutwak of the Graduate School of Nutrition at Cornell University became interested in this disease because he saw so much of it reported by physicians, with four times as much among older women as men. Naturally, childbear-

ing makes great demands on a woman's body for calcium. Dr. Lutwak made a study of 1127 men and women between 45 and 95 years of age. He found that X rays showed no bone loss until at least 30 percent of the calcium was withdrawn. It was clinically observed that those who developed abnormal porousness and enlarged canals of the bones, as well as those whose bones became soft, deformed, and brittle (as in osteomalacia) had less calcium in their diets than normal subjects of the same age and sex. As calcium was increased, together with adequate amounts of vitamin D, more of it was absorbed and the withdrawal from the bones was halted. This confirms many other studies which show that more calcium is absorbed when the diet has been well-balanced over the years, and deformity of bones is associated with a diet low in calcium over the years.

Tests on astronauts Gordon Cooper and Charles Conrad after eight days' confinement on space flights showed withdrawal of bone calcium amounting to 12 to 15 percent. This finding was significant for others as well, and prompted a study of

X-ray photo of hands shows rickets
(left) *and normal bones* (right)

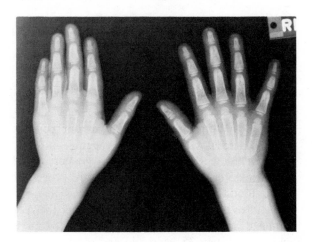

bones. Vertebrae of the spine may collapse, causing curvature of the back, and eventually loss in height.

There is a constant need for calcium in the unborn baby. When the mother's diet is balanced in food needed, both she and the baby are stronger and more attractive. (See Chapter 13 for further discussion of this topic.)

A Peace Corps volunteer helps a Hausa mother in Northern Nigeria feed her poorly nourished baby nonfat dry milk mixed with boiled water. This food will save his life.

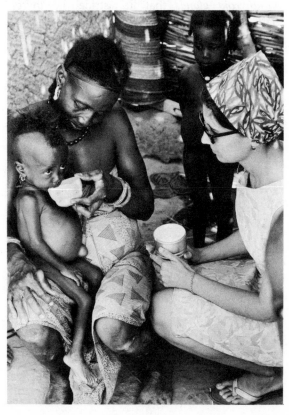

persons on earth in bed-rest positions. It was learned that there is a greater loss of calcium from bones when at bed rest than when the person is moving normally, and that the higher the amounts of calcium in the diet, the less loss. The test subjects' diets ranged from 300 (the amount found in less than one glass of milk) to 2000 milligrams of calcium.

Calcium reserve: asset in teen-age marriages

Girls who marry in their teens and become mothers at an early age are fortunate if they have built up a calcium reserve in their bones. When there is no reserve in the bones, studies show, the blood takes calcium from the spine and pelvic bones.

Girls who have calcium-poor bones when they begin pregnancy and who have poor eating habits get into trouble, though they may not know it. The body's adaptation to the need of the baby means that calcium is taken from the mother's

Calcium as part of a nutrient team

You recall from Chapter 2 that nutrients, hormones, and enzymes work together as a team to produce a high level of good nutrition. This is well illustrated in the use of calcium in the diet. Calcium must also be accompanied by phosphorus, magnesium, and vitamins D, C, and A to aid at one stage or another in its absorption and use by body tissues.

MAINTAINING CALCIUM LEVEL. The intelligence service that controls the level of the calcium in the bloodstream depends on a tiny pair of *parathyroid glands* that lie astride the thyroid gland. These little glands secrete a hormone that gives the signals to maintain calcium at a steady normal level. Hence they send the message to "rob the bones" when too little calcium is in the diet. When there is too much calcium, it is eliminated in the urine after all immediate needs and reserves

fig. 5–3 **THE PARATHYROID GLANDS**

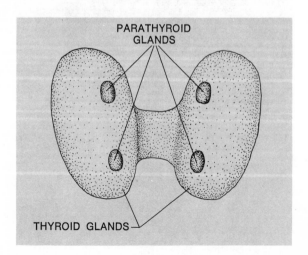

PARATHYROID GLANDS

THYROID GLANDS

are met. Few young people have much calcium reserve.

Decline in intake

Unfortunately, the 1965 National Dietary Survey revealed that the average family in our country used 10 percent less milk than the average in 1955. This decline was associated with a greater use of soft drinks, other beverages, and more processed snack foods. All girls and women nine years of age and over failed to eat a diet that met the recommended amount of calcium. Boys between 9 and 17 and men 35 years old and older also had too little of it. Such a condition leads to premature aging.

Calcium in the atomic age

Atomic explosions have introduced a new health hazard to pollute the atmosphere for mankind all over the world. Radioactive strontium 90 (**strän′ chē əm** or **stränt′ ē əm**) is one of the more serious elements. Along with other radioactive elements, it is released into the upper atmosphere and settles down on plants, soil, and water. Animals eat the plants. Man eats both plants and animals.

STRONTIUM 90 IN MAN. Strontium 90, like calcium, is deposited primarily in the bony structure of the body. High amounts in the body may cause bone cancer and leukemia (cancer of the blood that starts in the bone marrow). All of us on earth now contain some strontium 90 in our bodies. The younger the child, the more he contains in proportion to his body weight.

Authorities tell us that thus far the amounts found in man are quite small by comparison with what we can tolerate. More research is needed and is under way constantly to re-evaluate just what this level of tolerance is for us.

STRONTIUM 90 IN ANIMALS. One thing learned is that in experimental animals those whose diets contain the most calcium retain the least strontium 90. To pinpoint this, two groups of white rats were fed exactly the same diet with the same amount of strontium 90, except for one difference: Group A had 2 percent calcium in the diet and Group B had 0.5 percent, or a fourth as much. What happened? The animals with the larger amount of calcium in the diet retained 75 percent less strontium 90 than the other group.

Fortunately, strontium 90 is less effectively absorbed than calcium. It is also excreted more quickly.

STRONTIUM 90 IN FOODS. Chemists have measured strontium 90 in foods. They report 75 percent less in the meat of beef, for instance, than in the plants eaten by the animal, and 90 percent less strontium 90 in milk than in the feed cows eat. The cow seems to act as a filter for her milk.

"Of all food sources of calcium, the calcium of milk has the lowest strontium-90 content," reports R. F. Holland of Cornell University, adding, "This means that the more milk there is in the diet, the less strontium 90 per unit of calcium will be deposited in the body."

Phosphorus, an essential mineral

In 1968, phosphorus was added to the list of essential nutrients needed daily. This is required in about the same proportion as calcium. (See the RDA table on pages 446–447.) It had not been added before because it appears widely in food and there is not much chance of having a shortage of it.

Danger of excessive phosphorous

But there is a possible danger of having too much phosphorus, recent research is showing, especially when calcium is too low in the diet. Here is an example. Dr. P. Henrikson and Dr. Lennart Krook at Cornell University reported in 1968 that dogs fed a high phosphorus–low calcium diet developed troubles with their teeth, and the structures that support them. The bone was destroyed first and then the gums became inflamed, rather than the other way round, which is the view commonly held. The research team suggested that the diet of human beings, which is high in meat and low in milk, is also high in phosphorus and low in calcium. They infer that the adult loss of teeth and disease of gums are not only related to nutri-

These highly complex instruments are measuring the precise amounts of calcium, iron, sodium, potassium, and magnesium in foods.

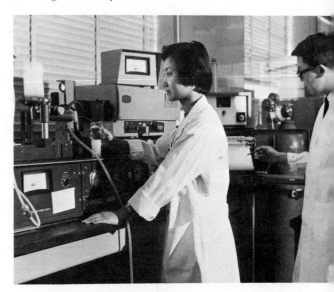

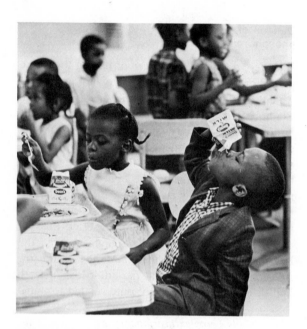

Milk is the best drink for all ages.

cium deficiency. Other symptoms are unusual sensitivity to noise, dilated blood vessels, and a rapid heart, which may cause convulsions. These symptoms are seen by medical men among those suffering from alcoholism, diabetes, parathyroid disease, and the protein disease kwashiorkor.

Magnesium and the bones

Magnesium is essential for life. It is a part of the bone framework and 70 percent of it serves on the team with calcium, phosphorus, and other nutrients in building bones. There is more magnesium in the soft tissues of the body than there is calcium, but less in the blood. When there is a deficiency of it in the diet, it, like calcium, is withdrawn from the reserve in the bones.

Magnesium as coenzyme

Magnesium, aside from helping build bones, acts as a coenzyme in building amino acids into body protein. It is thought that magnesium activates enzymes, contributes to muscle-nerve contractions, and helps regulate body temperature. When it is not in proper balance, the bones do not form normally. It is also needed for normal growth. When animals are fed moderately low levels of magnesium there are calcium deposits in the soft tissues. This increases a tendency toward cholesterol plaques in the arteries—a significant fact to note for further research on man.

Sources of magnesium

This mineral is present in a wide range of plant and animal foods—milk, meats, cereals, vegetables, and fruits. The richest sources are dried beans, peas, nuts, and whole-grain cereals. Fruits

tional deficiencies, but also specifically to too much phosphorus and too little calcium.

Phosphorus is a part of each living cell, we learn by tagging it with radioactive elements. Its primary functions were discussed in connection with calcium. It is richly found in meat, organ meats, fish, poultry, milk, cheese, cereals, legumes, and nuts.

Role of magnesium for life

In 1968, for the first time, the Foods and Nutrition Board included the mineral magnesium among the nutrients required daily. It is not likely that you will have too little of this mineral, if you eat a balanced diet. It is essential for all plant and animal life. When this mineral is deficient in man, extreme nervousness is present, as in severe cal-

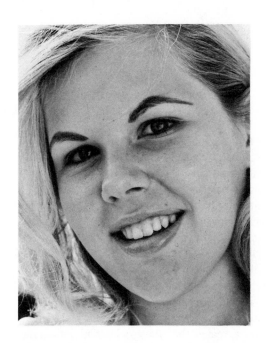

A healthy complexion, glowing hair, and vitality are the rewards when the diet is rich in riboflavin.

contain the smallest amount. See the RDA table on pages 446–447 for exact recommendations regarding the amount needed daily.

More research is needed on this nutrient, to guide us as to the ways we can improve our lives through a better use of food.

Riboflavin for good looks and long life

The exciting research on riboflavin, an important vitamin in the B complex, opens another vista on how milk as part of a balanced diet can help us achieve a better life. **Milk is our best common food source of riboflavin.**

Riboflavin and normal growth

Riboflavin was discovered as a growth-promoting vitamin. Without adequate amounts, animals studied in research failed to grow normally and eventually died. Riboflavin is needed from the first moment life begins until growth is completed. Human beings are stunted in growth when they do not have enough of it in the diet. But our need does not stop when we are grown.

Riboflavin and healthy complexion and hair

One of the reasons that milk helps make beautiful skin and hair is the enormous amount of riboflavin it contains, as compared with other foods we eat daily. When too little is in our diet, the skin is too oily around the nose and chin and the hair is also too oily. In severe deficiency, there is facial dermatitis. In animals the hair falls out. The tongue is red and sore. The lips crack at the corners and sometimes crust over.

Riboflavin and reproduction

It has been demonstrated that riboflavin in sufficient amounts is essential for normal reproduction. A shortage of it in lower animals causes such deformities as clubfeet, harelip, and cleft palate. Spontaneous abortion of the young may occur. In test studies, when mothers who had had deformed young were given a diet rich in riboflavin, their next litter was completely normal.

These same conditions have been observed in human babies, especially among teen-age mothers with a history of poor eating habits. And they are commonplace in developing countries where the diet is too low in this vitamin. No mother would willingly submit to an experimental deficiency diet, but many select one without knowing it.

Riboflavin as aid to vision

When there is a riboflavin deficiency, the eyes experience sensitivity to bright light. This is one reason many feel the need for colored glasses. Riboflavin also helps normal vision. Cataracts (kat′ ə rakts), cloudy white growths over the eyes, may eventually cause blindness in monkeys, mice, white rats, and chicks when there is a severe ribo-flavin deficiency in an otherwise balanced diet. In the white rat studied by one research group, when a cataract developed in only the left eye, large amounts of riboflavin were given immediately and regularly. The right eye was saved! Many of us know older people who have cataracts. With more research, we may have a clearer picture of the role riboflavin plays in helping our long-term vision.

A study of college girls and 15-year-old girls in Montana revealed that those who had inflamma-tion of the eyelids ate diets containing less ribo-flavin than those whose eyelids were normal.

Oxidation of nutrients

The chief function of riboflavin is to act with other B vitamins in the oxidation of food—protein, car-bohydrates, and fats—in cell tissue. Therefore, it is essential for life. It is a part of all cell tissues.

**Riboflavin and
the life span**

Dr. H. C. Sherman and his associates at Columbia University studied this vitamin through several generations in the white rat. He sums up their findings as follows: "A diet of higher riboflavin value [as compared with adequate] tends to result in better development, higher adult vitality, greater freedom from disease at all ages, somewhat longer life, and a longer 'prime of life.' " All of us are interested in retaining the prime of life as long as we can, and Sherman points out that what he found in lower animals in this respect is undoubt-edly true for human beings, too.

table 5–3   Riboflavin Content of Some Foods*

FOOD	MEASURE	RIBOFLAVIN (mg)
Beef liver, fried	3 oz.	3.56
Nonfat dry milk	1 cup	1.21
Sweetened condensed milk	1 cup, undiluted	1.16
Heart of beef, braised	3 oz.	1.04
Evaporated milk	1 cup, undiluted	.86
Cheddar cheese	½ cup, grated	.52
Baked custard	1 cup	.50
Cocoa	1 cup	.45
Skimmed milk	1 cup	.44
Buttermilk	1 cup	.44
Whole milk	1 cup	.41
Cottage cheese, creamed	½ cup	.31
Pork, roast	3 oz.	.78
Roast beef, relatively lean	3 oz.	.19
Salmon, canned	3 oz.	.16
Sirloin steak	3 oz.	.16
Chicken	3 oz.	.16
Eggs	1 whole	.15
Ice cream	1 3–oz. cup	.11
Turnip greens, cooked	½ cup	.17
Collard greens, cooked	½ cup	.19
Broccoli, cooked	½ cup	.18

*SOURCE: *Nutritive Value of Foods*, Bulletin No. 72 (Washing-ton, D.C.: USDA, revised 1970).

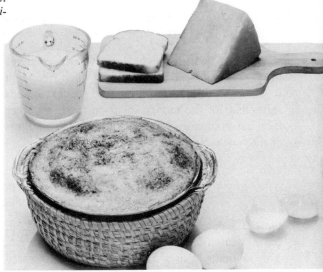

Cheese fondue, made with nonfat milk, cheese, eggs, and enriched bread is rich in riboflavin and other needed nutriments.

Food sources

Like calcium, riboflavin is not found in abundance in many foods. Milk is the best source that is practical to use in planning meals every day. This is illustrated in Table 5–3. While beef liver and beef heart are the best sources of riboflavin, we do not eat them often. Lean meat, dried beans, dried peas, green leafy vegetables, eggs, and cheese are fair sources. Other foods contain small amounts. Sugar and fats contain none.

Daily requirement

The daily requirements of riboflavin for the different age groups and both sexes are shown in the RDA table on pages 446–447. The need for this vitamin is related to body weight, naturally, as the more cells you have to supply with nutrients, the more riboflavin required. Hence more is also needed during growth, in proportion to weight, as new tissues are built.

One quart of milk provides 1.67 milligrams of riboflavin—enough to meet the recommended amount for all ages and both sexes (except women during pregnancy and lactation).

Nature of riboflavin

Knowing the nature of this vitamin helps us retain it in our food. It was discovered in 1879 by isolating a yellowish-green fluorescent substance from the whey of milk. But it was not until 1935 that it was synthesized by man. Research in the 1930's showed that there were several different parts to this vitamin, which was also called vitamin B_2, vitamin G, and the growth-promoting vitamin. These parts were all combined and given the name riboflavin, to indicate their chemical nature.

Riboflavin is soluble in water and reasonably stable to heat in the absence of light. But it is quite easily destroyed by sunlight, daylight, or even artificial light.

HOW TO PRESERVE RIBOFLAVIN. The practical point to remember is that milk must be kept out of the light and refrigerated, as more of this vitamin is lost when the food is warm and in the presence of light. To retain the maximum amount in cooking, the pan should be covered and the food served immediately or kept covered until serving time. Dark containers are better than clear glass to retain it. The larger the surface area exposed to light, the less riboflavin is retained.

It is clear that those who do not use milk in the daily diet are likely to be short in the riboflavin they need in meals. Since it is necessary for the oxidation of your food, it is easy to understand why the alcoholic who derives a large share of his calories from alcohol may also have a red nose or bloodshot eyes—an effort by the body to bring more blood with the nutrients needed for the tissues.

Desserts made with milk are excellent for rounding out meals or for snacks.

We can now better understand why the prime of life is prolonged and aging delayed when riboflavin is generously supplied in meals and snacks. Studies show that for the money spent on food, no other food can compare with milk for the large amounts of riboflavin and calcium provided.

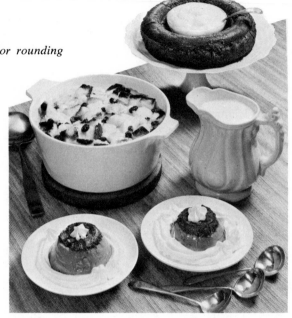

Protein: generous and perfect in milk

Only 3.5 percent of milk is protein, you recall, but a quart of milk yields 36 grams of protein. This amounts to over half the daily need for rapidly growing young people or for adults. This

Milk adds protein, calcium, riboflavin, and other important nutrients to any dish.

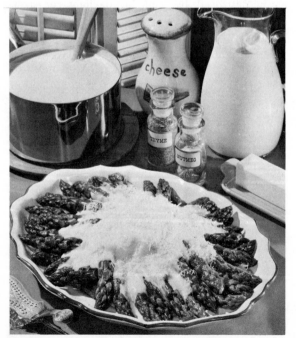

points up the importance of not judging a food by the percentages of nutrients without knowing what the figures mean.

Not only is the amount of protein in milk generous, but it contains all the amino acids required by the body, and each in about the right proportion. You may wish to reread Chapter 3, where we discussed the value of protein in your life. As a first food, milk is an excellent source of this nutrient. This is another reason that milk is recommended for all age groups. Fortunately, the protein in milk stays with the solids, and it is therefore abundant in all forms of concentrated milk, cheese, and ice cream. It is not associated with fat.

Other important nutrients in milk

While calcium, riboflavin, and protein are the primary contributions of milk to meals and snacks, a quart daily also supplies some quantity of all the known vitamins and a variety of essential minerals. It contains about a fourth of the thiamine and a third of the vitamin A recommended for adults. The latter is in the form of pure vitamin A (not carotene) and is soluble in the fat of milk ready to be absorbed. (See Chapter 7 for a discussion of vitamin A.)

Milk sugar valuable

The most desirable form of sugar found in any food is lactose, milk sugar. Although it requires only one step for digestion, lactose is slowly digested. This allows time for it to help promote the growth of a healthy type of bacteria in the intestinal tract and to check the growth of less desirable ones.

Lactose makes calcium more soluble, and thus increases its absorption. No other sugar does this. It encourages the growth of organisms that enable the body to make some B-complex vitamins right in the intestines.

Milk, a good snack food

Since snacks are providing an increasing amount of the food we eat, especially for young people, it is good to know that milk in one form or another is an excellent snack food. Aside from giving you a quick lift, it contributes richly to your required nutrients for the day at a low cost in calories.

The fat in whole milk or cheese, or in low-fat milk, as well as other fat, makes possible the absorption of all the fat-soluble vitamins (A, D, E, and K). This is important.

Weaknesses of milk

Low iron content

Even milk, the most nearly perfect food, is not perfect. It is low in iron, but the iron that it does

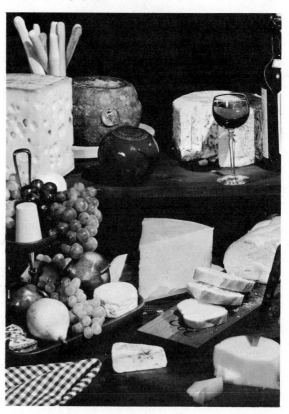

Cheese and fruit, a favorite Continental dessert and snack, is becoming popular in this country.

contain is excellently absorbed and utilized by the body. (For a discussion of iron in the diet, see Chapter 3.) The iron found in liver, egg yolk, red meat, shellfish, green leafy vegetables, potatoes, and whole grains or cereal-breads enriched with iron offsets this weakness in a balanced diet.

A full-term baby is born with about four months' reserve of iron. This tides it over until it can take iron-rich foods.

Type of fat

Another weakness of milk is the fact that its fat is of the "saturated" type that recent research shows to be less desirable than the "polyunsaturated." This is discussed in Chapter 11. You will see when you finish studying Chapter 11 that milk has had to bear an unfair portion of the blame for the "saturated" fat in our diets. Remember that nonfat milk in any form has all the benefits of fresh whole milk, except vitamin A, and 75 fewer calories.

In weighing the strengths of milk against its weaknesses, we see that our forefathers knew by experience what we have learned through the science of nutrition: that some milk in the daily diet is a very desirable food.

Meaningful words

acne
allergies
calcium
cataracts
coenzyme
cleft palate
clubfeet
fluorescent
harelip
lactose
leukemia
magnesium
osteoporosis
oxidation
parathyroid gland
phosphorus
prime of life
riboflavin
saturated
strontium 90
trabeculae

Thinking and evaluating

1. Summarize in your own words the reasons why milk and its products are outstanding foods for you. What are the weaknesses of milk? How can these be overcome?

2. What is the difference between whole milk and skim milk in calories? In nutrients? When would you use each? Why would you use milk in a weight-control diet?

3. Select three beverages and six foods that you like and eat, and compare them with milk as to calories and also as to the following nutrients: calcium, riboflavin, protein.

4. Explain how bones and teeth are formed. Why is milk so important in helping you attain a good posture? Healthy jaws? Strong teeth? In prolonging the prime of life?

5. Why is adequate milk so important in the diet of a pregnant woman? During lactation? In the diet of adults? In that of older persons? Young children? Teen-agers?

6. How does the body store calcium? What happens when the diet is too low in calcium?

7. The body maintains a constant level of calcium. Why?

8. Explain the importance of milk in regard to its riboflavin contribution to your diet.

9. Of what value is milk in this atomic age in relation to strontium 90?

10. What are some common misconceptions about milk? Have you believed any of these? Do you believe them now? Explain your answer.

11. How do you account for the fact that Americans used less milk and milk products in 1965 than in 1955? What can you do to remedy this? Why does it matter?

12. Do you consider the money spent on milk a good investment? Why?

Applying and sharing

1. Using the table of Nutritive Value of Foods, on pages 448-449, figure out how much calcium, riboflavin, protein, vitamin A, and fat is provided by
   a. 1 glass whole milk
   b. 1 glass nonfat milk
   c. ½ cup cottage cheese, creamed
   d. ½ cup ice cream
   e. 1 ounce cheddar cheese

2. Refer to the record you kept of the food you ate for seven days. Use it and the table of Nutritive Value of Foods in the Appendix to answer the following questions: How much calcium did your diet provide each day? Riboflavin? Protein? How does this compare with the amount recommended in the RDA table on pages 446–447 for your age and sex?

3. Plan balanced menus for meals and foods for snacks that you will actually eat, to provide the amount of milk or milk products you need for seven days.

4. Visit a dairy farm or pasteurizing plant in your community, if possible. Discuss what you learned there.

5. Visit a cheese store or the cheese section of a large supermarket. Learn the cost per pound of different varieties.

6. Share with your family what you have learned in this chapter. Make a plan as a family to improve your diet by increasing quantities of milk and milk products at each meal, if this is needed.

6

uses of milk
and milk products

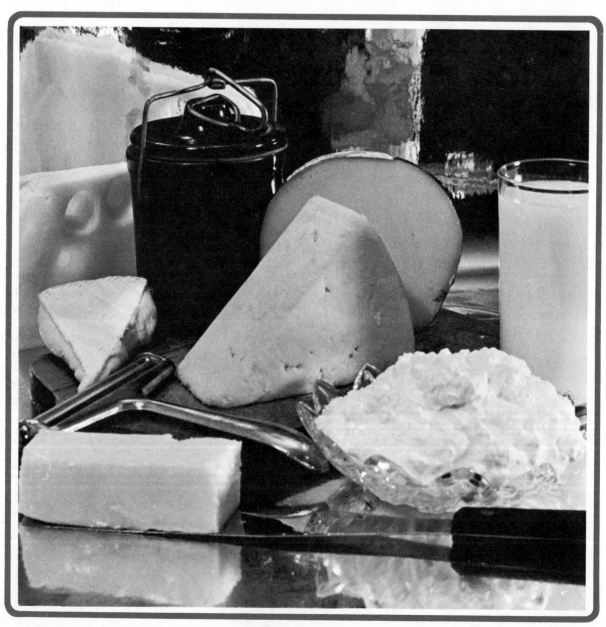

Milk is one of our most valuable foods in meals and snacks. You have learned how the nutrients it provides benefit our appearance and health. Let us now consider how to apply what we have learned about this food. This will affect our meal planning, food shopping, meal preparation, and meal serving. It is the true test of what we know.

Why milk is pasteurized

Milk is a highly perishable food as it comes from the cow. A new era for the good life was ushered in when, in 1895, Louis Pasteur, the eminent French chemist, discovered a process for partially sterilizing milk so as to destroy harmful bacteria. The process took his name. This discovery has improved the lives of the world's people beyond calculation, for it also opened the door to food canning.

Raw milk may become contaminated and cause a wide assortment of diseases and infections, including undulant fever, diphtheria, tuberculosis, dysentery, septic sore throat, salmonella, and typhoid fever. In ripening, cheese may develop a microorganism that destroys bacteria but most cheese, as well as milk, cream, butter, and ice cream, is pasteurized. There is no significant loss of the main nutrients—calcium, riboflavin, protein, or vitamin A—in the pasteurization process. There is some loss of vitamin C and thiamine. The protection to health outweighs this slight loss, which can be made up by other foods in a balanced diet.

Methods of pasteurization

More than one method of pasteurization is used. In the *hold* method, milk is heated to 143°F and held for 30 minutes. In the *quick* method, it is heated to between 163° and 175°F and held for 15 seconds. In each case, the milk is cooled at once. *Electrical shock* is a new method not widely used in the United States. Pasteurization by radiation is in the experimental stage, but has not been successful to date.

There are other reliable methods of pasteurization. For the family that uses milk from its own cows, a simple method is to bring the milk quickly to boiling temperature and then to cool it quickly in the refrigerator.

Varieties of milk in our markets

Our twentieth-century markets contain a remarkable variety of milks and milk products. This large family of foods includes whole milk; nonfat milk; frozen, canned, condensed, concentrated, cultured, dried, low-sodium, certified, fortified, and homogenized milk; yogurt; and milk in processed foods and flavored milk drinks. Ice cream, butter, and cheese are important dairy products. Figure 6–1 shows how our milk supply was used in 1969.

Do you know the differences among all the milks and understand how to buy the ones you need on the food budget you have? The price varies considerably, and so do the flavor and food value.

Raw milk

Raw milk is the unprocessed milk as it comes from the cow. It is often used by those who own their own cows and by some who are opposed to pasteurization. It is not sold commercially on a wide scale.

Certified milk

Certified milk is a form of raw milk that has a low bacterial count. It meets the high standards set by the American Association of Medical Milk Commissions. Because of the danger of transmitting disease through raw milk, most certified milk today is also pasteurized. Raw certified milk can be found in a few communities, but it is not a practical food—its high cost would absorb an unjustifiable share of the food budget and it deteriorates quickly.

Whole milk

Whole milk contains all the nutrients of milk. What we buy is a "pooled" milk from different

Pasteurization of milk in a large processing plant.

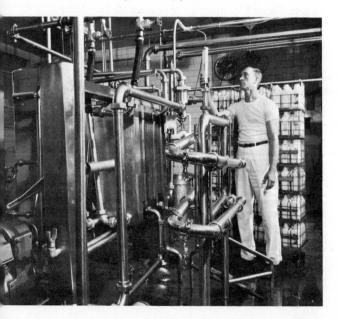

herds. The butterfat content is set according to state law and ranges from 2 to 4 percent. The proportion of milk solids (that is, the total nutrients other than fat) is also set by law and is usually not less than 8.5 percent. Such standards assure the consumer of not getting "watered" milk.

Read the label to determine whether milk solids are added. Unfortunately, the percentage of fat is usually not on the label. The consumer wants and needs to know the amount of fat a milk or milk product contains.

The cost of milk is lower when you buy it at the market, but some are glad to pay more for the convenience of home delivery. It costs less when sold in larger units, such as the gallon or half-gallon, but one must consider the storage space available when selecting containers. You get more riboflavin when milk is sold in containers that protect it from the light.

Homogenized milk

Homogenized milk is whole milk that has been processed to break the fat globules into a fine emulsion (one-tenth normal size) so that they are evenly suspended through the milk. The color is creamy, the texture is smooth, and the fat does not rise as cream.

Concentrated milk

Concentrated milk, marketed in various forms, is made by reducing the water content. The concentrated varieties include fresh, frozen, evaporated, condensed, and dried milk.

When buying any variety of concentrated milk, read the label to see what you are getting and what you are paying per quart when milk is reconstituted by adding water. All evaporated or dried milk is homogenized.

Fortified milk

Fortified milk is made by adding to whole or nonfat milk such nutrients as 400 International Units of vitamin D per quart. Vitamin A and milk solids may also be added. With a balanced diet, you will need no fortification besides vitamin D. If you are on a low-fat diet, however, you may need vitamin A.

Evaporated milk

Evaporated milk is produced by heating pasteurized homogenized whole milk in vacuum tanks to draw off 60 percent of the water in vapor. The milk is then canned, sealed, and immediately sterilized by heat. There is no loss of major nutrients. Vitamin C, vitamin B_6, and thiamine are reduced. Vitamin D is often added for nutrition.

Evaporated milk is used in the same manner as whole fresh milk when an equal amount of water is added. It is also used in concentrated form to provide more nutrients in such dishes as mashed potatoes, scalloped vegetables, creamed meats, gravies, and other foods.

Evaporated milk is sterile, has a soft curd, is emulsified, is easy to digest, and is therefore well suited to infant feeding. Cans are easily stored on the shelf, but once they are opened the contents should be refrigerated and treated as fresh milk.

Dehydrated milk

Dehydrated (dried) milk is produced by a process which removes all moisture, leaving essential nutrients in concentrated form. It is marketed in several forms: whole dry milk, nonfat milk, instant milk, cream, and buttermilk, all of which may or may not be fortified.

It may be packaged by the quart or in bulk. You pay more for extra packaging. Usually, the greater the amount, the lower the cost per unit. Read the labels and check the weight, then figure the price per quart to decide which is the most economical form for your needs, in view of your storage space.

Nonfat dry milk

Nonfat dry milk is the least expensive form. It contains all the nutrients of whole pasteurized milk, except fat and vitamin A, and it costs only about one-third as much, depending on the kind you

The dairy showcases of our supermarkets have a dazzling array of various types of milk and milk products.

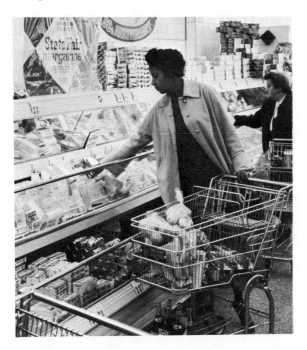

use. It can be added to other foods in dry form or mixed with water, or added as half-and-half with fresh fluid milk, lowering the fat and the cost. It is sterile, economical, nutritious, easy to digest, easy to store, and when reconstituted has a pleasant flavor as a beverage.

Dehydration gives a new dimension to milk. Nonfat dry milk may be added to the foods of people with poor eating habits, the sick, the fast-growing child, or those dieting to lose weight. The nutrients in the diet are thus increased without changing the flavor of the food and without adding many calories.

Buttermilk

Buttermilk is nearly always "cultured" milk, made from skimmed milk by adding a culture of lactic acid bacteria as a starter and then fermenting the mixture at about 70°F until milk sugar (lactose) is converted to lactic acid. Some of this lactic acid unites with a protein in the milk (casein). This forms a thick curd or gel called clabber. Many enjoy the sour taste and thick texture of this product. Commercial buttermilk usually has a little salt added to bring out its flavor. Sometimes a gum is added to prevent the whey from separating out.

Fermented milk has the virtues of the milk from which it is made, and it is more digestible because of the fine protein curd. Plain cultured buttermilk has 90 calories, or 75 less than whole milk, per 8-ounce glass. But when butter granules are added, as in the commercial product known as churned buttermilk, it has about 110 calories per glass.

Yogurt

Yogurt, another fermented milk, is usually made from whole homogenized milk, but it may also be

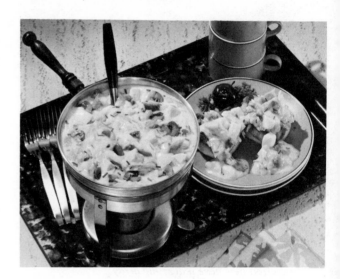

Nonfat dry milk added to a dish enhances its flavor and nutrients.

made from low-fat or nonfat dry milk. The microorganisms active in producing yogurt help prevent excessive intestinal putrefaction by changing the type of intestinal flora (bacteria). This type of intestinal bacteria aids in the formation of some B vitamins, it is thought.

Some antibiotics destroy useful bacteria in the intestinal tract. Yogurt is sometimes recommended by physicians as a restorative after the use of these drugs. However, some food fanatics have recommended yogurt out of proportion to its recognized value. In Turkey and other developing countries, yogurt is made at home and is used with meats, vegetables and cereals. It is also used as a beverage and as a dessert. As sold in our country, yogurt is an expensive way to buy milk. You can make it at home with nonfat dry milk for about ten cents a quart.

If a yogurt culture does not develop, or develops too slowly, it may be because the milk contains a trace of antibiotic or germicide, or because a bacteriophage (bak tir′ ē ə fāj), a virus that attacks bacteria, is present. The bacteriophage can be destroyed if you bring the milk to a quick boil and cool it to 100°F. Then add the yogurt culture and let it set to form a curd.

Condensed milk

Condensed milk (evaporated and sweetened) is about 42 percent sugar. It is used mostly for desserts, candy, ice cream, and beverages. It is no substitute for other forms of milk, but is a good food for desserts.

Milk drinks

CHOCOLATE-FLAVORED MILK. Chocolate-flavored milk is made with starch, gelatin, and gums to produce a thick texture and prevent the cocoa from separating from the liquid. It is higher in calories, costs more, and is less nutritious than plain milk. The butterfat content is usually about 2.3 percent and there are about 190 calories in 8 ounces.

FRUIT-FLAVORED MILK DRINKS. Remember to read the label on all flavored milk drinks. Some are made from skim milk, and water may be added. You can make your own flavored milk beverages. You will then know what is in the drink and it will cost less. To make it thicker and more nourishing, add one-third cup of nonfat dry milk to one cup of whole fresh or evaporated milk.

Cream

Cream is classified as:

1/Heavy, which is usually 35 to 40 percent fat and is used for whipping to top desserts, or as part of frozen and chilled desserts

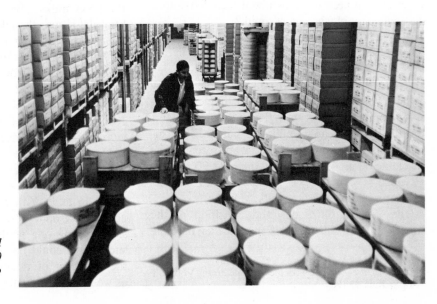

Cheddar cheese, in 41-pound wheels and blocks, takes 10 to 16 months of aging to develop its "bite."

2/Light, usually 18 to 20 percent fat and used for pouring cream

3/Half-and-half, which has a fat content of about 8 percent and is more popular as a pouring cream for coffee and cereals than light cream

4/Sour cream, which is fermented with lactic acid and is usually 12 to 18 percent fat and is used in seasoning vegetables, as an alternate for whipped cream in topping desserts, in salad dressing, and with meats

Measure for measure, cream contains far more calories and vitamin A than milk. Sour cream contains about 30 calories per tablespoon.

Milk substitutes

On the market today, and found in or near the dairy case, are "imitation" or "filled" milks that are sold as substitutes for milk, at a lower price. What do you need to know about these? Are they the equivalent of whole cow's milk?

Filled milk

Filled milk contains nonfat milk solids which may or may not equal those in natural milk, but generally compare well with it. This product contains vegetable oil instead of milk fat, but does not always contain vitamins A and D. Until recently, the vegetable oil used was coconut oil, over 90 percent of which is saturated, as compared with 60 percent saturated fat in whole milk.

The Council on Foods and Nutrition of the American Medical Association* reports that the

---

*Journal of the American Medical Association, Vol. 208, No. 9, June 2, 1969.

advertising is misleading. The facts are accurate, but the consumer is misled by such descriptions as "No animal fat," "No butterfat," "Only pure vegetable oil used," "High nutrient drink," and "High protein drink." The consumer who is looking for products with low animal fats is tricked into thinking that he is making a wise decision.

Again, the consumer has a right to demand that the actual ingredients be listed on the label by accurate names. Some manufacturers of this milk have changed from coconut oil to other oils containing polyunsaturated fats (explained in Chapter 11). Since these "milks" are promoted as substitutes for real milk, they should be equal to or surpass the nutrients milk contains. And a sanitary code should be required for them. Filled milks have a legal definition established by Congress in 1923.

Imitation milk

Imitation milks have no standard of identity or legal definition, though one has been proposed by the Food and Drug Administration. These milks contain water, vegetable fat, sodium caseinate (a milk protein) or soybean protein, and fat, frequently coconut oil. In 1969, this type of milk had 1 percent protein, as compared with 3.5 percent in whole milk. It may or may not contain the vitamins and minerals in milk.

Until the producer puts on the label what is in these imitations, one may pay less for a quart, but get more water and sugar and less of the nutrients found in milk. You need to apply all you know about milk and these substitutes when you consider buying one of them. A world standard for such milks could be set. This would greatly help the nutrition of people in developing countries, as well as in our own.

Ice cream

The Romans claimed they originated ice cream for the Emperor Nero and his court. Next it was mentioned as being served in the royal dining salons of France. First advertised for sale in our country in 1786, it is now our favorite dessert, with vanilla as first choice of flavors, chocolate next, and strawberry third. In 1969, 9.5 percent of all milk produced in the United States went into ice cream and other frozen dairy treats.

We lead the world in the production of ice cream. In 1969, for instance, we produced over 725 million gallons of ice cream. Russia was next, with one-tenth of our total production.

Today you may buy many types of frozen milk products, including ice cream, sherbet, and imitation ice cream, or ice milk.

Ice milk

Ice milk contains 2.7 percent fat, as compared with 10 to 14 percent in regular ice cream. While the calories and fat are about one-fifth as high as those in ice cream, the fat used in ice milk has usually been coconut oil. By consumer demand, this can and should be changed. This is another example of the need for accurate labeling. It is especially important for those requiring a low-fat,

Commercial ice cream, ice milk, or sherbet can be varied with different sauces or fruits.

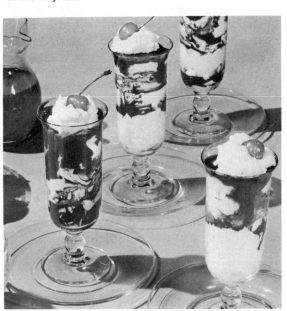

Homemade ice cream is a rare treat. When made or served with fresh fruit, it becomes a special delicacy that will appeal to all ages.

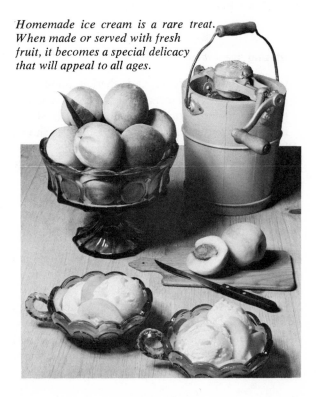

low-calorie diet to know the ingredients in products on the market.

Sherbet

Sherbet may be made with fruit or fruit juice, or coloring and flavoring. It contains 1 to 2 percent fat, 2 to 5 percent milk solids (as compared to 20 percent in ice cream and 11 to 15 percent in ice milk), and almost twice as much sugar as ice cream and ice milk. A half-cup serving contains 130 calories, while a half-cup of ice milk contains 100 calories. For this reason, the common belief that sherbet is a wiser choice in weight-control diets is false.

Storing ice cream

Commercial ice cream and sherbet should be stored in their containers in the freezer section of the refrigerator. Homemade ice cream is stored in tight freezer containers in the freezer. It should be used within a week after storage and not refrozen when it melts, unless it has just been freshly made.

Cheese

It is thought that cheese was discovered around 9000 B.C. Early records show that the Arabs were using cheese about 2000 B.C. This discovery seems to have been made by early Asian travelers who carried milk in containers made from the dried stomachs of animals. The enzymes (rennet) in the animal-stomach flasks acted upon the warm milk and converted it into curd and whey.

Kinds of cheese

There are over 400 varieties of cheese, known by more than 2000 names. Most cheese is made from cow's milk, but some is made from the milk of goats and sheep. Cheese is classified according to its degree of hardness or softness and whether its flavor is mild, medium, or sharp. Table 6–1 shows some of the more popular varieties of cheese used in our country.

Most cheese is made from the curd of milk, which contains most of the protein and fat. Some of the minerals and vitamins are in the curd, but, since they are water-soluble, most stay with the whey. In some kinds of cheese, the whey is evaporated and added back to it in the form of milk solids. This type is far more nutritious.

There is an increasing demand for nonfat cheese. Although the fat is what helps produce the delightful flavor, we can look for more nonfat and skim milk cheese on the market. For instance, the Scandinavian whey-type mysost cheese is now made in our country and sold under the name primost.

Cheese consumption

Cheese consumption in the United States has steadily increased as our interest in gourmet cooking and dining has increased. Over two billion pounds are made each year. This is a record-setting figure. Our most popular cheese is American cheddar, either natural or processed.

PROCESS CHEESE. Process cheese is a molded plastic cheese, made by mixing one or more varieties and adding not more than 3 percent (in terms of the total weight of the finished product) of an emulsifying mixture. It is pasteurized (as are most of our cheeses), molded, and sealed in packages that need no refrigeration until they are opened. Many processed cheeses have added milk solids and are therefore especially nourishing. Some homemakers prefer this type of cheese for cooking, because it costs less per pound, melts quickly, and blends smoothly.

There are numerous varieties of process cheese. Each one contains the food value of the cheese from which it is made. Milk solids may be added. If so, this will be indicated on the label.

CHEESE SPREADS AND CHEESE FOODS. Cheese spreads and cheese foods contain less cheese and more moisture than other types of cheese. Flavorings, such as pineapple, pimento, or pickle, are added. Cheese spreads have a smooth, soft texture and spread easily. They may or may not contain added milk solids.

All cheese and cheese foods should be stored in closed containers, in the refrigerator. For best flavor, they should be served at room temperature.

Standards for cleanliness in milk and milk products

Clean, wholesome milk is made possible through the observance of high standards at every step of production. Herds are carefully checked for health, fed a well-balanced diet, and kept in clean barns. Milk requires sanitary handling at all times. After milking, it must be quickly cooled to 50°F. It travels in refrigerated trucks or railway cars and is kept refrigerated until it is sold to you. Then its care is up to you.

Care of milk in the home

As soon as milk reaches the kitchen, wash the container and dry it with a paper towel. Then refrig-

erate it at 40°F. This keeps out light, thus protecting the riboflavin content, removes any surface contamination, and insures further protection of flavor and nutritive value.

It is a mistake to let a bottle of milk stand out on the table all during a meal. Bacteria grow quickly in milk or cream at room temperature. Milk can be contaminated in your kitchen by people sneezing or coughing, by dirty hands, or by the container into which it is poured.

Keep milk and cream covered, except when pouring it from the container. Learn to estimate the amount required for each meal. If what is left in the pitcher is poured back into the original container, the entire quantity can be spoiled. Every member of the family should cooperate to keep milk and milk products scrupulously clean, covered, cold, and out of the light.

Cooking with milk and cheese

A final step in preserving the good flavor and nutritive value of milk and its products is to prepare it properly when it is used in cooking. Milk scorches easily because of the sugar it contains. This creates a brown ring on the pan. To avoid this, cook milk and milk products at a low temperature in a covered pan, to keep out the light. This may be done in a thick-bottomed pan directly over the heat or in a double boiler. The first method is faster. The second avoids the danger of scorching, boiling over, or toughening the protein. It also assures a good flavor—and a simple clean-up job.

Covering the pan not only helps retain the riboflavin, but also prevents a "skin" from forming on top of the milk. Be sure to use a rubber spatula to scrape off all the casein (protein) that encrusts

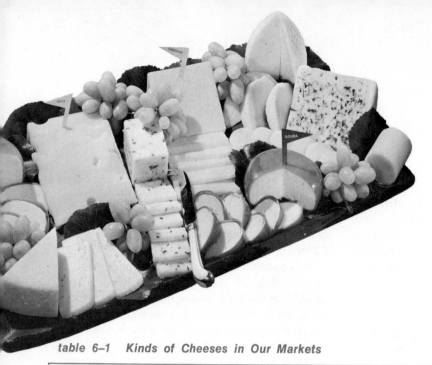

table 6–1 Kinds of Cheeses in Our Markets

CLASS	NAME	COUNTRY OF ORIGIN	FLAVOR AND USE
NATURAL For grating Ripened by bacteria	Parmesan	Italy	Sharp flavor; used as seasoning, for topping dishes
	Romano	Italy	Pungent flavor; used in cooking
	Sapsago	Switzerland	Aromatic; clover leaves added; made from skim milk; used in cooking
HARD To eat as is or use in cooking Ripened with bacteria	Cheddar	England	Mild, medium sharp, or very sharp flavor; used as is, in sandwiches, in cooking
	American cheddar	U. S.	Flavor mild to very sharp; our favorite cheese; same uses as cheddar
	Caciocavalle	Italy	Sharp, according to age; used as is, and as seasoning
	Edam	Netherlands	Cannonball shape, red cover; mild flavor; used as is, with fresh fruit, with crackers
	Gouda	Netherlands	Cannonball shape, red cover; mild flavor; mealy texture; same uses as Edam
	Swiss (Emmenthaler)	Switzerland	Medium flavor; has large eyes or gas holes; alternate use for cheddar
	Gruyère	Switzerland	Tiny gas holes or eyes; flavor milder than Limburger; used for dessert
	Provolone	Italy	Mild to sharp flavor; stringy texture in cooking; used in cooking
SEMISOFT To eat as is Ripened with bacteria	Brick	U. S.	Flavor mild to sharp; used for buffet and sandwiches
	Muenster	Germany	Mellow flavor; used for buffet and sandwiches
	Monterey, Jack	California, U. S.	Mild flavor; used for buffet and sandwiches
	Port du salut	France	Flavor mild to sharp; used for buffet and sandwiches
	Gammelost	Norway	Mild flavor; used for buffet and sandwiches

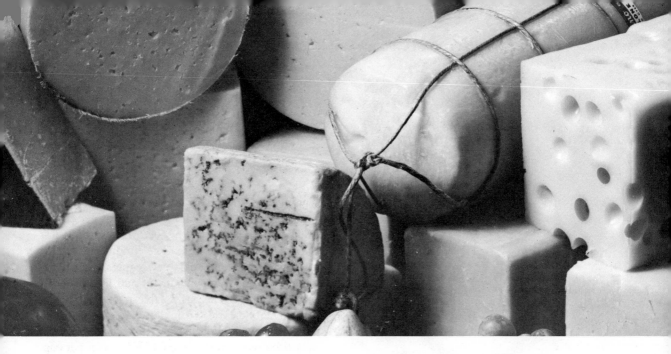

CLASS	NAME	COUNTRY OF ORIGIN	FLAVOR AND USE
SEMISOFT MOLD Ripened by bacteria Blue mold produced by *Penicillium Roqueforti*	Roquefort	France	Sharp flavor; used for salad, buffet, dessert
	Gorgonzola	Italy	Sharp flavor; made in cylinders 12″ in diameter; used for salad, buffet, dessert
	Bleu	France	Sharp flavor; used for salad, buffet, dessert
	Stilton	England	Sharp flavor; used in salad, buffet, dessert, cooked foods
SOFT Ripened	Bel Paese	France	Rich flavor; used for dessert
	Camembert	France	Rich flavor; used for dessert, served with crackers and fruit
	Brie	France	Rich flavor; used for dessert, served with crackers and fruit
	Neufchatel	France	Mild flavor; flavored with pineapple or other condiments; used as appetizer, in spreads
SOFT Unripened Made from skimmed milk but may have cream added	Cottage	Universal— Holland claims to have originated, but origin not certain	Bland flavor; a cottage or home-made cheese of all nations; used plain, for salads, cooking
	Ricotta	Italy	Mild flavor; used in cooking; similar to cottage
	Mysost Gjetost	Scandinavia	Light brown color; sweet, mild flavor; made of whey; buttery texture. Local name is *Primost*. Used as is, on crackers
	Cream	U. S.	Mild flavor; used in spreads, sandwiches, appetizers

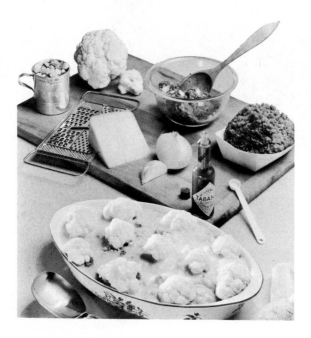

This tangy casserole combines ground meat, grated cheese, hot pepper sauce, milk, and cauliflower to tempt the appetite in cool weather.

the pan, and beat it into the milk along with the "skin," for both are good proteins.

Cook cheese at a low temperature, too, to retain good texture. High temperature causes the protein to become tough and stringy.

New technique of making white sauce

The proper technique of making white sauce is so basic that when you learn to do this you have the skill required for all top-of-the-stove cooking with milk. Furthermore, the recipe for white sauce

which you will find in the Cookbook section on page 418 uses only 1 tablespoon of fat per cup of milk for all types of white sauce. This is much less than is ordinarily used. The traditional recipe given in most cookbooks, newspapers, and magazines uses equal amounts of fat and flour. Thus a medium white sauce has 2 tablespoons of fat and 200 to 250 calories from the fat; a thick white sauce has 300 to 375 calories from fat; and a very thick one 400 to 500 calories from fat per cup.

Since the test of our knowledge of good nutrition is in practicing it, we do need to change some of our traditional recipes to fit our modern knowledge, if we are to enjoy the good health, long life, and fine appearance to which we are entitled. The basic recipes in this book do adapt recipes to conform to latest nutritional information.

The table of Nutritive Value of Foods in the Appendix shows that 1 tablespoon of butter or margarine yields 100 calories, 1 tablespoon of lard 115, and 1 tablespoon of oil 125. Fat is discussed further in Chapters 11 and 21.

USES FOR WHITE SAUCE. White sauce is basic in meal preparation. *Thin sauce* is used for cream soups and thin custards, such as blancmange, floating island, homemade ice cream, trifle, and other desserts. *Medium sauce* is used for Welsh rarebit, creamed meat, creamed vegetables, scalloped dishes, and many casseroles. It is also used with meat drippings for gravy and sauces. By adding sugar, eggs, and seasonings, we produce a mixture suitable for all types of cream pies and puddings. *Thick white sauce* is used for soufflés, croquettes and casseroles.

Thus we see that a soufflé that calls for 2 cups of thick white sauce has only 250 calories from fat in our recipe, but would have 750 calories from fat if the traditional recipe were used. This is applying what we have learned.

Consumption of dairy products

Despite an abundance of milk and milk products, the United States lags far behind a number of other countries in its use of these products. For example, we rate sixteenth in consumption of whole milk equivalent, with an average of 565 pounds per person in 1969. Finland ranks first, with 1363 pounds per person; Ireland is next, with 1307; and New Zealand third with 1219. The figures for these three countries are for the year 1968.

In the use of cheese, the United States is tenth, with an average consumption of 10.6 pounds per person in 1969, as against France with 28.8 pounds, Switzerland with 22.1, and Denmark with 20.6 pounds per person in 1968.

While there are no figures for nonfat milk, it is probable that the United States rates first in the use of this product. In 1969, we used 143 million pounds of yogurt, an increase of 30 percent over 1968.

The 1965 survey of American eating habits shows that our use of dairy products in general is decreasing. This is especially noticeable in the case of milk. On the other hand, the survey disclosed that more soft drinks were used than formerly. These too often replace milk in the diet.

Using milk and milk products to balance meals

You know the contributions that milk makes to a meal and to the day's diet. You also know its weaknesses. In planning meals, you now wish to use milk in balance with other foods for a tasty and healthful diet. The easiest way to get the recommended amount of milk is to drink some with a meal or snack. But this is not always desirable

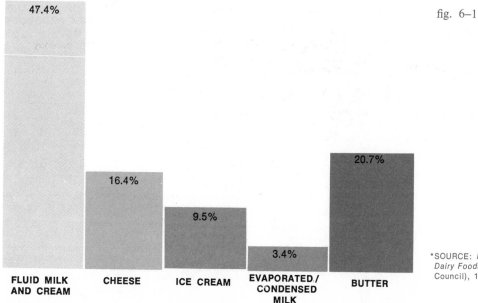

fig. 6–1 HOW AMERICANS USED THEIR MILK SUPPLY, 1969*

47.4%   16.4%   9.5%   3.4%   20.7%

FLUID MILK AND CREAM   CHEESE   ICE CREAM   EVAPORATED/CONDENSED MILK   BUTTER

*SOURCE: *How Americans Use Their Dairy Foods* (Chicago: National Dairy Council), 1970.

Chiffon pies made with nonfat dry milk add extra nutrition, few calories, and a delicious lift to a meal.

or possible. Hence the homemaker should include dairy products in her meals and snacks.

Milk in a balanced breakfast

Cereal cooked in water with nonfat dry milk added, and served with a glass of milk and a citrus fruit or juice, provides a simple, balanced breakfast. In many countries, bread and cheese is almost standard for breakfast. This is a custom Americans might adopt for variety. This meal, then, might consist of a glass of milk, a bread-and-cheese sandwich, and an orange—certainly well-balanced and quickly prepared, if a person is in a hurry.

Extra nutrition in other meals

Hot dishes using cheese, such as macaroni and cheese, Welsh rarebit, or cheese fondue, are easy

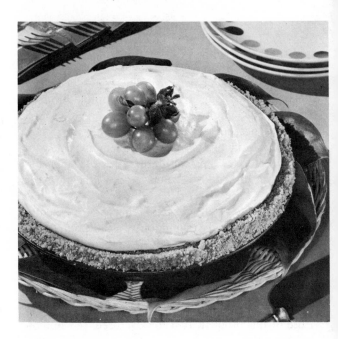

	1950	1969
FLUID WHOLE MILK	259 pints	220 pints
FLUID NONFAT AND LOW-FAT MILK	14.5	47.9
ICE CREAM	14.8 quarts	15.2 quarts
ICE MILK AND SHERBET	85	110
CHEESE	7.6 pounds	10.6 pounds
EVAPORATED MILK	18.5	6.0
NONFAT DRY MILK	3.5	5.1
WHOLE DRY MILK	0.3	0.3
BUTTER	9.1	4.7
COTTAGE CHEESE	3.1	4.8

fig. 6–2   **USE OF MILK AND MILK PRODUCTS IN U.S.***
(Per person)

*SOURCE: *How Americans Use Their Dairy Foods* (Chicago: National Dairy Council), 1970.

to make and inexpensive. If served with a cooked vegetable, a vitamin C-rich salad (such as cabbage or sliced tomatoes) or a citrus fruit for dessert, they constitute a meal superbly balanced in nutrients.

Foods may be cooked with whole milk or non-fat dry milk to augment a meal that may be low in milk's nutrients. For example, milk may be added to meat and eggs. Fish poached in milk is tasty when delicately seasoned with onion, parsley, black pepper, and lime juice or tarragon vinegar. Pork chops become tender, brown, and delicious when baked in milk. White sauce may be used as a base for creamed eggs, meat, fish, or ground meat to produce an enjoyable, nourishing main dish. Creamed chicken or turkey on toast, called à la king, is a dish fit for a royal palate.

Milk makes yeast breads and hot breads nourishing and moist. Spoon bread contains the most milk and is an excellent main dish for breakfast, lunch, or dinner—"different" in flavor and easy to prepare.

Cheese with crackers or fresh fruit is a climax that gives a gourmet touch to a good dinner. Ice cream and milk puddings have unlimited possibilities as desserts. They may be served alone or atop a piece of plain cake or pie, or with fresh, stewed, or canned fruit to make a festive and nourishing finale to a meal.

There are numerous other ways of using milk and milk products for all your meals and snacks. You can achieve a healthful and balanced diet with accurate nutritional information, ingenuity, and the will to use it.

Meaningful words

bacteriophage
casein
certified milk
churned buttermilk
clabber
concentrated milk
condensed milk
cultured milk
dehydrated milk
diphtheria
dysentery
emulsification
evaporated milk
fermentation
filled milk

Thinking and evaluating

1. Consider reasons why young people might not use the amount of milk daily that they need. Discuss how this may be overcome.

2. What kind of milk and cheese would you advise newlyweds to buy if their income is limited? If their food budget is liberal? Why?

3. What kinds of milk are on the market? What kind would you use for a low-cost diet? Which kinds of milk and cheese would you recommend for a low-fat diet? Why?

4. How are cheeses classified? Explain the difference between cheddar cheese, cottage cheese, and cream cheese. Recalling the preceding chapter on the fat in milk and cheese and using the table of Nutritive Value of Foods in the Appendix, which cheese would you choose on a weight-control diet? A low-fat diet? Why?

5. How many of the cheeses discussed in this chapter have you tasted? Can you cultivate a wider taste? Explain.

6. Explain how milk and its products should be cared for from the dairy to the home, and in the home, to retain the best flavor and nourishment.

7. What precautions should you take in cooking with milk or cheese?

8. What are the different ways that milk may be used in each meal?

9. Are you better prepared for the responsibilities of marriage as a result of your study of milk? Explain.

Applying and sharing

1. Using the table of Nutritive Value of Foods in the Appendix, compile a table of foods richest in calcium, listing approximately 20 different foods. Be prepared to discuss how this table may be useful to you in planning balanced meals that provide maximum nourishment.

2. Have the class form into groups of several members each, each group selecting a different form or product of milk for study. Have each group report on how to use the product or form chosen in planning breakfasts, lunches, dinners, and snacks.

3. What standards have been set up in your community to assure consumers safe, clean milk of acceptable quality? Do you consider the standards adequate? (If a summary of standards is not readily available in your library, apply to your local or state Public Health Department.)

4. Consult the seven-day record you kept of your eating habits. Did you meet your recommended daily allowance for milk? If not, make a plan that will provide one-fourth of your daily need at each meal and a fourth at a snack.

5. Share with your family what you have learned about milk. Decide what kind of milk each person needs and how much money to allow each week in the family food budget to obtain it.

6. Visit a dairy farm or pasteurizing plant, if there is one in your community. Discuss what you find out about the way milk is handled and processed.

7. Visit a cheese store or the cheese section of a large market. Learn the price per pound for different varieties. Using the table of Nutritive Value of Foods in the Appendix, figure out the amount of different nutrients per serving.

8. Plan balanced menus for one week around the milk dishes you have already chosen. These should meet the individual needs of each

member of your family and should be practical from the standpoint of the family food budget.

9. Prepare a balanced dinner in which you use cheese as a meat substitute.

10. With the class divided into groups, have each group plan and prepare a balanced meal in which some use is made of milk. Evaluate the results. Can your milk dish be improved? Does the meal planned by any one group show better balance than the others? Where can improvements, if needed, be made in the planning and preparation of meals as a whole? How skillfully was the work of your group managed?

11. With your mother's approval, prepare and serve at home a balanced breakfast using milk. A balanced lunch. A balanced dinner.

12. Plan balanced meals for two persons for one week, to include sufficient milk or cheese for a young couple on a low food budget, a moderate food budget, and a liberal food budget. Prepare one of the meals you planned and evaluate it.

7

vegetables and
fruits for fitness

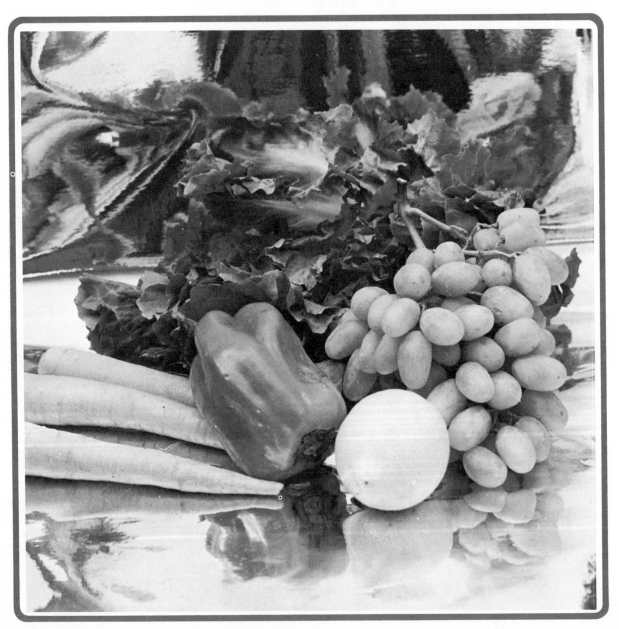

It was Socrates, the great Greek philosopher, who said, "It is a disgrace to grow old through sheer carelessness before seeing what manner of man you may become by developing your bodily strength and beauty to their highest limits." In this chapter, we shall consider the ways in which wisely chosen vegetables and fruits in your diet can help you develop "your bodily strength and beauty to their highest limits."

Though vegetables and fruits are too low in some of our diets, this is not due to lack of variety. Recently on the summer market over 200 different varieties of fresh vegetables and over 70 different varieties of fresh fruits were counted. This does not include the hundreds of processed ones—canned, frozen, dried, freeze-dried, pickled, preserved, and in the many convenience forms. As a group, all fruits and vegetables are valuable because of the nutrients they provide, but some are far more valuable than others.

We depend on fruits and vegetables to provide about 90 percent of the vitamin C and two-thirds of the vitamin A in our diet. They also help keep the chemistry of our bodies healthfully normal, provide the soft bulk that makes possible the natural elimination of waste from the alimentary canal, and help us achieve and maintain desirable weight, since they are the food group lowest in calories. They contain no cholesterol and (with the exception of olives, avocados, and coconut), no saturated fat (the latter is explained in Chapter 11). For these reasons they are key foods in helping prevent and control diseases of the heart and the circulatory system. This is a factor of great importance.

We are fortunate to have so many of these foods available in our country. But, unless we learn to know and use them in each meal, we are in reality among the disadvantaged.

How vegetables and fruits make nutrients

Vegetables and fruits draw sunshine, oxygen, and carbon dioxide from the air, and water, minerals, and nitrogen from the soil, to manufacture their own food in the leaf. They distribute the nutrients to tubers, roots, seeds, fruits, and flowers and retain high vitamins and minerals in the leaf. Scientists are constantly developing new breeds of these foods to provide larger amounts of nutrients, such as vitamin C and protein.

Vegetables and fruits for weight control

Problem of overweight

Overweight is a major health problem in our country. The cause and the cure, in most cases, relate directly to food and drink. When you understand how to use vegetables and fruits, they can help you attain and maintain throughout your life the slender figure you desire. The trouble is that too many people do not realize this fact.

They can also help you keep your family well and vigorous. Many men have a problem controlling their weight. Indeed, it is the mother or wife who all too often helps develop this problem by poor meal planning and poor cooking. You can avoid overweight through proper balance of nutrients in meals and careful food preparation.

It is important to know which vegetables and fruits are most valuable in balancing meals and to form the habit of eating them every day. The green leafy vegetables are especially good choices because they provide many vitamins and minerals and are low in calories, as you can see in the table of Nutritive Value of Foods, in the Appendix.

Yet how often do you eat them or find them on restaurant menus when you eat out? Raw lettuce and cooked greens are needed by all of us, especially weight-watchers.

A common mistaken idea is that potatoes are fattening. The table of Nutritive Value of Foods shows the wide variety of nutrients found in white and sweet potatoes, so that you can readily understand why they are recommended for all age groups, including those on weight-control diets. A potato weighing approximately five ounces contains 22 milligrams of vitamin C—almost half the amount recommended daily for females from age 12 on. Next to citrus fruits and tomatoes, potatoes provide more vitamin C for the money than any other food and the second largest amount of iron, rating next to dried beans and peas, the least expensive source. They yield more thiamine for the dollar than any other food. And all this for 80 calories!

If you wish to keep your figure consistently slender, it is desirable that you acquire the habit of eating generous amounts of the succulent vegetables, cooked and raw, at lunch and dinner and have a fruit or fruit juice at breakfast. In the day's diet, include a potato with only a small amount of fat—or learn to eat it without fat—and use fruit, preferably raw, as your dessert. When you are hungry between meals, fill up on raw vegetables, such as celery, carrot sticks, green lettuce, and others you like. Instead of drinking artificial or carbonated drinks, use your calories for needed nutrients and have a fruit juice. The habit of using vegetables and fruits generously in meals and snacks can help you keep slender and fit. Overweight is so important that an entire chapter (20) is devoted to it.

Vitamin C for survival

Discovery of vitamin C

Records show that scurvy existed at least 3500 years ago. Few diseases have struck at western man more savagely than scurvy.

fig. 7–1 **POTATOES/ A VALUABLE FOOD IN WEIGHT CONTROL DIETS***
Percent of food dollar spent and nutrients contributed in diets**

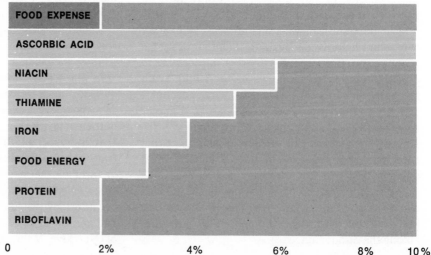

*SOURCE: Unpublished data on a 1955 Food Consumption Survey (Washington, D.C.: Household Economics Research Division, Institute of Home Economics, USDA).

**Estimated average cooking losses have been deducted.

| | FOOD EXPENSE |
| ASCORBIC ACID |
| NIACIN |
| THIAMINE |
| IRON |
| FOOD ENERGY |
| PROTEIN |
| RIBOFLAVIN |

0   2%   4%   6%   8%   10%

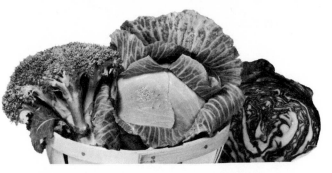

An American, Dr. Charles Glen King, has contributed much to mankind by his nutritional research and its practical application. He discovered ascorbic acid in 1931. (Other men in other countries made the same discovery at about the same time.) Dr. King has lived to see this vitamin synthesized inexpensively and used medically to help people all over the world. His discovery was a triumph. It opened a new field of knowledge by revealing the importance of fresh fruits and vegetables in our diet.

Conquest of scurvy

It seems incredible that some 400 years earlier it was found that green leaves could successfully cure scurvy. In Newfoundland during the winter of 1534–5, the French explorer Jacques Cartier was suffering severe losses from scurvy, which had already killed a fourth of his men and with which many more were afflicted. One day he noticed a healthy-looking Indian walking about and recalled that this man had had an advanced case of scurvy only a few days before. When he inquired how the sudden cure had come about, Cartier was taught how to make a brew from the green needles of evergreens. The scurvy-ridden men drank the brew and it was recorded that:

> It wrought so well that if all the physicians of Montpelier and Louaine had been there with the drugs of Alexandria [an early center of medicine] they would not have done so much in one year as that tree did in six days.

The men had been eating what they "liked"— meat, bread, cereals, fats, sweets, and drinks of different kinds. But their diet lacked "something" that the green leaves contained. Not convinced that anything so common as to come from green

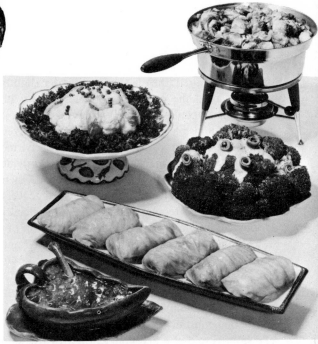

The many members of the cabbage family provide numerous vitamins and are low in calories. They may be prepared in many delicious ways.

leaves could bring about a cure so "miraculous," the physicians of Europe kept right on treating scurvy with drugs and continued to lose thousands of their unfortunate patients.

DIET AS KEY TO SCURVY. Some 222 years later Dr. James Lind, a British naval surgeon, confirmed the relationship of scurvy to diet. Having found drugs useless to save his men, he resorted to an experiment with 12 of them, all at an advanced stage of illness. Each of six pairs received identical diets except in one particular: one pair also received drugs; the second, a quart of cider daily; the third, 3 spoonfuls of vinegar; the fourth, 8 ounces of sea water; the fifth, a mixture of seeds, acidulated barley water, and gum; and the sixth, two oranges and one lemon daily. In six days, the two who had eaten the oranges and lemons were cured; the ones who had cider slightly improved, and the others remained seriously ill. The results were dramatically clear. "The most sudden and visible good effects were perceived from the use of oranges and lemons," reported Dr. Lind. He recommended that all ships provide lemon juice, fresh or in the form of syrup, to their crews. It was not until 1795, almost half a century later, that this recommendation was officially adopted. Gradually, perceptive physicians observed that scurvy was a "part of all diseases" and that "something" in oranges and lemons could free people from this scourge.

Most animals can manufacture vitamin C from other nutrients, but human beings, monkeys, and guinea pigs must depend on their daily food for it. The story is told of a pet monkey on a British ship that lined up with the sailors to get his share of citrus fruit or juice. The sailors were highly amused by his behavior. But it was no joke. We know today that he needed the vitamin C for survival.

Scurvy is not common in our country now, but it does occur and it is thought that many suffer slightly from it when they allow their diet to fall too low in vitamin C. Vanderbilt Medical School Hospital treated 103 cases of infantile scurvy between 1926 and 1954. In every case, the scurvy had resulted from long periods in which there was little or no vitamin C in the diets, and in every case the disease could be reversed in three to four days by the use of vitamin C or foods containing it.

Beneficial effects of vitamin C

What positive role is played by this vitamin, the absence of which is so destructive? How does it work for us?

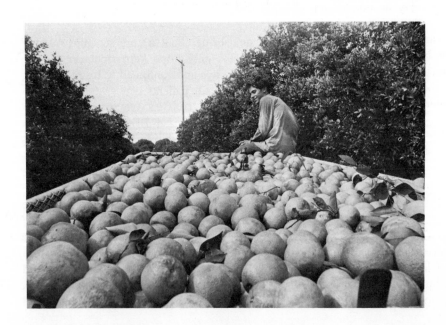

A carload of good health. Oranges are rich in vitamin C, which prevents scurvy and combats other ailments.

Functions of vitamin C

The broad role of vitamin C is to help form a gluelike substance called collagen, which holds all types of body cells together.

BUILDING, MAINTENANCE, AND FUNCTION OF ALL BODY TISSUES. It teams up with other nutrients, enzymes, hormones, and oxygen to perform these important tasks in producing a healthy body. This is one of many instances in which various elements work together for our good health and appearance.

BONY STRUCTURES. When there is too little vitamin C in the diet, the accompanying loss of body calcium results in thin, porous "honeycomb" bones, as illustrated in Figure 7–2. Bones in this condition are fragile and break easily.

FORMATION OF STRONG TEETH AND GUMS. When vitamin C is deficient, the teeth take shape in the mouth in irregular positions. Not all gingivitis (**jin jə vīt′ əs**) inflammation of the gums—is caused by vitamin C deficiency, but when this vitamin is too low, gums bleed easily when washed or when pressure is exerted.

TENSILE STRENGTH OF BLOOD VESSELS. When there is prolonged deficiency of vitamin C, the heart enlarges. In blood vessels, the lack of this vitamin is indicated by blue-yellow patches, likes bruises, beneath the skin, where tiny capillaries have hemorrhaged. These you can see. But you don't see bleeding that occurs inside body tissues or in organs such as the spleen, bladder, bone marrow, kidneys, adrenal and other glands, muscle tissue, and alimentary canal—hemorrhaging that occurs when cells "fall apart."

FORMATION OF RED BLOOD CELLS. Vitamin C works with a team of nutrients—iron, copper, protein, folic acid (a B-type vitamin, also called folacin), and others—in forming red blood cells in the bone marrow. This team also promotes the absorption of iron, and hence helps to prevent anemia, fatigue, and loss of energy.

NORMAL GROWTH AT ALL STAGES. When vitamin C is too low in the diet, your muscle tissue becomes soft and flabby, because the "intercellular cement" is too watery. This vitamin affects growth and well-being throughout life. It promotes the functioning of the sex glands and other glands and organs, and the development of firm, flexible muscles.

RESISTANCE TO INFECTIONS AND DISEASES. Vitamin C is helpful in preventing and healing respiratory illnesses such as colds and more serious ailments, like tuberculosis. Earlier

Green leafy vegetables can be used in many types of salad. They are valuable sources of vitamin C. How many can you identify?

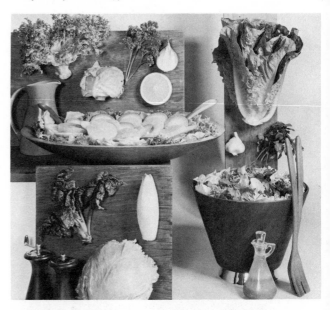

fig. 7–2 **BADLY FORMED BONE (HUMAN JAW)**

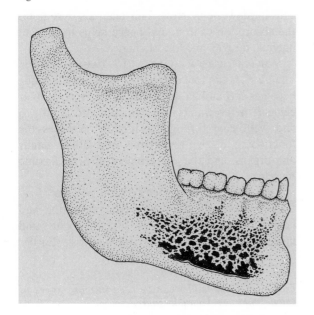

generations hit upon the use of hot lemonade in treating colds and other respiratory disorders. Today we know it helped because of the high vitamin C content of lemons, as well as the beneficial effect of fluids.

HEALING WOUNDS. It is common medical practice today to build up a patient to the point of vitamin C saturation (all that the tissues will hold) before and after surgery.

Some effects of vitamin C deficiency

Dr. J. H. Crandon reported in the *New England Journal of Medicine* the result of a self-imposed experiment. He ate a scurvy-producing diet for six and one-half months. After the first three months, a 2½-inch cut was made in his back. It

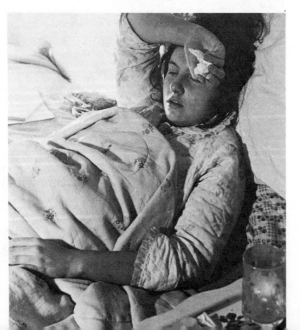

This vitamin also helps build resistance to infections and diseases.

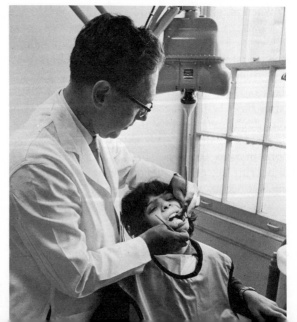

Vitamin C is important in the formation of strong teeth and gums.

healed normally in 11 days. Three months later, after he had been on the diet six months, a second cut was made. In 10 days, the wound had not even begun to heal. He stayed on the same poor diet but injected into his veins daily 1 gram (1000 milligrams) of pure vitamin C. The wound healed perfectly. When a new incision was made across the scar tissue, it also healed at once. Such healing does not occur unless there is sufficient vitamin C in the diet. It is known that healed scars break open in cases of severe deficiency of this vitamin.

There were two interesting side effects of Crandon's experiment: after 42 days on the diet, there was no vitamin C in his blood plasma, and in 122 days, the number of white blood cells, which help fight disease and infections, fell to zero. The experiment helps us understand that, when the diet is too low in vitamin C, many things occur that cannot be seen, of which we may even be unaware, but which may affect many of our vital needs.

Daily requirement of vitamin C

The table of Recommended Daily Dietary Allowances in the Appendix (pages 446–447) shows that our need for vitamin C depends on age, sex, size, height, and weight. A one-to-ten-year-old child needs 40 milligrams daily, as compared with an adult, who requires 55 to 60. Other factors include the amount of activity (the more activity, the more vitamin C is needed), temperature (a fever or a hot, humid climate that causes much perspiration requires an additional amount), and the state of health and nutrition (a person with a reserve needs less than a sick or poorly nourished one). Then there are individual differences. Because of inborn metabolic differences, some need more vitamin C than others.

Body storage of vitamin C

The reserves of vitamin C stored in the body are quite small. The largest amount is stored in the adrenal glands. When these glands (the adrenal cortex) secrete hormones, there is a sharp lowering of vitamin C and cholesterol in them. Smaller amounts are stored in the brain, the liver, and other glands and organs, and in the hemoglobin of the red blood corpuscles.

Vitamin C is absorbed from the small intestines and circulates to every tissue, so that each cell can use it to make the collagen that helps hold cells firmly together. When the body tissues and reserve depots are saturated, the excess is at once excreted in the urine as water and through the lungs as carbon dioxide. One cannot get too much vitamin C from food. The excess you eat at breakfast is disposed of before lunch (in less than four hours).

This is the basis for the recommendation that we have a source of vitamin C daily. Even better, distribute the foods that contain this nutrient among all three meals in the day.

You can understand, then, why breakfast skippers are likely to have a day's diet that is too low in vitamin C. Though we still have much to learn about this vitamin, we know enough now to improve the quality of life.

Sources of vitamin C

About 90 percent of the vitamin C in our daily diet must come from fruits and vegetables. Unfortunately, many staple foods we like contain none. This includes meat (except liver), eggs, dried legumes, nuts, fats, and sugars. There is only a small amount in milk. This explains why scurvy killed more people during the Crusades than the wars and why it was "a part of all diseases."

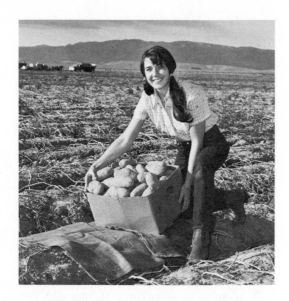

The potato is a very versatile food. It can be prepared in dozens of ways. This simple vegetable, with its rich vitamin C content, helped wipe out scurvy in Europe.

It was a lucky day for Europe when the Spanish explorers in America took back with them the white potato. Its vitamin C content wiped out scurvy. Some countries had to pass laws compelling the people to grow and eat it, for they resisted "strange food." But when they saw the "miracle" it performed for their health, they ate it and lived.

Importance of fruits and vegetables

The citrus fruits (oranges, lemons, grapefruit, limes, and others) and tomatoes are our best sources of vitamin C. Tomatoes in any form are excellent, because they, like the citrus fruits, protect the vitamin C with their acid content.

Other good sources are raw cabbage, strawberries, cantaloupe, green and red bell peppers, and papayas and properly cooked broccoli, Brussels sprouts, turnip greens, collards, kale, mustard greens, savoy cabbage, and potatoes, especially new ones. Consult the table of Nutritive Value of Foods in the Appendix for other good and fair sources to include in meals.

In buying fruit juices, compare the cost per serving to the amount of vitamin C contained in each. For instance, when vitamin C is added, you may think that the amount added is equal to that in a glass of orange juice, but this is not the case. Read the labels. Keep a notebook to record what you learn, and keep comparing the vitamin C content in various foods.

Studies in agriculture are making progress in producing vegetables with higher vitamin C content. One vegetable on which such work is being done is green beans.

How to retain vitamin C in food

Vitamin C is fragile and easily lost. It is soluble in water. Therefore, it is lost when foods soak in water, as when raw cabbage is crisped or potatoes are submerged to prevent darkening. Other ways in which vitamin C is lost in water are pouring the cooking water down the drain, using too much water in cooking, and discarding the liquid in canned vegetables and fruits.

To prevent these losses, vegetables and fruits should be cooked in a minimum of water for tenderness. The liquid left over from cooking or from canned fruits and vegetables should be used in soups or other cooking.

Vitamin C is easily destroyed by oxygen. The more surface exposed to the air, the greater the loss. The more bruised, wilted, or old the vegetable, the greater the loss by oxidation. Foods that are frozen and allowed to thaw before cooking lose a great deal of their vitamin C content. Therefore, buy and keep foods out of the sunshine or warm places, and store fresh ones in the refrigerator, frozen ones in the freezer, and canned ones in a dry, cool place. Cook vegetables whole when possible, or cut them with a sharp knife to prevent bruising. Research shows that there is less loss by cutting in cubes than in slices. Do not buy wilted or old vegetables and use those that you buy before they become wilted or old.

Heat also destroys vitamin C. Studies show that vegetables lose less of this vitamin if cooked in water that has been boiled one to two minutes to expel the oxygen. They should be cooked covered, as quickly as possible, and served immediately when cooked, to avoid loss of vitamin C. Leftovers should be stored at once in the freezer, and reheated quickly just to the boiling point and no more.

Alkali destroys vitamin C (and also thiamine and other vitamins). Therefore, don't add soda to green vegetables to retain the color, as is often done in public eating places and by unknowing homemakers. Contact with copper in cooking utensils also destroys vitamin C.

Over-ripening destroys vitamin C. Buy food at the peak for eating, and refrigerate it properly or otherwise store it to prevent over-ripening. Melons and fruits with skins on them do not lose as much vitamin C as succulent, exposed ones such as berries, beans, or shelled green peas.

Since very little vitamin C is stored in the body, and since we need it constantly, it is wise to include in each meal a food that is rich in this vitamin. Obviously, the meal skippers are hurting themselves by failing to provide foods that contain some vitamin C. Since it works on a team with other nutrients to do its jobs, it is best used as part of a balanced meal. Though we may not have scurvy in a definable form, we may feel and look the worse for it if there is too little vitamin C in the diet.

Vitamin A in the life of an attractive, healthy person

Discovery of vitamin A

In 1912, E. V. McCollum and his associates discovered vitamin A in butterfat. This started a search which resulted in the isolation of vitamin A in 1936, a quarter of a century later.

McCollum was puzzled. He had observed that a group of young cows that had been eating yellow corn and green corn leaves grew normally and produced healthy calves, while another group matured late and had calves that were born dead or died soon after birth. The latter group ate only the stalk and seeds of wheat. He concluded that it was an unknown nutrient in the corn which made the difference.

Vegetables should be handled carefully, to protect their vitamin C content.

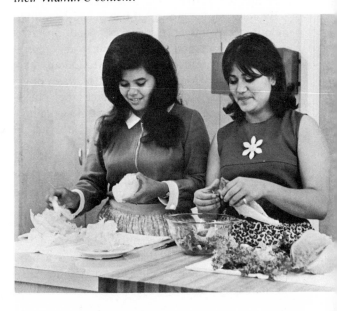

He requested a white rat colony with which to study this problem. The University of Wisconsin denied his request, on the ground that farmers would object to feeding pests that destroyed their grain. Since these animals complete their life span in one-thirtieth the time that man does (one year in their life would represent 30 years in ours), and they eat the same diet, they could help speed up the answer to this riddle. A private source provided the animals and facilities he had requested. Then McCollum began a series of experiments that stimulated research around the world.

He divided his animals into groups and gave them identical diets with identical calories—except that one group had butter, another lard, and another olive oil. Between 70 and 120 days—about 5¾ to 8 years in the life of a human being—the animals that ate the lard and olive oil stopped growing. Their physical appearance also changed. They developed rough, coarse hair, sore eyes, and poor humped posture, and soon died.

By contrast, the group fed butter had beautiful, smooth coats, bright clear eyes, good posture, excellent growth, and a lively manner and reproduced healthy, strong young. McCollum had found that the "something" in butter was not in the other fats. At about that time the Polish chemist, Casimir Funk, coined the word "vitamin," meaning "vital for life," and the nutrient McCollum had discovered was named vitamin A.

Later, H. Steenbock, also at the University of Wisconsin, isolated a new crystalline substance from carrots. When fed to animals, carotene, as he called it, gave the identical results as butterfat, cod-liver oil, or egg yolk had given in tests by other scientists in our country and abroad. In 1929, T. Moore found that carotene was a pro-vitamin A and could be changed to vitamin A by the animal and human body.

Vitamin A for a fuller, longer life

H. C. Sherman discovered in his studies of over 80 generations of animals that vitamin A may directly affect the length of life, extending it longer and in a more vigorous state. Let us consider its major contributions.

Effects on vision

Vitamin A is essential for good vision. The Egyptians knew by 1900 B.C. that there was a relation between vision and the food a man ate. Both the Egyptians and the Greeks advocated eating raw liver to prevent blindness and promote good vision.

Vitamin A helps prevent xerophthalmia (**zir äf thal′ mē ə**), sometimes known as "dry eye" (because the lachrymal gland, which normally secretes fluid to keep the eyes moist, does not function). With this disease, bacteria grow; pus forms; the lids stick together, becoming scabby and swollen, and may close completely. In advanced cases, blindness results. These conditions have been produced in animals by means of a diet deficient in vitamin A. Styes may be a minor manifestation of a deficiency of this nutrient.

TO PREVENT NIGHT BLINDNESS. Vitamin A helps prevent night blindness by combining with protein, cholesterol, and other nutrients to form "visual purple," a pigment essential for the retina. When you look at sunlight on water, snow, or chrome, or at the headlights of a car, or go from a dark room to a bright one, the visual purple changes first to yellow, then to white. In the change, vitamin A is used up. The brighter the light, the faster it is used. To make visual purple, the body must draw on the vitamin A from its last meal or from its reserves. Night blindness is responsible for many highway accidents.

For centuries, Newfoundland fishermen have said that if a man can't see at night, he should eat the livers of codfish. Fortunately, there have always been plenty of cod in their waters and abundant vitamin A in their fish livers.

Effects on growth, reproduction, and lactation

Vitamin A is essential for normal growth. It was the early researchers' efforts to determine why animals failed to grow that led to the discovery of vitamin A.

Reproduction and lactation are affected by the amount of vitamin A in the mother's diet, as we noted in discussing McCollum's work. Sherman

Night vision. (above) *After a car has passed, a normal individual sees a wide stretch of road.* (below) *A person deficient in vitamin A can barely see a few feet ahead and may not see the road sign at all.*

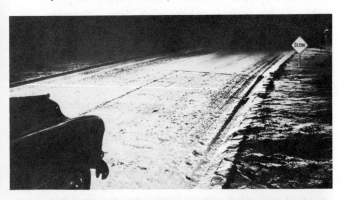

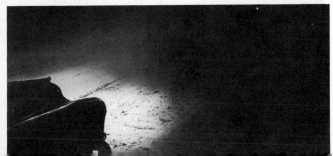

confirmed this in his study of over 80 generations of white rats. When their diet was high in vitamin A, the rats grew to full adulthood and produced normal young. When it was deficient in this vitamin, they grew to almost adult size, then stopped growing and could not reproduce young. In a USDA feeding experiment at Beltsville, Maryland, a vitamin-A deficiency caused degeneration of the testicular tissue in bulls and made them impotent. With vitamin A deficiency, cows could conceive but produced weak or stillborn calves.

Benefits for skin and hair

Vitamin A is beneficial for the skin and hair. One of the first symptoms of a deficiency of this vitamin is rough, dry skin, possibly with pimples. Ancel Keys and his coworkers at the University of Minnesota found that 24 of 31 persons on a low vitamin A diet (1810 I.U. daily) for 23 weeks showed skin eruptions, dry and scaly skin, and lusterless hair.

Animals on a vitamin A deficient diet for a long period lose their hair. It simply falls out. Thus vitamin A plays an essential role in promoting a healthy and attractive appearance.

Defense against infection

Vitamin A helps defend the body against bacterial infections and disease. The millions of tiny epithelial (ep ə thē′ lē əl) cells compose the epidermis or entire outer covering of the body. A healthy, unbroken skin protects us from invasion of some bacteria. Vitamin A has a major function in promoting the vitality of these cells. Similarly, they line the soft tissues of the mucous membrane of the entire respiratory tract, the mouth and alimentary tract, the urinary and genital tracts, the tear glands, and all other glands and organs in the body.

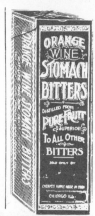

A turn-of-the-century catalogue ad

THE RESPIRATORY SYSTEM. To take one example of what happens when vitamin A is deficient, the cells that line the respiratory tract dry out and the mucous membrane becomes rough. The normal secretions disappear. Naturally, this makes one more susceptible to respiratory infections. Experience taught Northern Europeans that cod-liver oil could help prevent and cure respiratory diseases, even tuberculosis. We know in this case it was the vitamin A in the oil that gave such good results.

THE DIGESTIVE SYSTEM. When the mucous membrane of the digestive tract becomes clogged with dry, hard epithelial cells, obviously this interferes with absorption of the nutrients from digested food into the bloodstream. In lower animals, when such a condition exists, diarrhea and other digestive disturbances occur.

Furthermore, bacteria migrate in larger numbers through the alimentary canal to other parts of the body. To demonstrate this, typhoid-producing bacteria were inserted by a tube into the stomachs of two groups of white rats. In the group deficient in vitamin A, 93 percent of the animals soon had typhoid bacteria in the liver, lungs, kidneys, and spleen, as compared with only 38 percent of the animals whose diets had adequate vitamin A.

Effects on tooth formation

Vitamin A helps form teeth. The same epithelial cells that form outside and inside coverings of the body also help form the teeth. Before birth, these cells fold inward in the gums and form a cap over the bud of the tooth. Later this vitamin is a key nutrient in forming enamel on the teeth. When it and other required nutrients are available in sufficient amounts at the time they are needed, the enamel is laid down in closely packed, six-sided hard prisms, giving a smooth, attractive surface. When it is deficient, the prisms do not fit tightly together. Pits form. Food lodges in these pits and ferments. This may cause further etching

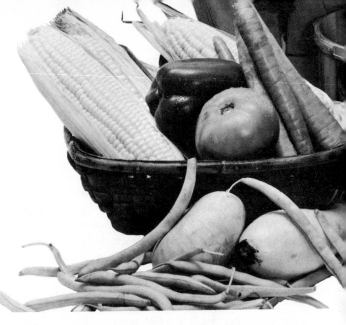

or eroding of the teeth, leading to decay. Poor diet and illness of the mother during pregnancy influences the development of "baby" teeth, which are formed before birth, and "permanent" teeth, which form in the bud behind the baby teeth.

The final laying down of enamel occurs during the first ten months after the birth of the baby. It is estimated that about two-thirds of the pitting that occurs in poor enamel takes place during these first ten months, although it may not show up until later.

Thus, from the beginning of life, the future appearance and soundness of your teeth are affected, first, by your mother's diet, and second, by your own eating habits. Vitamin A works for your teeth and other cells in your body in cooperation with other vitamins, minerals, and protein, as well as enzymes and hormones. This underscores once again the need for a balanced diet.

Role in kidney disorders

It has also been observed that vitamin A helps prevent the formation of kidney stones. A pioneer medical nutritionist in India, Dr. R. McCarrison, described kidney stones as the poor man's disease. It was a logical name for a condition so prevalent among the poor, whose diet consisted mostly of cereal, especially wheat. McCarrison fed to white rats the same diet as was eaten by his patients who had kidney stones. He found he could produce the identical condition in these animals in three months after weaning. Then he prevented the formation of the stones in other groups on the same diet by adding either butter, whole milk, or cod-liver oil, all rich in vitamin A.

Further studies indicate that many kidney ailments afflicting people of middle and old age can be traced to earlier minor infections. These may recur many times before a condition of obvious disease sets in.

Nature of vitamin A

Pure vitamin A is colorless, though the carotenes from which it is made are deep yellow. It is an odorless, needlelike crystal. It is resistant to heat, but may be destroyed by oxygen in long, slow cooking at low temperatures. Little is destroyed when it is cooked in the absence of oxygen, as in a pressure cooker. Vitamin E also protects it from oxidation—another example of teamwork in nutrients. It retains its values better in vegetables and fruits that are cool and moist.

It is not soluble in water, but needs some fat in the meal to enable it to be absorbed from the digestive tract and the bloodstream into tissues. Unfortunately, vitamin A and the other fat-soluble vitamins—D, E, and K—are absorbed by mineral oil. These vitamins are all eliminated in evacuation of wastes, along with the mineral oil. For this reason, mineral oil is not a desirable laxative.

Vitamins A, D, E, and K are measured in terms of International Units, referred to in tables as I.U. or U.S.P. (United States Pharmacopoeia). There are four and one-half million I.U. in each gram of pure vitamin A.

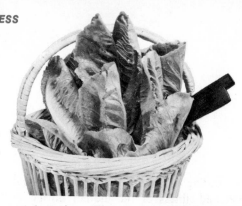

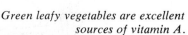

*Green leafy vegetables are excellent
sources of vitamin A.*

Unlike vitamin C, about four months' supply of vitamin A may be stored in the body. About 95 percent is in the liver, one reason why liver is so valuable in the diet. Small amounts are stored in the lungs, kidneys, and fatty tissue. Vitamin A accumulates gradually to a peak of reserve in adulthood. Young animals and children have little or no reserve. A reserve is a great advantage when there is a shortage in the diet or when illness occurs.

It is considered desirable that we get about one-third of our vitamin A in pure form from animal fat, and two-thirds from the carotenes in fruits and vegetables. It is best to keep our reserves of this vitamin high, and for that reason to include deep green leafy vegetables or yellow vegetables and fruits in the day's diet or, as a minimum, every other day.

Can you get too much vitamin A?

No, not from food. But you can from vitamin pills, unless they are taken under the direction of a physician. Some pills are quite concentrated in vitamin A. Well-meaning mothers may give their children 40 to 50 times the recommended amount daily. If prolonged, this can cause a condition known as hypervitaminosis—meaning an excess of vitamins—with loss of appetite, changes in skin pigmentation, itching and dry skin, loss of hair, and fragility and pain in bones. Here is a strong reason for depending on foods for our vitamins, not on pills.

How much vitamin A is needed daily?

The table of Recommended Daily Dietary Allowances in the Appendix shows the recommended amounts for different age groups and for preg-

nancy and lactation. The recommended amount for both sexes, age 12 and upward, is 5000 I.U. daily. This is about twice as much as is needed to prevent a deficiency disease. There are individual differences in ability to absorb this vitamin, dependent on the state of health and the balance of the total diet.

The amount of carotene changed into vitamin A varies with the food. Cooking carrots, for instance, makes more vitamin A available. Carotene may pass directly into the bloodstream or be changed

*A green salad helps you meet your
daily requirement of vitamin A.*

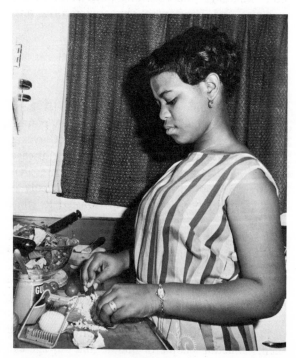

into vitamin A in the mucous membrane of the intestines or liver. Some ailments, therefore, such as diarrhea or liver disease, interfere with its absorption.

Sherman points out that it is scientifically sound to include generous amounts of vitamin A-rich foods in the diet, because this vitamin is involved in so many different functions and in so many major and minor ills. He suggests that 6000 to 12,000 I.U. of vitamin A daily would be more logical than the recommended 5000 I.U., would allow for individual differences, and would promote "higher health and longer life."

Foods rich in vitamin A

The best foods for vitamin A are the deep green leafy vegetables, the deep yellow vegetables and fruits, and liver. Thus color is the clue to this vitamin. Vitamin A is made from the provitamin or the yellow carotenes. The carotenes occur in the red and deep green foods, but the stronger colors hide them.

By using the table of Nutritive Value of Foods, you will observe that a half-cup of cooked green leafy vegetable, such as spinach, turnip greens, mustard greens, collards, or kale, contains from 4060 to 7290 I.U. of vitamin A. You will also find that a half-cup of carrots, winter squash, pumpkin, and sweet potato, and half a cantaloupe range from over 4000 to over 8000 I.U. of vitamin A. This is important information for meal planning and shopping.

Folacin for a vital life

Folacin, a B vitamin, has been included in the table of Recommended Daily Dietary Allowances since 1968. This is because research shows that it performs vital functions for life. We know it is essential for human growth, reproduction, lactation, and the normal formation of red blood cells.

Discovery of folic acid

Folic acid was discovered in the spinach leaf in 1943–44 by two laboratories working independently of each other. Like vitamin B_6, it exists in several forms in food, and like B_6 and some other vitamins, it is fragile. It is soluble in water and quickly destroyed by heat in an acid solution. As

Deep green and deep yellow vegetables are necessary in each day's diet for their vitamin A content.

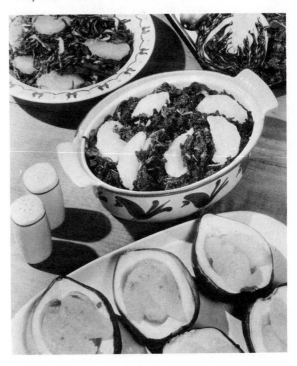

much as 65 percent of the folacin in food may be lost when food is cooked at normal cooking temperature for 10 minutes and 70 percent is lost when fresh leafy greens are stored for three days at room temperature.

Unlike most other vitamins, it is more stable in a neutral or alkaline solution. Only a small amount is needed daily, ranging from 0.1 milligrams at age 1 to 0.4 milligrams at age 10 and beyond. During pregnancy, the need is 0.8 milligrams. Though the amount is small, it might be said that seldom does so little do so much.

How folacin helps us

FOLIC ACID AND ANEMIA. When too little folacin (also called folic acid) is in the diet, anemia develops. This is a special kind of anemia, found most often in pregnant women and infants. It is called macrocytic (mak rō sit′ ik) or megablastic (meg ə blas′ tik) anemia. This means that the red cells are far too large and too few in number, and contain too little hemoglobin. It would seem that the body tries to compensate in size for lack of quality. When the condition exists, if folacin is taken by mouth or by injection, normal blood cells are made immediately and the person is cured, so long as the required amount of folacin is supplied. As many as 50 percent of the pregnant patients in some New York City hospitals were found to have macrocytic anemia.

Folacin works on a team with vitamin B_{12} in helping prevent and cure pernicious anemia. This was discussed in Chapter 3.

FOLACIN IN BODY TEAMWORK. Another way it helps us is in acting as a coenzyme, as do other B vitamins. But folacin has its own special part to play. It works with a team of nutrients, including amino acids, to make the nuclei (centers)

of all cells. Since cells divide for growth, each new cell has a new nucleus. You can now understand why folic acid is essential for pregnant women in larger amounts than other adults, and why infants need it so much. It is also easier to understand why anemia develops when this vitamin is in too low supply during pregnancy and infancy.

As a coenzyme, it is known to be essential for the breakdown and use of some specific amino acids and is believed to be probably needed for all of them. Continued research will shed more light on how this vitamin can help us. It has been helping right along, though we were not aware of its help. This teamwork illustrates vividly once again why we need to eat a balance of foods, and particularly green leafy salads.

Sources in food

The richest sources of folacin are liver, yeast, and green leafy vegetables. Some of the vegetables should be eaten raw in salads, since this vitamin is easily destroyed by heat.

Good sources are other green vegetables, dried beans, peas, nuts, and whole-wheat foods. Bread made of whole wheat and yeast are more valuable than refined breads, for folacin is lost in the refining process.

Brewer's yeast is the richest source of folic acid. In cereals, this vitamin is concentrated in the bran and germ. Table 7–1 gives the values of folic acid in various foods.

Value of minerals

Animals, poultry, and fish get minerals from the plant foods they eat. Some are used to meet their needs. Others are passed on to us when we eat them: calcium in milk, iron in liver and lean meats, iodine in seafoods. But we, too, can get much of our mineral requirement directly from plants, which provide iron, calcium, copper, potassium, magnesium, and small amounts of other minerals.

Sources of iron

You will note by studying the table of Nutritive Value of Foods, in the Appendix, that the green leafy vegetables, dried legumes, and some nuts are good sources of iron and fair sources of cal-

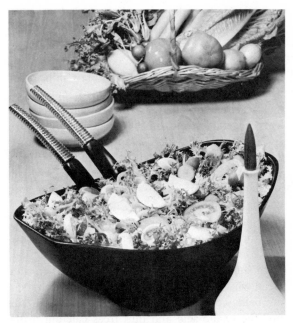

When green leafy vegetables are eaten raw, in salads, they retain the valuable folacin, which is easily destroyed by heat.

table 7–1   *Sources of Folacin*

FOOD	AMOUNT (Micrograms)*
Brewer's yeast, 1 T.	2022
Cow peas, cooked, ½ c.	439
Rice germ, 1 oz. (in brown rice)	430
Wheat germ, 1 oz. (in whole wheat)	305
Liver, 2 oz.	294
Wheat bran, 1 oz. (in whole wheat)	195
Rice bran, 1 oz. (in brown rice)	146
Asparagus, 3½ oz.	109
Walnuts, 8–15	77
Greens, cooked, 3½ oz.	42–77
Whole wheat, cooked, ½ c.	49
Oatmeal, cooked, ½ c.	33
Brown rice, cooked, ½ c.	20
Oysters, 3½ oz.	11.3
Beef, lean round, 3 oz.	10.5

*A microgram is 1/1000 of a milligram.

cium. Copper and folic acid are also present in green leaves and these aid iron and other nutrients in building red blood cells.

It was found in 1963 that vegetables and fruits contribute 20 percent of the iron in the diet. Green leafy vegetables are highly important, not only for the iron they yield, but also for the favorable conditions they provide for its absorption.

Sources of calcium

Next to milk, vegetables and fruits are our best sources of calcium. A half-cup of cooked collard greens provides 236 milligrams of calcium, as compared with milk, which provides 288 milligrams per 8-ounce glass. A cup of cooked dried beans yields 176 milligrams of calcium; a half-cup of raisins, 50; a half-cup of cooked rhubarb, 106.

In nations where little milk and few milk products are available, it is possible for people to get their calcium by eating larger amounts of green leafy vegetables and other vegetables and fruits. In Northern Italy, for example, one may see an adult eating 1 to 1½ cups of cooked green leafy vegetable, dried beans, and a large green salad, and capping the meal with cheese—providing about one-half or more of the daily calcium need.

Some leafy vegetables (spinach, Swiss chard, beet tops, and most wild greens) and rhubarb contain oxalic acid, which combines with some calcium and is eliminated as waste. However, if a clean whole egg is placed in the pot in which these are being cooked, the calcium from the shell "ties up" the oxalic acid and thus frees calcium in the vegetable. The cooked egg may be used as a garnish.

Acid-alkaline balance

The chemistry of the body normally is slightly on the alkaline side. We have a built-in buffer system to keep it that way: when the blood tends to be too acid, the body releases alkaline minerals to "buff down" the excess. When food is oxidized by the body, the ash that remains is minerals.

Some minerals, such as phosphorus, chlorine, and sulfur, are acid-forming. These predominate in meat, fish, poultry, and eggs, and are somewhat high in cereals and flour and foods made from them. However, when one eats a balanced diet, vegetables and fruits furnish calcium, potassium, magnesium, and other minerals that are alkaline-forming. Only in cases of starvation, severe diabe-

tes, and some other diseases is this ability to maintain the proper chemistry lessened or impaired.

If a person says, "I can't eat tomatoes or citrus fruits, because they are too acid," you may be sure it is a whim and is contrary to scientific fact. (Some people, however, do have genuine allergies to these foods and must avoid them. This is an entirely different matter.) The citric acid in these foods is quite mild. By contrast, the gastric juice in the body is a highly concentrated hydrochloric acid. When we take as much as 40 grams of pure citric acid (about 1½ ounces), less than 5 percent appears in the urine, indicating that most of it is changed to water and carbon dioxide.

NATURAL ALKALINE. We are so constructed by nature that, if we eat wisely enough to keep fit, it is not necessary to waste money to alkalize ourselves artificially. It is important to understand that the vegetables, fruits, and milk in your meals provide the natural alkaline you need. If you need help beyond what a balanced diet can give you, then you need your physician to prescribe it. Actual harm can be done the body by overuse of nostrums urged upon you to "counteract acid."

Table 7–2 gives the foods that are potentially alkaline (base), potentially acid, and neutral. By proper choice of foods, you can maintain a balance between acids and alkalis.

Natural laxative foods

The diet that keeps us fit is the best laxative, and vegetables and fruits are best for this purpose. The undigested cellulose serves as a soft mechanical bulk, to push the food mixture against the soft villi in the intestinal tract, where the nutrients are absorbed. The waste is now pushed on to the large intestine, which eliminates it.

Vitamins C, A, and the B group, along with other nutrients, build a strong intestinal tract so that the peristaltic waves, basic to good elimination, are powerful and can do their job well. Prunes, figs, rhubarb, green leafy vegetables, and raw fruits and vegetables are excellent as natural laxatives.

Causes of digestive problems

Dr. M. M. Kirshen points out in an article in *The American Journal of Proctology* that it is the poor habits of eating too many refined foods containing little roughage and using drugstore laxatives that have caused constipation to become a common condition. He further states, "It is not unfair to say that our enormously developed food industry, which is often more interested in the outward appearance of a product than its wholesomeness, has contributed a great deal to this trend."

Aids to vitamin production

Vegetables and fruits, along with milk, help provide a healthful type of bacteria in the intestinal tract which aid the body in making some vitamins there. These vitamins include vitamin K, folic acid, biotin, choline, B_6, and possibly fragments of some others. Bacteria produced from eating meat, fish, poultry, and eggs are the putrefactive

table 7–2 *Acid-Base Reaction of Foods*

BASE OR ALKALINE ASH POTENTIAL	ACID OR ACID ASH POTENTIAL	NEUTRAL
Vegetables (all except corn and lentils)	Meats, poultry, fish, shellfish	Butter
Fruits (all except cranberries, plums, and prunes)	Bread-Cereals of all types	Margarine
	Macaroni-noodle products	Cooking fats and oils
	Cakes, cookies	Sugar
Nuts: almonds, coconut, chestnuts	Eggs	Syrups
Milk, all kinds	Cheese, all types*	Starches
Molasses	Cranberries, prunes, plums	
Honey, jams, jellies	Corn, lentils	
	Nuts: walnuts, peanuts, Brazil nuts, filberts	

*Much of the calcium mineral which is found in whole milk is lost with the whey in making cheese, leaving predominately acid-forming elements.

Vegetables and fruits provide roughage and are thus excellent laxatives.

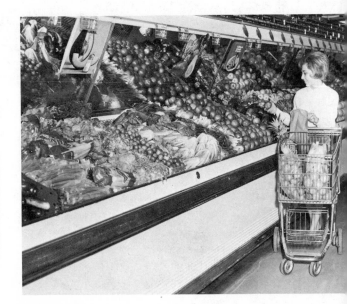

type, and they need vegetables and fruits to counterbalance this weakness.

Legumes: low-cost source of protein, iron, and B vitamins

Legumes—dried beans, peas, lentils and peanuts—are those plants that can take nitrogen from the air, as well as from the soil, and lay it down as protein in the seeds. They are the only group of vegetables, with the exception of nuts of all kinds, that are important for protein. When used with cereal grains, legumes (which have been called the poor man's meat) provide the major amount of protein in the diets of about two-thirds of the people in the world. Fresh beans and peas have 4 to 6 percent protein and dried ones about 7 to 8 percent. Soybean flour has 10 to 15 percent pro-

tein of good quality. Vegetables other than legumes have 1 to 4 percent protein, and most fruits from 0.05 to 2 percent.

In the "Basic Four" guide for planning daily meals (Table 2–2), legumes are placed with the meat group. Since they are plant foods and lack completely or have insufficient amounts of some of the essential amino acids, they are not "complete," and are thus "limiting" protein foods. However, when supplemented with some milk, cheese, meat, or eggs, their protein is well used by human beings, and at low cost.

Soybeans and peanuts almost approach meat in quality of protein. Oriental people use the soybean in many ways as food—soy milk, cheese, flour, and sauce, as well as dried beans and fresh, either plain or sprouted.

Research in the United States has produced peanut butter with 26 percent protein content. Its use

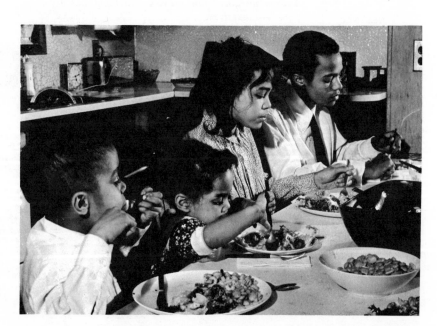

A family that eats legumes occasionally as a meat substitute gets protein, iron, and B vitamins at low cost.

increased about 60 percent in the decade between 1955 and 1965. Soybean products are being produced as meat substitutes with the taste of bacon, steaks, chops, chicken, corned beef, frankfurters, and many other foods we enjoy. It is a fascinating thought that research will help solve the protein problem for an expanding world population by improvement in the use of legumes. An acre of ground in the United States can produce about 450 pounds of protein from soybeans. The same ground would yield 43 pounds of protein from the meat of animals that eat plant proteins in pasture.

Through UNESCO, the United States has helped finance a pilot project in Nigeria, for example, where groundnuts (peanuts), a major export crop, are pressed into a cake, removing the oil. The dry cake becomes a high-protein meal that helps balance the diet when mixed with the staple dish of yam, gari, or a mixture of cereal grains. When powdered dry milk is added, it becomes a food that can save the lives of thousands of infants and young children. In tropical Africa, crushed peanuts are added to stews and top many dishes as we do with cheese.

While nuts average 16 percent protein, they are also high in fat and hence in calories. They are generally expensive, too. In our country we grow peanuts, almonds, walnuts, filberts (hazelnuts), pecans, hickory nuts, chestnuts, macadamia nuts, and pinenuts. Nuts keep better in their shells, and should be stored in the refrigerator or freezer after shelling. The nutrients in nuts are more available to the body when they are finely chopped or ground, or when cooked to soften by moisture.

The USDA reports that for a dollar spent on any food, legumes and nuts rank first in the amount of protein, iron, and niacin contained, and third in thiamine content. Potatoes rank first in thiamine, second in vitamin C and iron, and third in calories. Citrus fruits and tomatoes are first in vitamin C, third in vitamin A, and fourth in thiamine. Dark green and deep yellow vegetables rank first in vitamin A, second in calcium, and fourth in iron. As a food group, they are well worth your dollar.

Meaningful words

acid-base balance
adrenal cortex
adrenal glands
alimentary canal
ascorbic acid (vitamin C)
capillaries
cellulose
choline
citric acid

Thinking and evaluating

1. In your notebook, list the vegetables and fruits you like best and those you like least. With the aid of the table of Nutritive Value of Foods, in the Appendix, evaluate them for nutrient content. For cost. Think of your past experiences and analyze what influenced you to like or dislike these foods. What can you do to overcome your dislikes? How would you help a young child do this?

2. Of vegetables that you find in the market, which have you eaten? Which have you not eaten? Make a plan to broaden your taste for vegetables and fruits that are

   a. low in calories, as compared with other foods;

   b. high in vitamin C and vitamin A.

Meaningful words

epithelial cells
folic acid (folacin)
genital tract
gingivitis
hydrochloric acid
hypervitaminosis
intercellular cement
lachrymal gland
legume
mucous membrane
nostrum
oxalic acid
pathological
peristaltic waves
potassium
provitamin
respiratory tract
starch
subacute infection
urinary tract
xerophthalmia

3. Why are sweet potatoes and white potatoes good foods on a weight-control diet? Which vitamin C-rich foods would you select on a low budget? A moderate budget? Which for vitamin A?

4. What are the broad contributions made to the diet by vegetables and fruits?

5. Why is it desirable to have a source of vitamin C in each meal? What are the factors that destroy vitamin C? How may these factors be eliminated in your home? What is meant by "saturation" of body tissues with vitamin C? How may a generous consumption of vitamin C-rich foods in your diet help you now? In the future?

6. In what ways can vitamin A help the way you look and feel now? Later? What are the richest food sources of this vitamin?

7. What is the meaning of the terms carotenes, provitamin A, ascorbic acid?

8. Which vegetables are especially important in attaining and maintaining desirable weight?

9. Explain why vegetables and fruits help keep the chemistry of the body normally alkaline. Why they assist in normal elimination of waste.

10. Explain why it is important to understand the nutrient values in different fruits and vegetables in order to make wise selections when you plan and prepare meals at home. When you eat out.

11. In what ways can the practice of making wise choices in the fruits and vegetables you eat help your life? Help in the appearance of your skin, hair, teeth, bones, eyes, figure? Your resistance to disease and infections? Resistance to fatigue and anemia? General feeling of well-being? How can it help you when you marry and have your own home?

Applying and sharing

1. In your library, look up journals or books that show examples of extreme deficiencies in vitamin C and vitamin A. Can you see these in animal experiments?

2. Using the table of Nutritive Value of Foods in the Appendix, compile a table of richest sources of vitamins A and C.

3. Make a trip to the market where you shop and take with you your table of best sources of vitamins C and A. List in your notebook the following and make a copy for your kitchen pegboard:

   a. Best sources of vitamin C in fresh, frozen, and canned forms, with the price of each per serving.

   b. Best sources of vitamin A (include dried forms).

   c. Foods and beverages "fortified" with vitamin C, with cost per serving.

4. Analyze advertisements of products with added vitamins C and A. Are the claims justified? The price?

5. Keep a record of the total food you eat and drink for three days.

   a. Analyze your eating habits to determine your intake of vitamins C and A. How do they compare now with the first record you kept?

   b. Are you getting the recommended amount of vitamin C and vitamin A daily? In which meals or snacks? From what sources? How could you improve this?

6. Plan menus for three days with a good source of vitamin C in each meal and one source of vitamin A in each day's diet, choosing foods you enjoy and can afford. Save all these menus and calculations. Total the calories for each meal and snack, and for the whole day. Does the total fit your need for weight control? How would you alter it to fit your needs more specifically, yet retain the adequate balance of each meal?

7. Share with your family what you have learned, and see if you can interest them in taking part with you in any of the above experiences.

8

vegetables and fruits in meals

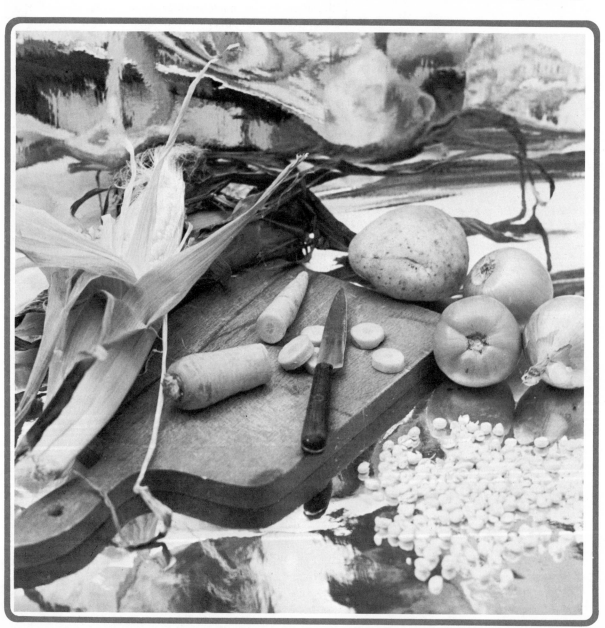

Many homemakers are praised for their skill and artistry in cooking meats and preparing desserts, but when you are lauded for the way you prepare the vegetables in your meals, you have received the greatest compliment.

Consumption and cost of living

It is most unfortunate that, as the cost of living has risen, vegetables and fruits have become inadequately represented in menus in American homes and in public eating places. When they are included, they are often cooked in such a way that they are neither enjoyable nor nutritious. You will not make this mistake, for you know how important these foods are in the daily diet. In this chapter you will learn how to prepare them for enjoyment and for retention of the maximum health values.

We consumed 9 percent less of this food group in 1965 than in 1955. The cost rose 14 percent, because of a general price rise and a shift from fresh produce to the higher priced canned and frozen varieties.

Best buys

The fresh fruits and vegetables in season were least expensive. The canned cost about 25 percent more per pound than the fresh. The frozen rose from an average of 34 cents per pound to an average of 39 cents per pound in 1965, as compared with a price rise from 14 to 18 cents per pound for the fresh form.*

---

*USDA Survey, 1965.

Classification of vegetables and fruits

Vegetables and fruits, along with cereal grains, are those parts of plants that we eat. The edible part may be in any of nine forms: the green leaves (such as spinach, turnip greens, the various forms of lettuce, and green onions); flowers (such as cauliflower, broccoli, asparagus tips, squash, pumpkin, tomato, and all fruits); stems (such as celery, asparagus, and leeks); fruits (including tomato, pumpkin, and squash, which are both flower and fruit, and cucumbers, watermelon, green peppers); roots (such as carrots, beets, sweet potatoes, and turnips); tubers (Irish potatoes, peanuts, and Jerusalem artichokes, for example); bulbs (such as onions and garlic); seeds (such as green beans, beans, corn, dried beans, peas, nuts, and some fruits); and fungi (mushrooms).

Fruits differ only slightly from vegetables. They are the seed-bearing parts of plants. Some are firm and fleshy, like apples, peaches, and pears; some are soft and succulent, like berries; others are quite juicy, like the citrus fruits. Botanically, cereal grains, nuts, and legumes are also fruits. Fruits have less starch and more sugar (in the form of fructose) than vegetables, little protein or fat, and more pectin.

Since the studies of 1965 indicate that our diets were more deficient in vitamins C and A than in 1955, and since we depend on vegetables and fruits to provide most of these nutrients, let us examine the factors that produce the greatest amount of these vitamins, so that we can become more skillful in using fruits and vegetables daily to balance our meals. Studies show that you get from one-fourth to almost one-half more return on the dollar spent for this group of foods in fresh

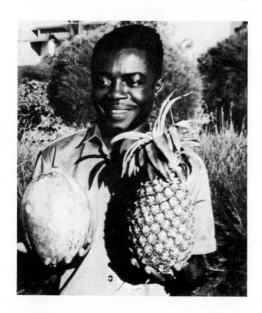

This Nigerian displays native papaya and pineapple. His people eat fruit as a snack, not for meals.

form, if wisely chosen, than from the same foods either canned or frozen. This is quite significant, especially for those on a low budget.

Judging quality in fresh vegetables and fruits

An untrained homemaker is often bewildered by the many forms of fruits and vegetables. She wonders, "What is the best to buy, the fresh or the processed?" The array of canned, frozen, dried, freeze-dried, pickled, spiced, smoked, and waxed ones can present quite a problem.

Standards for judging quality

In judging quality in fresh vegetables and fruits, watch for freshness, maturity, size, weight in relation to size, and natural color for its kind. Some of these characteristics affect the flavor, nutrients, and cost. Others affect the cost but not the nutrients.

FRESHNESS. Lettuce and cabbage should be crisp, firm, tender, clean, and untrimmed. The latter point is important, because the outside leaves protect the food against loss of vitamins, protect freshness, and provide vital nutrients. All fruits and vegetables should be free from soft spots or brown, black, yellow, or dark spots on the leaves. There should be no withering.

MATURITY. Green vegetables (all leaves, peas, green beans, asparagus, and hybrid sweet corn) and root vegetables (such as carrots, beets, and parsnips) are of higher quality when slightly undermature. When these get old, they become tough and woody and have less flavor and nutrients. Mature fruits have the best flavor. Mature but green tomatoes or hard fruit should be ripened at room temperature, out of the sun. Green mature tomatoes have more vitamin C than red gas-ripened ones. Old, withered vegetables or fruits are low in flavor and nutrients.

SIZE AND WEIGHT. In general, medium size is a good choice. Overlarge carrots, turnips, and beets may be woody. Overlarge white potatoes may have a hollow center or wireworms, with black streaks. Small oranges may have more juice, less thick skin, and more nutrients than overly large ones. A small, hard, firm head of cabbage is likely to have fewer worms, less residue from spray, and less loss of vitamin C than a large, loose head. Select the size to suit your planned use for the food and the price. Weight is a better indicator of quality than size. Heavy weight for size indicates high quality and much juice.

COLOR. The color should be characteristic for its kind. The color of fruits and vegetables relates to their freshness. Green vegetables should have deep color, not fading into yellow-greens. This color should be uniform and free of dark colored spots. Yellow vegetables should be deep yellow. Cauliflower and white potatoes should be a clean white. A green underskin on a potato means the presence of a toxic chemical, solanine. Such potatoes are not a bargain, even at a low price.

Prepackaging

ADVANTAGES. When food is prepackaged, it is protected from dirt, germs, and withering (oxidation). There is less bruising because of handling by customers. It is possible that a higher quantity of vitamin C is available.

DISADVANTAGES. Prepackaged potatoes may be green-skinned. To protect them from turning green, potatoes are now being packaged in dark-color plastic. Some packaging has the food placed

In judging quality of fresh vegetables and fruits, check for freshness, maturity, size, weight, and color.

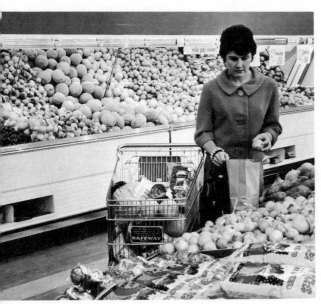

in such a way as to hide blemishes or spoilage, and the consumer must examine prepackaged produce carefully. The dripping of juice in a fruit package indicates poor quality.

Processed vegetables and fruits

Advantages

The lean winters of our forefathers are gone, thanks to the new technology in canning, freezing, and drying fruits and vegetables and their juices. Formerly, in the early spring and summer, after a long, hard winter, there was a high incidence of pneumonia, respiratory diseases, and other sickness. Few people associated this with the fact that fewer vegetables and fruits were eaten in the winter. Now we know that the fruits and vegetables that provided the diet with vitamins C and A, and other vitamins were scanty in winter. The reserves of these vitamins were lowered, and in some cases depleted. Naturally, with weaker cell tissues, people were then and are now more predisposed to sickness and infections.

Processed foods help make a good diet available all year round. Then, too, they are convenient, clean, and ready to be quickly prepared for a meal. Dried and canned forms are easily stored and transported.

CANNED FOODS. Canned food is sterilized, cooked, and ready to eat. Some vegetables need a little seasoning. Just before serving, heat them to below the boiling point. Further cooking is undesirable, lest you destroy texture and vitamins.

Canned varieties of food approximately equal fresh foods of high quality in nutrients, if each food is properly handled. They may be less pleasant in taste and color than the fresh, especially the

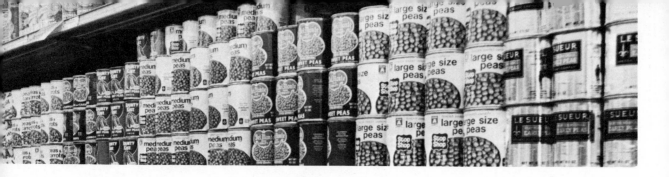

green leafy ones. However, spot checking reveals that people accustomed to eating canned peas, for instance, prefer the flavor to that of fresh or frozen peas. In this study, you will broaden your taste for vegetables.

FROZEN FOODS. Frozen foods are not sterilized, but there is no growth of microorganisms if they are kept frozen until you are ready to cook and eat them. Frozen foods should be stored at 0°F. They often cost more per serving than other types, for it costs more to store them. The color, flavor, and nutrients of frozen foods are as good as those of first-quality fresh ones.

Time saved in preparing and cooking processed vegetables and fruits frees the homemaker to use her time for other purposes, as these foods provide built-in maid service, which women appreciate.

CONSUMPTION. In 1965, the quantity of vegetables processed was eight and one-half million tons. Between 1953 and 1965, the per capita annual use of citrus fruit increased from 40 to 50 pounds a year, and that of all other fruits from 48 to 53 pounds. This was an average of one-quarter pound of fruit used per day per person.

Disadvantages

The chief disadvantage of canned and frozen foods is that they cost more per pound than high-quality fresh ones in season. This is a point of great importance to those on a low-cost food budget. It would be foolish to buy either canned or frozen potatoes or carrots, for instance, if you are on a low-to-moderate budget and the fresh ones cost less. On the other hand, canned or frozen peas might be lower in cost than fresh ones. Thus you must determine how much you can afford to pay and investigate for yourself the foods that cost less per serving in your markets at different seasons.

Another disadvantage is that because the volatile acids cannot escape from canned foods, green vegetables turn olive or a pale color that is less appealing to us. However, this does not affect the nutritive value or taste of the food.

Canned nonacid vegetables that are held too long in storage or at too high a temperature (above 65°F) lose vitamins—up to a fourth of the thiamine, also vitamin C and some vitamin A. This can be avoided by not overbuying and by using what you buy in order of purchase, within four to six months. However, canned citrus and acid fruits may be kept in the home for a period up to a year without loss of vitamins.

Frozen foods often cost more per serving than the fresh or canned, because storage costs more. They are, however, convenient and of good quality.

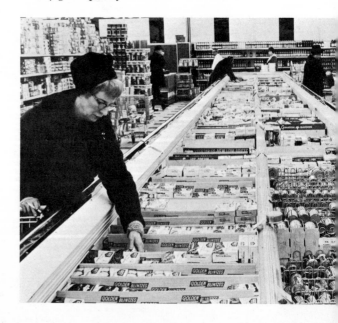

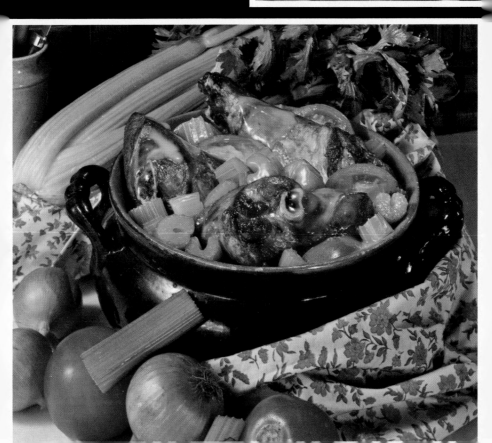

crisp vegetables for a satisfying winter meal.

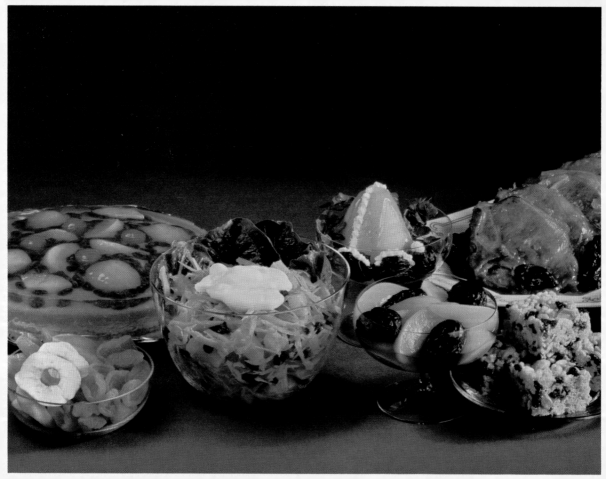

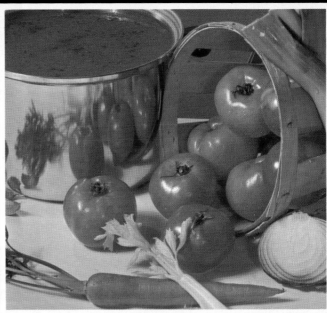

(top right) *Homemade tomato soup tempts any appetite on a blustery winter day.*

(top left) *Chili con carne, gazpacho, and corn pudding are Mexican favorites that are becoming popular in this country.*

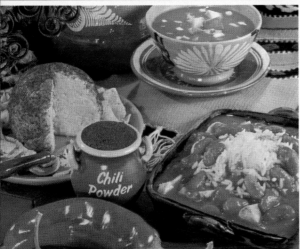

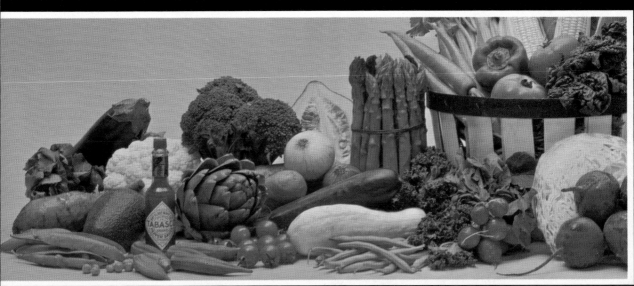

Strawberries and cream is one of the easiest and most luscious of desserts. (top right) This appealing display of party snacks is doubly attractive: it is delicious and low in calories.

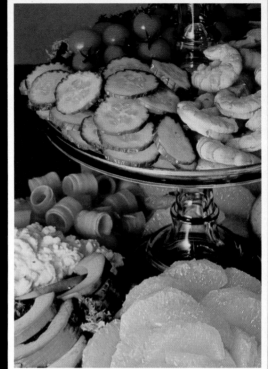

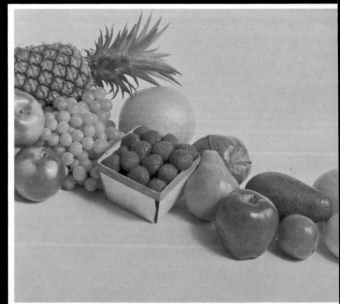

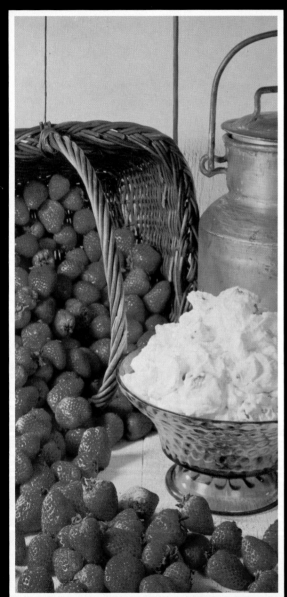

Canned vegetables and fruits are available the year round. They come in many varieties and can sizes to suit the needs of the homemaker.

Canning and freezing foods

Speed of processing

Commercial processors use the same first steps, whether canning or freezing. Plants are located in the heart of the district where food is grown. The food is whisked from harvest to plant, often in a flume of water on a conveyor belt. Then it is prepared and is canned or frozen within minutes after harvest. Unless they have their own gardens, few homemakers have a chance to be so prompt in the use of fresh varieties. This is particularly significant for the leafy and succulent vegetables and fruits that deteriorate quickly.

Nutrient loss

However, there are two disadvantages to processed vegetables and fruits that fresh varieties do not encounter when properly prepared. Studies show that the flume of water in which the food is moved to prevent wilting and deterioration causes loss of water-soluble vitamins and minerals, and the blanching process by which the food is dipped in boiling water or exposed to steam, then dipped in cold water to cool, causes further loss. Steam is the better method of blanching. Blanching is essential to stop enzyme action within the food, which would cause rapid deterioration after harvest. This technique will surely be improved to provide a minimum loss of nutrients. Commercially, as well as at home, the more that is known and practiced in preparing foods to eat, the better the retention of nutrients and flavor.

Research has shown that well-equipped plants that apply our latest knowledge lose as little as 5 to 10 percent of the water-soluble nutrients.

Others less well equipped and less knowledgeable lose 40 to 50 percent! As a guide in this respect, when you buy canned vegetables and fruits, note the name of the processor, for well-established firms take pride in the highest quality product and have good, modern equipment.

Canning methods

New methods of canning far surpass the old-time "boil-and-can" method. These include pressure canning, "flash" canning, and some methods now under study, that will undoubtedly be tested and adapted for general use.

Within a few hours after they are picked, fresh Florida oranges may be sent to machines like this extractor, which squeezes the fruit rapidly and in large volume. The juice may then be canned, frozen, or bottled for immediate use.

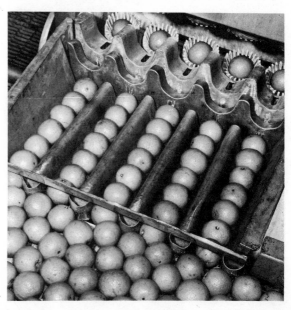

PRESSURE CANNING. Pressure canning, the first improvement, uses six pounds of pressure for vegetables to reach a temperature of 230°F and destroys all harmful bacteria. The food will keep.

"FLASH" CANNING. HTST (high temperature-short time) is a new method of "flash" canning. The food reaches a temperature of 285°F in a flash and is held only seconds or a few minutes at most. Then, in an aseptic (germ-free) chamber, it is canned, sealed, and quickly cooled. Juices, baby foods, peas, corn, and all small unit foods are canned by this method.

Other methods under study or in use include:

1/High-frequency electronic heating

The canning process.

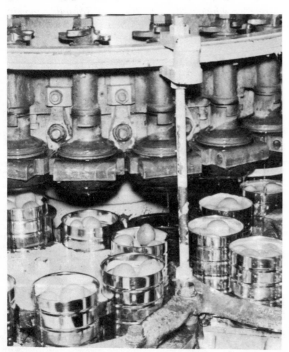

2/The addition of antibiotics, such as nisin and subtilin

3/The addition of chemicals, such as propylene oxide, hydrogen peroxide, and others

4/The mechanical shaking of the containers to circulate heat and decrease cooking time

Freezing method

Fresh vegetables and fruits are quickly frozen and held at 0°F until they are used. When frozen food thaws, it should be used at once. Refreezing causes rapid deterioration of all aspects of high quality (color, texture, flavor, nutrients) and could allow harmful microorganisms to develop.

Drying fruits and vegetables

There are many advantages to dried fruits and vegetables. This is man's oldest method of preserving them. They are a concentrated source of nutrients and energy, as the table of Nutritive Value of Foods in the Appendix shows. Fruits that are dried are allowed to ripen more before harvest than those picked for canning or for the fresh food market. They keep well for long periods when stored in a cool, dry place and the moisture is reduced to 18 to 24 percent. It is impossible for microorganisms to grow without adequate moisture.

Dried foods cost less per serving than the same kind if fresh, canned, or frozen. With the weight and bulk reduced, they are inexpensive and easy to package, transport, and store. For example, it takes 6 to 8 pounds of fresh apricots to make 1 pound of dried ones. They are available all year round, keeping well for long periods unless recontaminated with moisture. In dry places, like the tombs of Egypt and the caves of New Mexico,

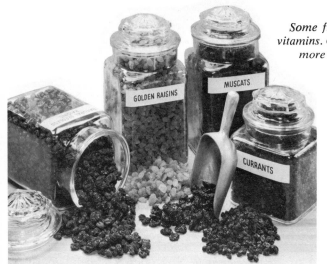

Some fruits are rich in iron and vitamins. One cup of raisins yields more than four times as much iron as a cup of grapes.

dried vegetables and fruits have been found that are of ancient origin.

In the dried form of fruits and vegetables, the carbohydrate and protein, along with iron, make significant contributions to the diet. One cup of dried raisins contains over four times as much iron as a cup of fresh grapes and a cup of uncooked dried apricots almost seven times as much iron and four times as much vitamin A as a cup of canned apricots. It is smart to give children dried fruit to eat as a sweet instead of candy or rich cookies. The calories in dried fruits carry more than their weight in meeting the day's total nutrient needs, and they are a tasty snack for anyone.

Light-colored fruits are sulfured to help retain color. Studies have been made on the effects of sulfuring on nutrients. At Stanford University, it was found that about three-fourths of the thiamine in light-colored fruits is lost in sulfuring, as compared with the dark-colored unsulfated fruits, which lost only 20 percent. However, sulfating tends to protect vitamin C.

Freeze-drying

Modern man is finding new ways to dry more foods. In freeze-drying, research is combining some of the best features of freezing with the drying process. Fresh frozen food is dried in a vacuum. Weight and bulk are reduced in some foods by half or more. Others keep their original size but weigh much less—a freeze-dried strawberry has one-sixteenth the weight of a fresh one. Texture and nutrients in such foods are retained but, unfortunately, the flavor and aroma of fresh fruit are lost. Research is under way to solve this problem.

The first foods successfully freeze-dried were peas, carrots, potatoes, apples, apricots, boysenberries, and cherries. Fruits used for "fresh fruit" pies are frozen in large quantities by this method. At present, the cost per serving for this type of dried food is high for family use.

Storage of vegetables and fruits

Canned and dried foods

It is good management to have a variety of dried and canned vegetables and fruits on hand. A reserve helps you quickly and inexpensively prepare an emergency meal for family or guests. These foods should be stored in cool, dry, dark areas below 65°F and above freezing. Once foods are dried, the nutrients remain stable. In hot, humid weather, however, dried fruits may ferment and spoil or mold. Not so with canned foods, but there is a gradual loss of vitamin content, as you may recall. Cool temperatures delay this loss and higher temperatures accelerate it.

Frozen foods

Frozen foods are maintained at a temperature of 0°F or lower, to maintain highest quality in flavor, color, and nutrients. To know when to remove the frozen strawberries without having the whole ones collapse, make note of the time required to thaw them and other fruits in the refrigerator. If you fail to remove frozen fruit from the freezer in time, let it thaw at room temperature, but do not heat it. It is better to have underthawed fruit than that which has stood too long after thawing.

Fresh vegetables and fruits

Most produce has been exposed to insecticides, sprays, sand, dirt, insects, and microorganisms from air and human beings. Even canned and packaged food is exposed to fallout and other contamination in the air and from other sources (see Chapter 16). For this reason, cans should be washed and then dried with a paper towel before they are opened. Unused food, except citrus and acid foods, may be stored in the can in the refrigerator when the can has been washed and dried before opening. Any unwashed food placed in the refrigerator contaminates other foods.

WASHING. Sort vegetables and fruits and, with the exception of berries, wash all of them thoroughly and dry them before storing. Fill the sink two-thirds full of water, changing water as often as necessary so that all the foods are washed in clean water. Scrub root vegetables, celery, asparagus, and the like with a brush. Wash green leaves a few at a time and drain them in a colander or wire basket made for the purpose. Shake off the surplus moisture.

STORAGE. Wrap fresh produce in old, clean towels or paper towels for best keeping quality and store it in the crisper drawer of the refrigerator. For best storage, the crisper drawer should be only two-thirds full. When packaged in plastic bags to prevent dehydration, fresh produce may be stored on the refrigerator shelves.

Store foods with a strong odor, such as onions, cantaloupes, or pineapple, in tight bags so that the odor does not affect other foods. All fruits and vegetables stored in the refrigerator retain moisture and crisp freshness better if each kind is packaged or wrapped, even in the hydrator.

ORDER OF USE. Use the ripest, most perishable fruits and vegetables first. Therefore, these should be stored in the front part of the refrigerator. Fresh green leaves are more likely to spoil than carrots, corn than potatoes, green onions than dry, mature ones. Late-crop potatoes keep better than new and early ones and are better suited to long-term storage. Potatoes lose about

Why would you open the lettuce so that each leaf is thoroughly washed?

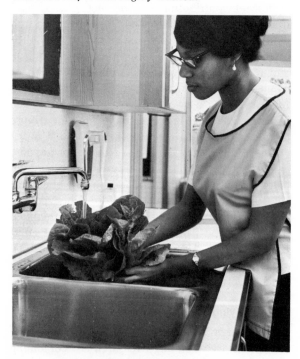

half their vitamin C after three months' storage, but they provide other important nutrients.

Good management in shopping

With your background of information, you are now prepared to do an excellent job in making choices among the vegetables and fruits. Effective food shopping is discussed in Chapter 19. Here we shall consider specifics for vegetables and fruits.

For best value and highest nutrition, vegetables and fruits should be purchased when they are fresh and in top condition. The following principles can serve as a buying guide for you, not only for fresh produce but also for the canned and frozen varieties.

1/Buy fresh vegetables and fruits at a market that has a rapid turnover and good refrigeration, including store air-conditioning—unless you can buy at a genuine farm market where foods are harvested just before marketing.

2/Avoid stores that display fresh produce in the sun and those that overwater fresh vegetables to give them an appearance of freshness. These practices cause deterioration and loss of water-soluble vitamins and other nutrients.

3/Shop for fresh produce on the days when it is freshest, but at a time when you do your other food shopping.

4/Observe good shopping manners. Examine fresh fruits and vegetables for weight and quality, but do not squeeze them, as this causes bruise and rot and increases spoilage. You may be sure the loss on such produce is included in the price. In the end, we all pay for poor shopping manners.

5/Buy vegetables and fruits in person for best choices and lowest cost.

6/The lowest-cost fresh vegetables and some fruits are often sold in bulk, not in packages. By buying in bulk, you can personally select each piece of produce, assuring high quality and uniform size. Often small potatoes cost less and, if not withered, are good boiled in the skin. Bulk greens enable you to avoid old ones that are deteriorating.

7/Large sizes of canned foods cost less per serving than small cans. Even a young couple can

Open-air displays of fruits and vegetables are tempting to passers-by. However, the nutrients are best preserved when these foods are in a cool atmosphere, away from the sun.

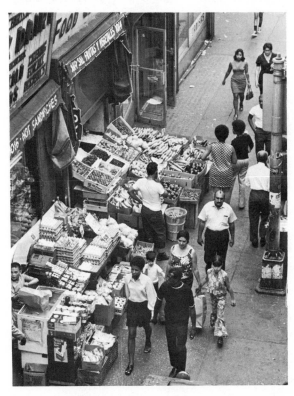

use a large can of tomatoes, juice, and most fruit, when they store these foods properly in the refrigerator. For instance, peaches or applesauce may be used plain at the first serving; next time, topped with a scoop of ice cream; and the third time, placed in a pan, topped with crumbled cookies and dotted with nutmeg, margarine, and brown sugar and browned quickly under the broiler.

8/Large packages of frozen vegetables in cellophane usually cost less than those in smaller amounts. When the large package is used without deterioration, it is the best buy. But weight and cost must be checked and compared with those of smaller packages, as "tricks" are practiced by some processors in different types of packaging (see Chapter 17). The consumer has found that on some occasions the larger package may cost more than the average size.

9/Compare the cost per serving of different kinds of processed foods with that of fresh ones. Buy what you need in the form that costs the least per serving. Dried beans and other legumes cost about a fifth or a tenth as much per serving as canned cooked beans ready-to-eat. Yet you may need some canned beans as a reserve. Canned tomatoes are often less expensive per serving than fresh ones, as are citrus fruits when the fresh ones are out of season.

10/Buy canned or frozen food in quantity to save money when sales are on. These usually occur at harvest time, when the new crop is ready for canning or freezing.

11/Buy processed food by descriptive labeling, rather than grade, as the grade refers to uniformity of size, color, and density of syrup. The higher grade costs from 1 to 4 cents more per pound, yet is not more nourishing. Grade A is fancy, B is choice, and C is standard. Descriptive labeling

tells you if the beans are "Whole," "Tender," "Very young," or "Mature." This is helpful in making a choice. See Chapter 17 for further details on what to look for on labels.

When you make your menus and shopping list, first study the vegetables and fruits in the table of Nutritive Value of Foods (in the Appendix), checking those that are rich in vitamins A and C. This can help you take advantage of seasonal prices and provide the nutrients you need for healthy, tasty meals. When you are familiar with the foods that are rich in these vitamins, you can make decisions quickly and wisely.

Shop for fresh produce on days when it is freshest, and examine it carefully.

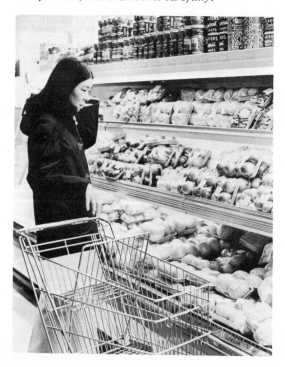

The concept of the salad

The new concept, based on research cited in Chapter 7, is that a green salad in the daily diet and/or some raw fruit is required to help us achieve our potential in appearance and vitality.

Equipment for salad making

A girl looking forward to marriage can list a number of items to help her enjoy the art of making salads. A friend might give her a "salad shower." A variety of bowls is useful. This might include a large wooden one and/or pottery, ceramic, clear glass, or crystal in different sizes to suit the taste and purse. A pepper mill, mortar and pestle, and oil and vinegar pitchers or a cruet set are all useful and beautiful to see on the table. Salad forks with four tines are ideal, and a set of salad plates is needed. See Table 19–1 for a list of basic equipment needed for meal preparation.

Purpose of the salad

The major function of the salad is to add contrast in texture (between soft, cooked foods and firm, crisp ones), in flavor (between bland foods and those enlivened by a nippy salad dressing slightly on the sour side), and in color, to make a meal attractive. Another purpose is to balance the meal nutritionally in vitamins, making up in the raw vegetables or fruits for nutrients destroyed by heat or other processes of preparation. The salad also helps control overweight by adding very few calories—ranging from 5 to 15 with a lemon dressing and increasing according to the kind of salad and the type and amount of dressing used. In Chapter 11 we consider why the vegetable oil itself is an important part of the meal.

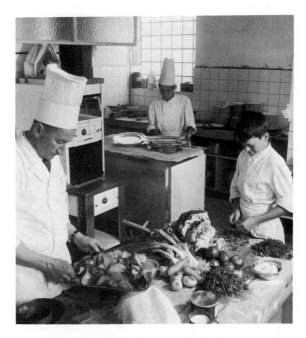

The salad chef plays an important role in a fine French restaurant.

Kinds of salads

Salads fall into several classes. They may be used as a first course accompanying a meal, as a separate course after the main one, as the main course, and as dessert.

The tossed green salad may be one kind of lettuce with French dressing, or several kinds combined. A variety of fresh or canned fruits or a combination of fresh and canned fruits may be used on a bed of green lettuce or watercress with a generous mound of cottage cheese in the center, as the main course of a meal. Grapefruit and orange arranged in sections on lettuce make an appetizing first course, and avocado adds flavor, texture, and color contrast with an elegant note.

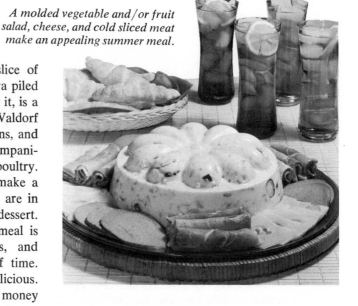

A molded vegetable and/or fruit salad, cheese, and cold sliced meat make an appealing summer meal.

Apple and pear slices may be used. A slice of fresh or canned pineapple with diced papaya piled in the center, with lime juice sprinkled over it, is a luxury salad as first course or dessert. Waldorf salad, using apple or pear with celery, raisins, and peanuts is easy to make and a favorite accompaniment for any type of meal, especially poultry. Strawberries circling a slice of pineapple make a salad that is moderate in price when both are in season—and beautiful to see or eat as dessert. A delicious accompaniment to a holiday meal is chopped or ground cranberries, oranges, and apples, which may be prepared ahead of time. Melon balls or cubes are beautiful and delicious. Take advantage of seasonal fruits to save money and add exciting variety to salads.

MAIN DISH OR CHEF'S SALAD. This has a base of tossed greens and one-third cup of meat, poultry, or seafood per serving. The meats should be in large enough pieces to let you see what you are eating. Diced sharp cheese may also be used. Eggs are used stuffed as part of the salad or in sections or slices to garnish it. The meat may be prepared ahead of time and allowed to marinate with the dressing for best flavor. Greens may be ready to toss. Potato salad, hot or cold, is a main dish when ham, cooked frankfurters, eggs, or cheese is added as a source of protein.

GELATIN SALADS. Gelatin is used as a base to incorporate either raw or cooked vegetables or fruits, meats, fish, cheese, or poultry. The shape of the mold and the color of the salad are important. The gelatin salad has the advantage of sealing in the foods so that there is no loss of vitamins from oxidation when it is made ahead of time. It is well suited to small children and elderly people, especially when raw food, such as carrots, needs to be ground. When made with fruit, it can serve as a salad-dessert.

Preparation of the salad

The selection of ingredients and the preparation of the salad are important for its success. Remember four easy basic points about salad ingredients: they should be fresh, clean, cold, and crisp. The salad is no better than the quality of lettuce and other ingredients that make it.

Assemble your equipment and all ingredients before you begin. Do much of the work ahead. The greens and other fresh ingredients should be washed, cold, crisp, and ready for use.

Tear the greens in bite-size pieces just before using them. Cutting bruises the edges, if the greens must wait as long as an hour before being served. All foods are more attractive when the pieces are large enough to retain their shape without mashing together, and not so large as to be unmanageable for eating.

SALAD DRESSING. The salad dressing can't make a good salad out of poor-quality ingredients, but it can bring out the delicious flavor of high-quality ones. There are basically three kinds of dressings, each with variations:

1/French dressing, which is oil, vinegar, and seasoning

2/Mayonnaise, which consists of oil, egg, and seasonings whipped to a smooth, stiff emulsion

3/Cooked or boiled salad dressing

Favorite herbs and spices, bleu or Roquefort cheese, or chili sauce may be added to French dressing or to the other dressings for variety. When you are in doubt as to the kind to use, of the many ready-to-use or ready-to-mix dressings, French dressing is a good choice. Oil and vinegar or lemon or lime juice looks better on greens than other

Orange and onion circles on lettuce are delicious with a baked bean or spaghetti main dish. Why do you need milk or cheese to balance this meal?

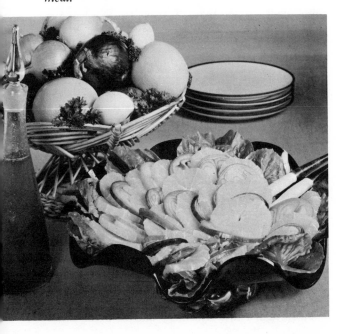

dressings. A basic French dressing* is simple to make. Keep a pint of it on hand in the refrigerator and add vinegar or lemon juice as needed. It can be made so much less expensively at home than the commercial type, and you can choose an oil high in linoleic acid to give the individual touch and the greatest nutritive value. Lemon and lime juice impart high vitamin C, as well as a piquant flavor. Wine and tarragon vinegars alter the flavor, too. Add chili sauce to mayonnaise and you have Russian dressing. Add diced pickle or horseradish for tartar sauce to use with fish.

Remember that the ingredients in a salad are low in calories, but oil contains 125 calories per tablespoon and mayonnaise 100. In French dressing, if you use two parts vinegar or lemon juice to one part oil this reduces calories by two-thirds.

TOSSING THE SALAD. This is a feat in fine restaurants and adds an artistic note to the meal at home. The ingredients, accompaniments, and equipment are brought to the table. The making and tossing of the salad are as beautiful to watch as the carving of a fine roast or fowl.

For a gourmet touch, try herbs, such as mint, chives, and rosemary for fruits; chives, parsley, basil, or tarragon for greens. Peppercorns, toast cubes with garlic and sharp cheese seasoning, bits of bleu cheese or crisp bacon crumbles add flavor to mixed vegetables. These may be added last, before the tossing begins. (See Table 22–1, pages 396–397, for other herbs to use.) The seasoning mixture is poured over the bowl of ingredients, then lemon juice or vinegar. Now you take the fork and spoon from below and come up through the ingredients and over, tossing ever so gently until

*For an easy basic recipe for French dressing, see *You and Your Food* by Ruth Bennett White (Englewood Cliffs, N.J.: Prentice-Hall, Inc., 1970), p. 430.

all is moist, but glistening and firm. Use only enough dressing to coat the salad, leaving very little in the bowl. Spoon it lightly onto the salad plates and serve. This can all be done in the kitchen, but to share it at the table makes eating an art, whether the meal is served to the family or to guests, whether it is a simple snack on the patio or a feast at an elegant table.

Salad in the menu

When the salad is a separate course, serve it with crisp crackers, hot, thin toast, or bread. Select the salad to fit into the whole menu. If you are serving fresh fruit and cheese for dessert, omit the salad. When the meal is a festive occasion, keep the salad low in calories, bright in color, and contrasting

A vegetable or fruit salad with cheese sandwiches is a popular luncheon menu. How do you rate this meal? Why?

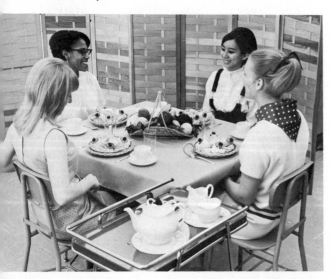

in texture and flavor—a good idea for everyday meals, too.

The art of making a fine salad is learned. Experiment and practice. When you succeed, you have gained another achievement that will help you be a gifted and popular hostess.

Cooking vegetables and fruits

Reasons for cooking

As you recall, we need some raw fruits and vegetables to provide the nutrients easily destroyed by heat. However, there are a number of important reasons for cooking these foods on occasion.

1/Humans are not as well equipped to digest and absorb as much raw vegetables as cooked ones. Besides, we prefer the taste of some vegetables, such as potatoes, asparagus, beets, kale, turnip greens, collards, rhubarb, and others, cooked, rather than raw.

2/Cooking reduces the bulk, especially of the green leafy vegetables, and enables us to consume larger amounts.

3/The cellulose and protopectins are softened when cooked, making possible a more complete digestion and absorption of the nutrients. The protopectins have a cementing effect on the structure of fruit cells. Ripening and cooking change protopectins to pectin.

4/Some research has indicated that the pectins combine with cholesterol and eliminate it—thus pointing toward another value of fruit in preventing and treating heart-circulatory disease.

5/Cooking destroys molds, yeasts, and microorganisms that cause food to spoil. Spoiled food, if eaten, can cause dysentery and other diseases.

Many vegetables are better digested and absorbed when served cooked. These are among the most popular.

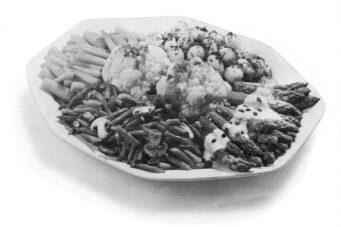

When living in places where sanitary conditions are poor, as you may if you travel or work in developing nations, it is safer to eat hot, cooked food or raw food that can be peeled.

6/Young children, older people, and those with some types of disease require the nutrients from fruits and vegetables but cannot digest or absorb them in the amounts required, unless they are cooked.

7/Proper cooking improves the flavor of many vegetables and adds untold pleasure and variety to meals.

Basic principles for cooking

Vegetable cookery often sinks to the lowest standard in cooking of any food group. It need not be

For peak flavor, crisp texture, attractive color, and highest nutrients, vegetables should be cooked in little water for a very short time. Why?

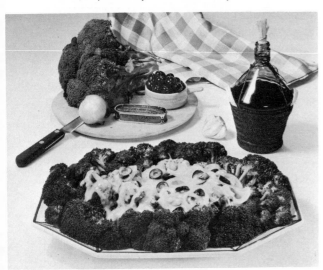

so. Many homemakers, chefs, and institutional cooks fail in this branch of cooking, but you can succeed.

The aim in cooking vegetables is:

1/To attain tender, yet firm, crisp texture that is neither soft and soggy nor tough and hard

2/To retain the best color consistent with saving food values

3/To retain the maximum nutrients at the lowest cost

4/To achieve full peak flavor

All these aims may be achieved, whether the vegetables are boiled, steamed, panned, simmered, or cooked in waterless or pressure saucepans. The method for all is virtually the same, though the timing varies. Special instructions for pressure cooking are given with the pressure cooker, though in general the times stated are too long. For all cooking of vegetables and fruits, experience will teach you the correct timing for each. The texture of the food should be neither too firm nor too soft. The following principles will serve as a guide for most successful cooking of this important food group.

1/Use as short a time as possible. This will assure maximum flavor and nutrients, as well as the color of the cooked product.

2/Cook in a thick, flat-bottomed pan with a tight-fitting lid, to keep out oxygen from the air. The bottom of the pan should be the same size as the heat unit, and the pan should be the correct size for the amount of food to be cooked.

3/Use as little water as possible, and only water that has been boiled for two minutes to expel all oxygen. This will keep vitamin C loss to a minimum. The amount of water clinging to spinach or Swiss chard is sufficient for cooking. In general, use one-fourth to one-third cup of boiled water per pound for root and tuber vegetables. More is needed for potatoes and less for carrots. Frozen vegetables require less water than most packages suggest, but you may be guided by the package directions until you find the right level for your taste and equipment. Dried beans, peas, and lentils require three cups of water per cup of dried food, except when a pressure saucepan is used. In the latter case, use two cups of water per cup of food.

4/Cover the pan, bring it to a boil quickly, and then lower the heat until bubbles just form and break. Water will not boil above the temperature of 212°F, no matter how much heat you apply or how hard the pot boils. Cook the food until it is just tender, and serve it at once.

5/Use all the remaining liquid. Our pioneer forefathers enjoyed dipping bread in the "pot liquor," a habit that helped them retain all the nutrients released from the food into the liquid. The cooking liquid can be used as the base of a soup or a sauce and achieve the same results for us.

PANNING VEGETABLES AND FRUITS. Place a small amount of fat in a firm, shallow, broad-bottomed pan, such as a skillet (with a lid), a chicken fryer, or an electric skillet. Add the fresh or frozen vegetable, season it, and stir until each piece is coated lightly with fat. Little or no water

Panned vegetables are especially popular in the Orient and gaining favor in this country. Why is this method recommended?

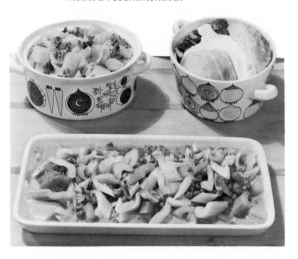

is needed. The thin coat of fat helps the vegetable retain its flavor and vitamins. Cover the pan. Cook only until the vegetable is just firm-tender, stirring at intervals to hasten cooking on all sides and to prevent loss of color (three to five minutes).

The following vegetables and fruits are well suited to panning: green beans, green peas, summer squash, spinach, cabbage, endive, eggplant, onions, fresh apples, pineapple, and peaches.

IMPORTANCE OF TIMING. Accurate timing is essential for good flavor, color, texture, and retention of nutrients. Table 8–1 gives the approximate cooking time for 33 vegetables. The time required depends on the size of the pot, the size and state of maturity of the food (small pieces and young, tender vegetables require less time than large pieces or old, tough vegetables), and the form (whether the food is fresh, frozen, or dried). Frozen foods take less time than fresh, and fresh less time than dried. Overcooking produces a soft, unattractive, less tasty, and less nourishing food.

table 8–1   Approximate Timetable for Cooking Vegetables*

VEGETABLE	BOILING** (Minutes)	STEAMING** (Minutes)	PRESSURE SAUCEPAN** (15 Pounds Pressure) (Minutes)	BAKING** (Minutes)
Artichokes, Jerusalem, whole	25–35	35		30–60
Asparagus, tips	5–15	7–15	½–2	
Beans, lima, green	20–30	25–35	1–2	
Beans, snap, whole, or 1-inch pieces	15–30	20–35	1½–3	
Beets, new, whole	30–45	40–60	5–10	40–60
old, whole	45–90	50–90	10–18	40–60
Broccoli, stalk and buds	10–20	15–20	1½–3	
Brussels sprouts, whole	10–20	10–20	1–2	
Cabbage, green, quartered	10–15	15	2–3	
shredded	3–10	8–12	½–1½	
Cabbage, red, shredded	8–12	10–15	½–1½	
Carrots, young, whole	15–25	20–30	3–5	35–45
mature, whole	20–30	40–50	10–15	60
sliced	15–25	25–30	3	
Cauliflower, whole	20–30	25–30	10	
flowerets	8–15	10–20	1½–3	
Celery, diced	15–20	25–30	2–3	
Chard, Swiss	10–20	15–25	1½–3	
Collards	10–20			
Corn, on cob	5–15	10–15	0–1½	
Eggplant, sliced	10–20	15–20		
Kale	10–25			
Okra, sliced	10–20	20	3–4	
Onions, small, whole	15–25	25–35	3–4	
large, whole	20–40	35–40	5–8	50–60
Parsnips, whole	20–40	30–45	9–10	30–45
quartered	20–30	30–40	4–8	
Peas, green	8–20	10–20	0–1	
Potatoes, white, medium, whole	25–45	30–45	8–11	45–60
quartered	15–25	20–30	3–5	
Rutabaga, diced	20–30	35–40	5–8	
Spinach	3–10	5–12	0–1½	
Squash, Hubbard, 2-inch pieces	20–40	25–40	6–12	40–60
Squash, summer, sliced	10–20	15–20	1½–3	30
Sweet potatoes, whole	25–35	30–35	5–8	30–45
quartered	15–25	25–30	6	
Tomatoes	7–15		½–1	15–30
Turnips, whole	20–30		8–12	
sliced	15–20	20–25	1½	

*Adapted from Handbook of Food Preparation (Washington, D.C.: American Home Economics Association, Terminology Committee of the Food and Nutrition Division, 1958).
**The time for any method cannot be given exactly, because it depends on the variety and maturity of each vegetable and the size of the pieces into which it has been cut. Use the shortest time possible to obtain the desired results.

Retention of color

GREEN VEGETABLES. Green color is the most fragile. Heat decomposes the green chlorophyll. Harmless acids, which turn deep green to a drab olive green, are released. You may have noted this when you added vinegar to hot, wilted lettuce salad. Since green is more appealing to our appetite and sense of beauty, let us learn how to retain it.

Though soda, added to green vegetables, helps retain the green color, it destroys some of the many B vitamins and vitamin C and gives an unpleasant flavor. It is not necessary to resort to soda to retain green color when you cook properly.

Cook green vegetables quickly until they are just tender and remove them quickly from the pan to serve at once. The pressure saucepan is the best piece of equipment to accomplish this goal, when properly used. Most frozen vegetables or fresh green ones are tender before the chlorophyll is broken down.

Stop the cooking in a pressure saucepan at once by running cold water from the tap over the lid of the pan. Remove the lid to let volatile acids escape. Serve green vegetables immediately. If you use a regular pan with a lid, leave the lid slightly ajar to emit the volatile acids and help retain the green color.

Panned green vegetables should be cooked just before serving. Otherwise, they may lose the green color while waiting.

WHITE VEGETABLES. Add one teaspoon of vinegar to the cooking water of white vegetables, such as cauliflower, onions, celery, turnips, white cabbage, or white potatoes, to help retain the whiteness. If it is desirable to peel potatoes ahead of time, wrap them tightly in plastic and store them in the hydrator in the refrigerator to prevent darkening.

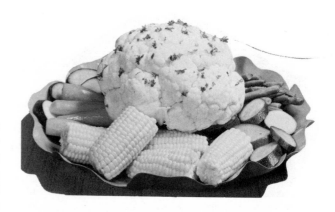

RED VEGETABLES. When vinegar is added to red cabbage or beets, the color is deepened by acid. Alkali (hard) water turns red foods a blue-purple color.

PEELED LIGHT FRUITS. To prevent darkening of peeled light fruits by oxidation, dip them in lemon or lime juice or use a commercial preparation that contains vitamin C. This applies to pears, peaches, apples, bananas, and avocados.

How to save nutrients in cooking

Vitamins, minerals, amino acids, and good flavor are concentrated in or near the skin, seeds, and darkest green of the outside leaves of vegetables and fruits. Cook these foods in their skins, when possible. When it is necessary to peel or trim them, use a peeler or pare thinly with a sharp knife to retain the maximum nutrients. The less surface exposed, the greater the retention of vitamins and minerals. Table 8–2 shows the amounts of nutrients lost by vegetables and fruits in their preparation and cooking.

Further hints on saving nutrients in vegetables and fruits include the following:

1/Stir in as little air as possible while food is cooking. Whipping air into hot foods destroys vitamins, especially C. When you serve whipped potatoes, remember to serve coleslaw or another good source of vitamin C, as well.

2/Blend or sieve vegetables or fruits when they are cold, as there is less destruction of vitamins by oxygen.

3/Cook frozen vegetables straight from the freezer. Thaw fruits in the refrigerator. Observe and record the cooking time, for further reference. This is good management.

4/To help retain maximum nutrients in canned vegetables, pour the liquid from the vegetable into the cooking pot and boil it down to about one-fourth cup. Then add the vegetable and the seasonings. Heat to boiling, but don't cook, the vegetable, as it is already cooked and further heat destroys its quality. Drink the liquid of fruits or add it to breads, gelatin salads, or desserts.

If you observe the precautions given in Chapter 7 for retaining the maximum amount of vitamin C in foods, you will retain the maximum of other nutrients and flavors, too.

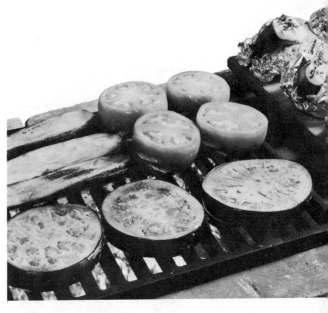

Whenever possible, vegetables should be cooked in their skins. This method helps retain their maximum nutrients.

Seasoning fruits

Fruits are so delicate in flavor that to add much seasoning may detract from the taste of many of them. Few require sugar, even when eaten raw. Dried fruits need no additional sweetening. Many canned fruits have too much sugar added. A heavy syrup helps preserve the shape of the fruit. However, in our calorie-conscious world, requests from many homemakers for less sugar have helped bring about the use of lighter syrup with fewer calories.

Orange or lemon improves the flavor of mild fruits, such as pears, when slices are added dur-

table 8–2 *Loss of Nutrients During Preparation and Cooking of Vegetables and Fruits*

FOOD GROUP	THIAMINE	RIBOFLAVIN	NIACIN	VITAMIN C
		Percentage		
Citrus fruits, tomatoes	—	—	—	15
Leafy green and yellow vegetables	45	40	40	50
Potatoes, sweet potatoes	25	20	20	35
Other vegetables and fruits	20	20	20	25

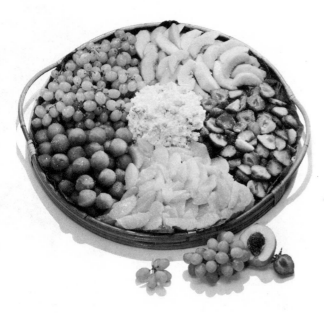

Few fresh fruits require sugar, even when eaten raw. With cottage cheese, fresh fruit makes a low-calorie, attractive, and delicious buffet meal.

ing cooking, and to such vegetables as sweet potatoes, yellow squash, carrots, beets, and rutabaga.

A mixture of fresh, frozen, canned, or stewed fruits creates a pleasant compote. Europeans use spices, such as cinnamon, nutmeg, ginger, allspice, and cloves, to season fruits and vegetables. Some herbs (mint, rosemary, and sesame seeds) are also used for variety. Many American homemakers experiment with these, especially gourmets.

Seasoning vegetables

No amount of good seasoning can make up for poorly cooked vegetables. But well-selected sea-soning can make well-prepared vegetables a gourmet's delight.

Basic seasonings

Salt, fat, and pepper are three basic seasonings.

SALT. Salt substitutes have been made by chemists for those on a low-sodium diet for health reasons. Vegetables taste flat without salt or its alternate. Worcestershire sauce, celery, onion, and garlic salts, dried parsley, soy sauce, and prepared mustard all contain generous amounts of salt to bring out flavor.

FATS. The fats used for seasoning vegetables are vegetable oil, margarine, butter, pork or other meat drippings, and sweet and sour cream. The kind of fat used greatly affects the taste of the vegetable. For instance, green or dry beans, lentils, and peas, and fresh cabbage or green leafy vegetables are much tastier when seasoned with brown pork drippings from a roast, chops, ham, or bacon than with plain fat. If a vegetable oil is preferred, remove all fat, but use the tasty brown meat drippings with the vegetable oil. Such a combination will bring you compliments for the fine flavor.

Butter has been considered the aristocrat of seasonings for vegetables. Because of the saturated fatty acids in butter, as well as the high price, the trend is now away from it. Sour cream has only 30 calories per tablespoon and a small amount is used to top baked potatoes, cabbage, cauliflower, and other vegetables, as well as salads.

Modern research is showing that the most healthful fat to use in seasoning is vegetable oil high in linoleic acid. (For details, see Chapter 11.)

PEPPER. Pepper—hot or sweet, black, white, green, or red—is a favored seasoning for many cooked vegetables and for salads. The amount you add depends on your taste. In some parts of the world, especially hot, tropical countries, a great deal of pepper is used. It is possible that this habit stems from the need to hide the unpleasant flavor of foods that could not be refrigerated—one of the initial reasons for the use of many spices in foods. Today, we use pepper to bring out the flavor of food, not to hide it.

ONION. Whether fresh, in salt, in dried flakes, or frozen, onion is universally prized for adding savor to a dish. It enhances green leafy vegetables, green beans, other vegetables, soups, stews, casseroles, and salads. We use over two billion pounds of onions a year.

GARLIC. Garlic in cloves, salt, dried flakes, or juice is used with vegetables in small amounts to give a distinctive savor. A light touch is needed in its use.

SPICES. Spices, along with the peel and juice of lemons and oranges, give a gourmet taste to some vegetables when properly used. Try a few whole allspice in lentil soup to give an elusive, mellow flavor. Nutmeg, added to carrots with a little honey, makes them especially delicious. Cinnamon sticks added to homemade French dressing lend a tantalizing flavor. The addition of nutmeg, cinnamon, or ginger, along with pineapple chunks or pieces of orange or lemon, produces a nippy flavor. Try different spices or herbs with beets, carrots, parsnips, turnips (white or yellow), pumpkin, tomatoes, eggplant, squash, and other vegetables. (See Table 22–1 for spices and herbs to use for seasoning vegetables.)

HERBS. Herbs may be grown in pots in a sunny window of the house or in a border or corner of the yard. Growing them is a good hobby. They can add delightful flavors to fruits and vegetables. Experiment and discover the fun of adding an individual touch to your cooking through skillful use of herbs.

Mix and match vegetables and fruits

Vegetables and fruits may be mixed in a number of combinations to produce an interesting variety in your meal planning. For example, two or more green leafy vegetables may be mixed, as blending or harmonious flavors. The addition of ham or bacon bits sparks up the flavor of these and other bland vegetables and the legumes. Onion may be served together with virtually any vegetable, and adds sharp contrast especially to bland-tasting vegetables. In general, the vegetables should complement each other, or provide contrast in color, flavor, and texture.

The same is true of fruits. Pineapple, for instance, is a very versatile fruit and may be combined with almost any other fruit for brisk, tart flavor contrast. It is also added to carrots and sweet potatoes in holiday and special-occasion dishes.

Using vegetables and fruits to balance the daily diet

Fruits and vegetables are useful additions to all meals and snacks and add not only valuable nutrients but also flavor and variety. Fruit and cheese are an excellent team at any time. Vegetables and fruits may be used as appetizers, in beverages, as garnishes for meat and other dishes, in baked foods, in salads, and in soups. Fruits by themselves form a delicious dessert.

Meaningful words

carbohydrate complex
chlorophyll
electronic heating
fallout
freeze-drying
nisin
pectin
propylene oxide
protopectin
solanine
subtilin
volatile acids

Thinking and evaluating

1. Why do you consider the money spent on vegetables and fruits well spent?

2. How would you judge the quality of fresh vegetables and fruits? What are the advantages and disadvantages of using the fresh ones, as compared with the frozen, canned, or dried?

3. What is meant by a processed food? What are its advantages? Disadvantages?

4. What is the cost of fresh vegetables and fruits in your market, as compared with that of the various processed forms of potatoes, peas, carrots, sweet potatoes, green leafy vegetables, and other vegetables? What do you conclude from this comparison?

5. What are the basic methods of cooking vegetables and fruits? Do you think we use these methods well? Explain. Which methods are used most in your home? Give examples of foods suited to each method. How many have you tried?

6. How would you summarize the things that a wise shopper for fruits and vegetables needs to know and practice?

7. Explain why it is important to wash raw fruits and vegetables thoroughly before they are eaten raw or cooked.

8. Describe how to store the following kinds of fruits and vegetables: fresh, frozen, canned, dried.

9. Explain the steps in making a good salad; the function of the salad in the meal. What foods lend themselves well to salads? To finger salads? What salads are suitable for a first course? As a main dish? As accompaniment to the main course? As dessert?

10. Which raw vegetables have you tried as snack foods? Why are they well suited for snacks if you wish to control weight? Which fruits are suitable for this purpose? List the different foods you would like to try raw as snacks and with meals.

Applying and sharing

1. Keep a record of the vegetables, fruits, and juices you eat at meals for three days. How can you improve each meal? Your snacks? Using the table of Nutritive Value of Foods (in the Appendix), figure out the number of calories from these foods each day. List separately the calories from the salad and the salad dressing.

2. Visit a supermarket near your home. Write down the following:
   a. The green leafy vegetables, yellow vegetables, and fruits available in each season of the year; fresh, frozen, canned.
   b. The cost per serving of the fresh, canned, frozen, and dried fruits and vegetables.
   c. The fruit or vegetables that give the most economical use of your money in different seasons. Of your time and energy.
   d. The vegetables you enjoy eating most; those your family likes. Which should you eat more often?

3. Examine vegetables on cafeteria steam tables and on restaurant menus. How do you rate them, from best to poorest? Give reasons. Do the same with salads. Compare it with your home cooking.

4. As you observe what other shoppers select in buying vegetables and fruits, do you think they understand how to use their money wisely? Explain. Do you think they show poor manners in handling foods? What are good manners in shopping for these foods?

5. Consult with mature people who in your opinion do a good job in helping their families enjoy the vegetables they need to eat. Find out what guides they use. Decide whether they have modern information or not. How do you think they can improve?

6. Suppose you were a bride and wanted to serve a balanced diet each day on a low-cost food budget.
   a. Plan the daily menus for one week to meet your total nutrient needs and provide variety in vegetables and fruits within your budget, and to maintain desirable weight.
   b. Underscore twice the foods rich in vitamin C in each meal; underscore once the foods rich in vitamin A; underscore three times those under 50 calories per serving.
   c. Give two or more ways to prepare each vegetable and fruit dish in each meal. Indicate which seasonings you would use.
   d. If you had a husband who did not like spinach, how would you supply alternates that he likes?

7. With the class divided into groups, let each group plan balanced menus that you can prepare at school using the most needed fruits and vegetables. Have a tasting session for comparison.
   a. First try different methods of cooking the same leafy vegetable, yellow vegetable, white and sweet potatoes, beans, and another vegetable in season.
   b. Try different forms (fresh, canned, frozen) of the same vegetable, each group using a different form. Compare results.
   c. Try different seasonings with the same vegetable, varying the amounts. Compare results. Record what you liked best.

9

bread-cereals, the staff of life

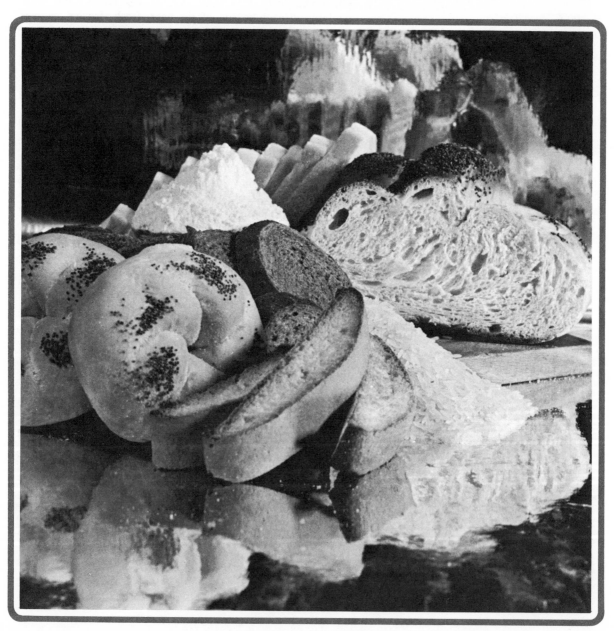

Cereal grain in the culture of a people

Corn: the New World's cereal

The culture of people in different lands is shaped, to some extent, by the cereal grains which are the basic food in the diet. Corn is the cereal of the New World. One of the first things our ancestors were compelled to do was change their eating habits. They were people who had eaten wheat, oats, and rye. But on this continent it was corn that helped them survive the first rugged years.

Anthropologists have found that the Maya Indians in Mexico grew corn over three thousand years ago. Their high regard for it as the staff of life is manifested in a mural in the National Museum of Anthropology in Mexico City. Corn is portrayed with reverence, along with the sun, as the symbol of life. The word "corn" is similar in all the dialects of that country to "source of life." It is the preferred cereal of Mexico and Latin America to this day.

It was corn that the pioneers took with them as they moved west to settle our country. The Indians had taught them to use it in many ways. They made it into bread and baked it on hot rocks or hot ashes and called it corn pone (from the Indian word "appone" or "apan") or hoecake (because they removed it from the hot fire with a hoe). Two months after the seeds were planted, they could boil it young and tender on the cob. In four months from planting time, the mature corn could be boiled as hominy. They mixed it with beans, green or dry, and called it succotash (from the Indian "misickquatash"), and the resulting combination produced a far more nourishing dish than either ingredient alone. These dishes became standard in various parts of the country.

Today we grow more corn than any other nation—70 percent of the world's supply. It leads all our crops in acreage and money value, and from it we obtain many products besides bread.

Rice: the most widely used cereal

Rice, the grain of the Orient, is the world's most abundant cereal, furnishing the basic food in the diet of over half the world's population. The Pharaohs of Egypt ate rice, as did the early Greeks, Turks, and Arabs. When the Moors left Africa for Spain in the Middle Ages, they took rice with them, and its use then spread over Europe. By accident, a ship laden with rice was blown off its course from Madagascar and landed at Charleston, South Carolina, in 1694. Thus began the cultivation and enjoyment of rice in our country. While the Orient grows 95 percent of the world's rice, we grow some of the highest quality.

Wheat: the most balanced cereal

Wheat, the cereal grain of western man, is the best-balanced in nutrients. By enlightened plant breeding, we now produce wheat with larger amounts and better quality of protein then ever before. In the United States we eat about five times as much wheat as corn, and twenty-four times as much as rice. We also use oats, rye, and barley, but in much smaller amounts.

Bread is the most important food made from wheat. Most pastries and sweet baked foods, as well as macaroni products, are made from wheat flour. When wheat is mixed with other cereal grains for baking, it produces a lighter, more tasty, more attractive, and more nutritious bread.

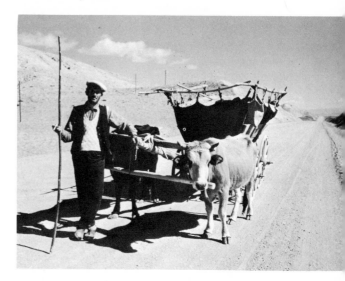

On the road from Ankara to Istanbul, Turkey, this farmer hauls his wheat in a cart made of black goatskins and drawn by oxen.

Why bread is called the staff of life

There is no mystery as to why earlier man called bread the staff of life. Cereal grains have been in the diet of mankind for some 15,000 years, according to geographers. Within this century, nutritionists and chemists have unlocked the secret of the power that lies within cereal grains, which are all similar but differ in the amount of nutrients they contain.

Nutrients in cereal-breads

As a group, cereal-breads yield:

1/Carbohydrates—the body's preferred source of energy.

Corn, the cereal of the New World.

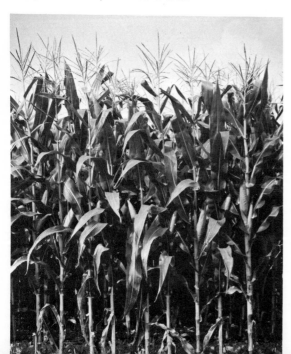

2/Protein—"incomplete," but providing almost a quarter of the protein in our diets, and a far larger share in the diet of developing nations.

3/B vitamins in the whole grains and the enriched.

4/Iron, phosphorus, and other minerals in smaller amounts.

5/Fat, low in amounts to balance a high-fat diet, and containing the important linoleic fatty acid to balance the animal fat in the diet. Fat occurs in the germ of whole grains. Associated with fat are vitamins A and E in wheat germ and vitamin A in yellow corn.

Advantages of cereal-breads

In practical use, cereal-breads have many advantages.

1/They are low in cost and easy to grow quickly; meat takes much longer and is more expensive.

2/They are compact and easy to transport; they store and keep well.

3/They may be cooked with a small amount of fuel and equipment.

4/The bland flavor enables one to eat them at every meal without monotony.

5/They may be used in many different ways for variety.

With these assets, it is not difficult to understand why cereal grains are the basic foods in the diet of two-thirds of mankind today, or why earlier man depended on them so completely.

This bakery window in New York's Lower East Side shows some of the rich variety of cereal-breads that bring enjoyment and nourishment to people of all ages.

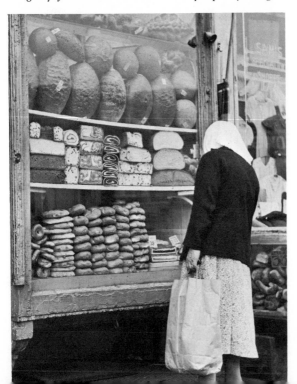

Carbohydrates and cereal-breads

The calorie fallacy

In our time, the problem of controlling overweight has caused us to develop a keen consciousness of calories. But the knowledge we assume we have is often confused, misleading, and prejudiced. For example, some people will not eat bread or potatoes, although they are recommended for a balanced diet. They say these foods are "too high in calories" and "too starchy." They think that starch is a fattening nutrient and that if they eat more meat and less of these foods they will not get fat. In reality, as you recall, the protein in meat contains the same number of calories (4 per gram) as the starch in carbohydrate foods, and the fat in meat contains two and one-quarter times as many calories (9 per gram). Yet people do not refrain from eating meat because of calories. All foods have calories. No one food is fattening.

Calories and energy

Calories are units of energy. Energy is the first need of all human beings. If your eyes were as powerful as supermicroscopes, you could look at the human body's trillions of cells (no larger than 1/1000 of an inch in diameter) which are the efficient engines that select oxygen and nutrients from its capillaries. With these two ingredients, aided by enzymes and coenzymes (vitamins), a remarkable "explosion" takes place: energy is released. The waste product that follows at once is heat, not energy, but it serves a useful purpose along with energy, for it warms the body.

When you feel cold, you shiver. This burns energy, for you are moving muscles and the heat that follows the release of energy warms you. You feel hotter when you run hard than when you walk, for you are burning more energy and heat accumulates more quickly than you can eliminate the waste product as carbon dioxide and water. The water may be eliminated through the skin as perspiration and the carbon dioxide through the lungs.

IMPORTANCE OF CARBOHYDRATES. Scientists have learned that the nutrient the body prefers to use as a source of energy is carbohydrate. You recall from Chapter 2 that carbohydrates are broken down from starch and sugar and are absorbed as glucose. The normal, healthy body maintains a relatively constant level of glucose in the blood, so that the cells can burn their energy from this nutrient. Tiny fatty acids and amino acids pass in and out of the cells, which trap the glucose to burn as energy.

When you do not include sufficient carbohydrate in the diet, the body reserves from the liver and tissues are first exhausted. This takes less than 24 hours. Fat is the next nutrient to go, and protein last. This fantastic engineering design further illustrates the marvel of our body in using food to preserve life. Reserve energy is stored in the form of fat. Most of our reserve protein is in the form of live, working tissue. When fat is exhausted as a source of energy, the body destroys itself by burning tissue protein to maintain the functions essential for life, such as the heartbeat, respiration, circulation, and the like.

CARBOHYDRATE AND FAT. Studies show that carbohydrate is essential for the complete oxidation of fat. When there is no carbohydrate, or too little, the fat is not all burned. The leftover part is harmful. This substance is called ketone (kē′ tōn) body. When ketones accumulate in the blood,

the urine becomes too acid and the amount of sodium is reduced. This, in turn, reduces the body's ability to carry off the waste product, carbon dioxide. When this condition is severe, the person goes into a coma. This may occur in a diabetic whose body can't use carbohydrate normally. It occurs during starvation. It also occurs in self-selected reducing diets that either restrict all food or restrict carbohydrates too severely and too long. Fad diets that emphasize fats and restrict or eliminate carbohydrates follow a path of danger. The so-called drinking man's diet, popular in the mid-60's, is an example of this type of diet, that bobs up repeatedly under new names.

A further need of carbohydrate in the diet is to spare protein from having to be used for energy. This saves money, as animal protein is costly.

Role of cereal-breads

Where do cereal-breads fit in the picture? Along with potatoes, they are the richest source of carbohydrates. This amounts to about 75 percent of the calories in flour, meal, and cereal, most of which is starch. Cereal grains have been among the most important foods for the survival of man throughout the world. In developing nations to this day, many people get 60 to 90 percent of their calories from carbohydrates, mainly from starch. In the United States, we get slightly less than half of our calories from carbohydrates, with 75 percent of this amount from starch and 25 percent from sugar. In this century, the national diet has shown a decrease in the number of calories derived from potatoes and cereals and an increase in the amount from sugar. This is undesirable.

STARCH VS. SUGAR. The reason that the trend toward decreased intake of starch and increased intake of sugar is unwholesome lies in the nature of the two nutrients. Starch is a "complex" carbohydrate. It takes longer to digest but, more important, it is associated with protein, fat, vitamins, minerals, and cellulose. Sugar is a "simple" carbohydrate. It is digested quickly, yields calories for energy, and nothing more. That is why its calories are referred to as "empty."

STARCH AND CHOLESTEROL. Recent research indicates an added superiority of carbohydrate as a source of energy. Two groups of animals were fed identical diets, with exactly the same number of calories from carbohydrates, except that one group's calories were from starch and the other's from sugar. The group that ate starch had lower blood cholesterol than the group that ate sugar. While more research is needed before final conclusions are drawn, this subject is so important that an entire chapter (12) is devoted to a discus-

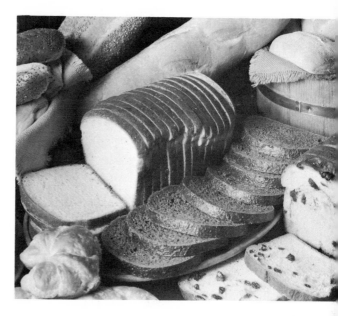

Cereal-breads are the richest source of carbohydrates, which are essential for energy.

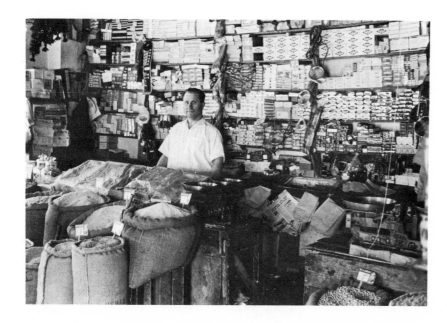

Cereal grains are sold from open sacks in this general store in Turkey.

table 9–1   *Comparison of Nutrients in Wheat Flour and Wheat Bread*

ONE POUND	PROTEIN (Grams)	FAT (Milligrams)	CALCIUM (Milligrams)	IRON (Milligrams)	THIAMINE (Milligrams)	RIBOFLAVIN (Milligrams)	NIACIN (Milligrams)
Minimum and maximum enrichment levels for the three B vitamins—thiamine, niacin and riboflavin —and iron are given in the table below							
FLOUR							
Unenriched (all purpose)	47.6	4.5	73	3.6	.28	.21	4.1
Enriched (all purpose)	47.6	4.5	73	13.–16.5	2.–2.5	1.2–1.5	16.–20.
Whole Wheat	60.3	9.1	186	15.0	2.49	.54	19.7
BREAD							
Unenriched (white) (3 to 4% nonfat dry milk)	39.5	14.5	381	3.2	.31	.39	5.0
Enriched (white) (3 to 4% nonfat dry milk)	39.5	14.5	381	8.–12.5	1.1–1.8	.7–1.6	8.–12.5
Whole Wheat (2% nonfat dry milk)	47.6	13.6	449	10.4	1.17	.56	12.9

SOURCES: *Composition of Foods . . . Raw, Processed, Prepared,* Agriculture Handbook No. 8 (Washington, D.C.: USDA, revised 1963) and *Definitions and Standards,* Part 15, "Cereal Flours and Related Products" and Part 17, "Bakery Products" (Washington, D.C.: Food and Drug Administration, U.S. Department of Health, Education, and Welfare).

sion of sugar and its possible connections with health disorders.

NEED IN MEALS. It is wise to include some starch in each meal, even in diets that are planned for weight reduction. In the normal diet, three to four servings of bread-cereal, amounting to no more than 150 to 200 calories, help provide balance for the whole day's diet. If one needs to reduce the total intake of food, then a smaller serv-

ing of bread-cereal is appropriate. The table of Nutritive Value of Foods (in the Appendix) shows the calories in different cereal-breads. This may help you select and use those that fit your calorie need. Note that one slice of whole wheat bread has only 55 calories, while a corn muffin has 150, and one cup of macaroni, cooked firm, has 190. Table 9–1 gives the nutrients in different flours and breads on the market.

177/

Protein and cereal-breads

Protein is provided in generous amounts in cereal-breads, with slightly less in the refined ones (see Table 9–1) than in whole wheat or enriched ones. Cereal grains vary in the amount of protein they contain, ranging from about 6 percent of their calories in refined ones to 18 percent in improved breeds of whole grains. Grains grown in soil with adequate nitrogen are found to contain more protein than grains grown in soil deficient in this chemical and grains grown in a hot, dry climate have more protein than those grown in a humid climate. Geneticists have developed breeds of rice, wheat, and other grains that are higher in protein than we have formerly known. Legumes and cereal-grains are now being used to provide a more nutritious diet for those on low incomes.

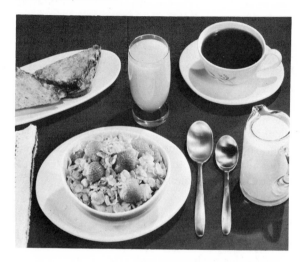

Milk supplies protein to enhance the nutrients in cereal and make it an ideal breakfast dish.

How proteins in cereal-breads are balanced

We have already learned from studies that, though cereal-breads contain incomplete protein when eaten alone, when we mix the cereals we balance the amino acids in one against the weaknesses in another. For instance, wheat improves the protein in any cereal. A cup of wheat flour mixed with a cup of cornmeal in making corn bread enhances the protein value of the bread.

You recall that milk balances the weakness of cereal-bread in amino acids and enables the body to use the generous amount of protein in these foods to build and repair body tissues. Meat (in any form) and eggs also supplement cereal-breads. Hence the homemaker who makes bread with eggs and milk is adding to the protein and the health value of the meal. While the added ingredients

increase the cost slightly, in the long run she is saving money by cutting down on possible future doctor bills and drugs.

Pouring a generous amount of milk over cereal converts it into an excellent main dish for breakfast. A one-cup serving of oatmeal yields 5 grams of protein when cooked in water, and acquires 9 additional grams of protein when cooked with one-third cup of nonfat dry milk per serving. If you use part of a glass of milk on this and drink the remainder, you add another 9 grams of protein. The whole adds up to 23 grams of protein in your breakfast main dish. This meets a generous third of the day's protein need for a normal adult. The most important benefit of this is that you can be sure that the protein in your cereal is well used. If you add an orange to the meal, you have a well-balanced breakfast containing only 400 calories. This will fortify you well for the morning.

The principle of proteins supplementing one another works with your two slices of bread in a sandwich of meat, cheese, egg, or peanut butter at lunch. It also applies to the cheese on a macaroni or pizza-type dish; to meatballs with rice, bulgur (cracked wheat), or spaghetti; to chicken or fish with noodles; to meat in soups and stews. To improve the flavor of main cereal dishes, cooks of every nation have used small amounts of meat, fish, poultry, beans, milk, cheese, eggs, or nuts, when they were available. And experience showed them that they became healthier and survived better, though they did not know it was due to a better use of the proteins.

Iron and B vitamins in grains

Iron in the whole grains and enriched cereal-breads helps each of us meet our daily iron need.

The people of India enjoy rice with most meals. In the East, it is the staple food in the diet.

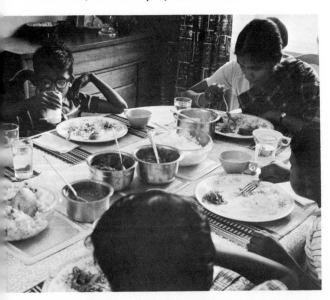

Although .6 milligrams in a slice of enriched white bread or 1.4 milligrams in a cup of cooked oats or macaroni may seem a small amount, three slices of bread and one cup of cooked cereal add up to 3.2 milligrams, more than one-sixth of a woman's daily need of 18 milligrams.

B vitamins are an important contribution of whole-grain and enriched cereals to the diet. Some of these were discussed in preceding chapters. Here, let us consider thiamine (vitamin B_1) and vitamin B_6.

Thiamine, the first vitamin

DISCOVERY OF THIAMINE.   Thiamine was the first vitamin discovered. It was found in rice in 1926. It is almost shocking to think that almost 50 years elapsed from the time the first clue to its vital role in the diet was discovered to the time it was identified and utilized. Between 1878 and 1883 Dr. B. K. Takaki, a physician in the Japanese Navy, proved by a carefully controlled experiment with navy personnel at sea that the eating of white polished rice as a major food staple led to the disabling disease known as beriberi. Then, in 1897, Dr. Christian Eijkman, a Dutch physician in Java, noted that his patients who ate white rice got the disease, but the poorer people whose main food was unpolished brown rice did not get it. By feeding white rice to ducks, chickens, and pigeons, he produced in them the same symptoms as those exhibited by his patients. Then he fed the sick birds natural brown rice and cured them.

Eijkman misinterpreted the results. Those who had beriberi had a stiffness in the ankles, with neuritis in the feet and legs. In severe cases, this resulted in paralysis, in retention of fluid (edema), in heart disease, and often in death. Eijkman thought these symptoms were due to the larger amount of starch in the white rice, which he believed poisoned the nerve cells. He concluded that the antidote for the "poison" lay in the polishings of the brown rice.

The latter half of his assumption was correct. In 1901 another Dutch physician, G. Grijns, gave the correct interpretation—that beriberi in man or birds was caused by the absence of some nutrient found in brown rice but lost when rice was refined.

Chemists all over the world set to work to find this substance. In 1911 the Polish chemist Casimir Funk, working in London, obtained a crystalline product from the brown polishings of the milled white rice. It was he who then coined the word "vitamin" (originally spelled *vitamine*) and called this substance the antiberiberi vitamin. He was bold enough to predict that other diseases might be caused by a shortage of similar substances in the diet. This led others to realize that **food could help prevent disease.** In 1926 two Dutch scientists, C. P. Jansen and W. P. Donath, discovered what is now called thiamine, the first of many B vitamins.

The curiosity of an American, R. R. Williams, prompted him to use his "spare" time for a quarter of a century to work on the problem. In 1936 he and his colleagues worked out the chemical formula for vitamin B_1. This is now made inexpensively, and saves pain and thousands of lives when used to fortify refined cereal grains.

But there is a gap between knowledge of what food can do for us, and the application of that knowledge. For instance, 11 years later—in 1947 —there were 24,000 needless deaths from beriberi in the Philippines. Our government took part in an experiment there which reduced beriberi by 89 percent, simply by "adding back" thiamine to the polished white rice.

HOW THIAMINE HELPS US. Thiamine helps us maintain a good appetite, digestion, elimination, relaxation, and memory. It works with a team of other B vitamins as a coenzyme to help the body burn glucose to release energy. It also is needed for the utilization of protein. It is essential for growth at every age level and has positive benefits for nerve cells and the circulatory system.

Beriberi is no threat in the United States, although 25 deaths from it were reported in 1956. These were among alcoholics, whose diet is greatly deficient, especially in thiamine. Many people, however, may have minor symptoms if they have had a prolonged mild deficiency in this vitamin. It may be manifested by depression, nervousness, a poor memory, anger, irritability, low tone of the gastrointestinal tract, fatigue, and general indifference to things that matter.

Chemists have found a test for deficient thiamine by determining the amount of pyruvic (pī rü′ vik) acid that accumulates in the blood and tissues. When sufficient thiamine is present in the diet, this acid does not pile up. The practical meaning for us is that for general good health and well-being, we need thiamine in our diets every day.

NATURE OF THIAMINE AND HOW TO RETAIN IT. If you understand the nature of thiamine, you can learn to retain the maximum amount in foods. Like vitamin C and other B vitamins, thiamine is soluble in water, but it is stable in dry form and in the presence of acid in foods. Like vitamin C, it is easily destroyed by alkali and, for this reason, we should eliminate from our files all recipes that call for a large amount of soda in baking. Prolonged exposure to heat destroys it, and so do high temperatures. When bread is toasted, there is a loss of 15 to 20 percent of the thiamine. This illustrates that the loss is greater in thin, small baked foods. There is less loss in loaves of bread,

Cooked breakfast cereals retain most of their thiamine.

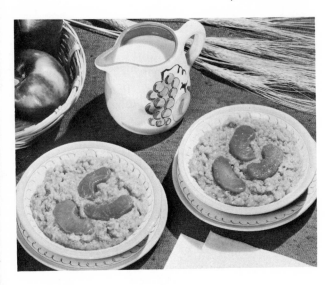

as compared with rolls, or in roast meat, as compared with steaks and chops.

Studies show that cooked breakfast cereals retain most of their thiamine, but 15 to 20 percent is lost in baking bread and 25 to 50 percent in cooking meat. The lower figure is for the large size or for meats that have been broiled or roasted. When the drippings from meat are used, three-fourths of the original thiamine is retained. When use is made of the water in which vegetables are cooked, less thiamine is lost.

CAN YOU GET TOO MUCH THIAMINE? Not from food. Only a few weeks' supply is stored in the liver, heart, muscles, brain, and kidneys. When your reserve supply is sufficient, if you have more than you need in the diet, thiamine is quickly eliminated in the urine and cannot be stored for future use. Thus it is wiser to distribute thiamine intake among all the day's meals and snacks than to take a vitamin pill and consider your needs met. The muscles give up their reserve of thiamine

first and the brain holds fast its supply to the last. This indicates how important this vitamin is for the brain. It may also account for weakness and muscle pains in the legs, when the diet is deficient in this vitamin. The body has built-in safeguards to protect us at the most vital points. But we can help it by developing eating habits that provide the nutrients we need in the required amounts.

DAILY NEED AND FOOD SOURCES. The allowance of thiamine for different age groups is shown in the table of Recommended Daily Dietary Allowances, pages 446–447. Table 9–2 gives the amounts found in different basic foods.

The amount needed daily depends on the number of calories consumed. Naturally, this is affected by age, growth rate, and activity. The requirement increases from infancy to the growth spurt in the teens, when the body's demand is greatest. When full growth is reached, slightly less is needed, for the calorie need also decreases. In a hot, humid climate, or where there is strenuous exercise or labor, more thiamine is required, especially if there is profuse perspiration and great activity. As with other nutrients, the need increases for a girl or woman during pregnancy or lactation, as the RDA shows.

Vitamin B$_6$ (Pyridoxine)

The discovery that vitamin B$_6$ was essential for life seemed like an accident. Actually, it is an example of how research dovetails with clinical experience of physicians. Babies six weeks to six months of age were having unexplained twitching of the muscles, irritability, and convulsions. Though these were found in different parts of the United States, and the symptoms were identical, there seemed to be no explanation for the condition at first.

table 9–2 *Best Food Sources of Thiamine*

	FOOD	SIZE OF SERVING	THIAMINE (mg)
MEATS	Pork, lean	3½ oz., roasted	0.60
	Pork liver	3½ oz., fried	0.34
	Calf liver	3½ oz., fried	0.24
	Lamb, lean	3½ oz., roasted	0.14
	Oysters	5, raw	0.14
VEGETABLES	Green peas, fresh	½ cup, cooked	0.28
	Green peas, frozen	½ cup, cooked	0.27
	Dried soy beans	½ cup, cooked	0.21
	Asparagus spears	½ cup, cooked	0.16
	Collards	½ cup, cooked	0.14
	Navy beans	½ cup, cooked	0.14
	Lima beans	½ cup, cooked	0.13
	Okra	½ cup, cooked	0.13
	Tomato juice	1 cup	0.12
FRUITS	Orange juice, fresh	1 cup	0.22
	Watermelon	1 slice	0.13
CEREAL-BREAD	Rice, brown	1 cup, cooked in water	0.23
	Rice, white, enriched	1 cup, cooked in water	0.23
	Oatmeal	1 cup, cooked in water	0.19
	Wheat cereal, dry, enriched	1 cup	0.19
NUTS	Nuts, average	16–24	0.18

SOURCE: *Composition of Foods . . . Raw, Processed, Prepared*, Agriculture Handbook No. 8 (Washington, D.C.: USDA, revised 1963) and *Nutritive Value of Foods*, Bulletin No. 72 (Washington, D.C.: USDA, revised 1970).

A research worker in the Food and Drug Administration observed that these symptoms in the infants were identical to those in baby rats fed a diet deficient in vitamin B₆. This vitamin, at his suggestion, was added to the babies' diets, and immediate relief resulted. Investigation brought out the fact that all the babies had been taking the same canned baby food, though the dry food manufactured by the same company did not produce these symptoms. Since 1951, when this occurred, vitamin B₆ has been added to canned baby food by all companies.

VITAMIN B₆ EASILY DESTROYED. Vitamin B₆ cannot help us if it is destroyed. This happens quite easily when a food is exposed to heat, light, and air, especially in a neutral or alkaline solution.

Seventy-five percent of B_6 is lost in the milling of white or refined cereals, and highly refined cereals have almost none, unless it is added back. Up to 50 percent may be destroyed in cooking. Vitamin B_6 was discovered in 1938, but we didn't know it was essential for human life until the 1951 incident with infants. Hence it was not added back in the enrichment of bread-cereals. Some food industries have taken the initiative and have added it to food. It is listed on the label when added to a food.

HOW VITAMIN B_6 HELPS US. When there is not enough of B_6 in the diet, the symptoms are similar to those in other B-vitamin deficiencies—rash and oiliness of the skin, sore mouth, dizziness, nausea, mental confusion, nervous disorders, failure to grow, loss of weight, anemia, convulsions, and kidney stones. All these symptoms, with the exception of kidney stones, are immediately relieved upon the addition of sufficient B_6 in the diet. When the diet regularly contains a sufficient quantity of vitamin B_6, the positive conditions of health are present.

Another important function of this vitamin is as a coenzyme in the use of food by cells. What is a coenzyme? It is a helper to the enzymes, that enables them to bring about a biochemical change in each special cell tissue. Without these partner B vitamins, normal metabolism (the building and repair of tissues and destruction and elimination of old, worn-out ones) is upset and nutrients wasted. Symptoms of illness follow which are often not recognized for what they are. An example of how B_6 works as a coenzyme is in joining with the amino acid tryptophane to make the B vitamin niacin. It is also thought to be important in the body's use of linoleic fatty acid to form another "essential" fatty acid which is discussed in Chapter 11.

table 9–3   **Best Sources of Vitamin B₆ (Pyridoxine Compound)***

FOOD SOURCES		TOTAL B_6 CONTENT mg per 100 gm
GRAIN	Wheat germ	1.31
	Wheat bran	0.82
	Buckwheat flour	0.58
	Soya flour	0.57
	Brown rice	0.53
	Corn	0.48
	Wheat	0.41
	Whole-wheat cereal	0.40
	Barley	0.39
	Popcorn	0.37
	Whole-wheat bread	0.20
	Rice cereal, dry	0.14
	Oatmeal	0.12
MILK	Canned, evaporated	7.50
	Cow's, fluid	0.10
MEAT	Liver	1.42
	Ham (cured and fully cooked)	0.70
	Salmon, canned	0.28
	Frankfurter, cooked	0.16
	Beef, ground, cooked	0.10
VEGE-TABLES AND FRUITS	Lima beans	0.60
	Bananas	0.32
	Carrots	0.21
	Frozen peas	0.11

*Most of these values are taken from M. M. Polansky, E. W. Murphy, and E. W. Toefer, "Compounds of Vitamin B_6 in Greens and Cereal Products," *Journal of the Association of Official Agricultural Chemists*, 47:750, 1964.

DAILY NEED AND FOOD SOURCES. The recommended daily need is given in the RDA table in the Appendix. This amounts to 2 milligrams daily for girls aged 14 and over and for boys and men aged 16 and over. Table 9–4 indi-

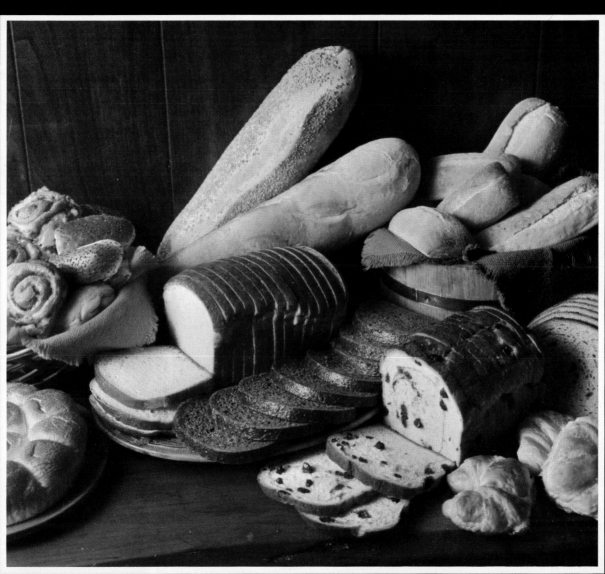

The tempting variety of bread—crunchy or soft, tangy or sweet—can stimulate and satisfy every appetite.

(top left) *Rice, the staple food of the Orient, is the world's most widely used cereal grain.* (bottom left) *Macaroni salad is a good accompaniment for meat, substituting for potatoes to vary the diet.*

Pamper your sweet tooth and reap extra nourishment with desserts made from dried fruits.

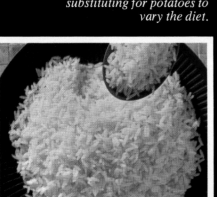

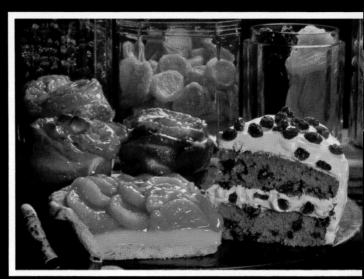

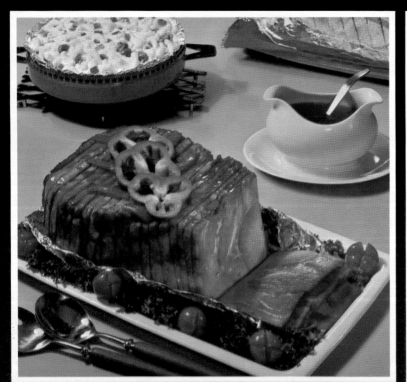

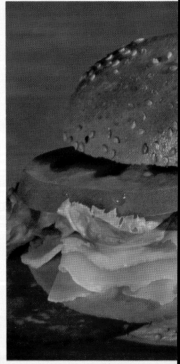

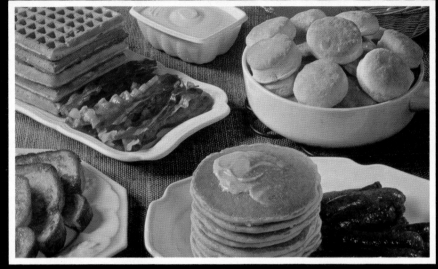

(left) *Breakfast won't be a skipped meal in your home if you serve tempting pancakes, waffles, French toast, or hot biscuits with bacon and sausages.*

This giant sandwich by any name (hero, submarine, hoagie, Poor Boy) is a great favorite everywhere.

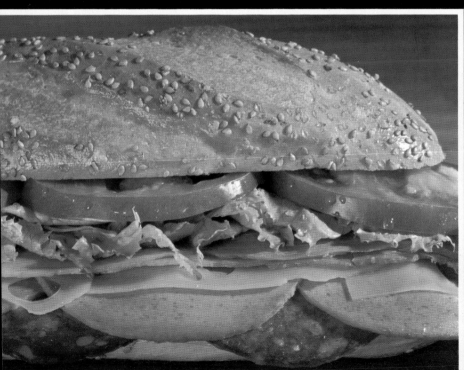

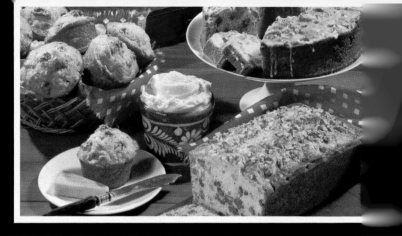

(right) By adding raisins, walnuts, candied fruit, or dried fruit, you can produce a delicious variety of cakes and muffins from a home-made quick-bread mix.
(below) Add a little spice to your menu with macaroni chili and see how quickly the bowls are emptied!

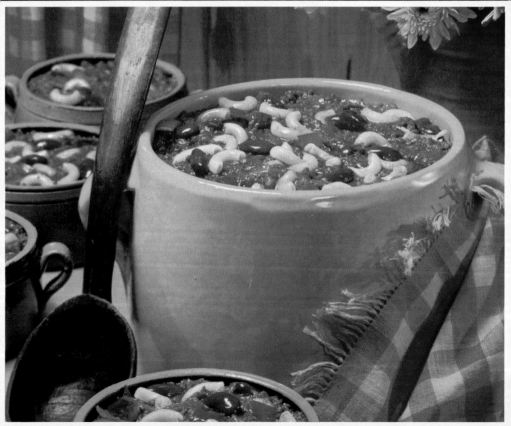

cates that this vitamin is found in about the same foods as other B vitamins, the richest source being liver of all kinds (1.42 milligrams per 3½-ounce serving). Wheat germ, wheat bran, whole wheat, yeast, and red meats are good to fair sources. Among vegetables and fruits, it is found in the green leaves, white and yellow potatoes, fresh and dried beans and peas, carrots, winter squash, bananas, avocados, pineapples, and other foods. One quart of milk contains 0.4 milligrams, or about a fifth of the daily need for a young person.

Those who eat a balanced diet will get all the vitamins B_6 they need, if they exercise care in the selection, preparation, cooking, and serving of their food. There are no known widespread deficiencies of this vitamin in our country. It has been helping us in our diet right along, though we did not know it until the 1951 incident. This is further encouragement for us to depend on food for the known and as yet unknown nutrients our bodies need, instead of vitamin-mineral pills with only the known ingredients.

Enrichment of cereal-breads

The enrichment of bread-cereals with thiamine, riboflavin, niacin, and iron that became mandatory for the whole nation in January, 1943 was a significant step forward for better health through improving the nutrients in a basic food. This is also a fine example of how the government, nutritionists, public health officials, and food industries can cooperate for the benefit of the consumer. This teamwork came to light when the legislation expired in October, 1946. The industries concerned volunteered, in many instances, to carry on with enrichment. Today, between 80 and 90 percent of refined bread-cereals are enriched, though only 30 of our 50 states have enacted legislation requiring it.

Meaning of terms

ENRICHED. The terms for enrichment have been confusing. Enrichment means that some of the thiamine, riboflavin, niacin, and iron removed in the milling to make "refined" cereals, flour, or meal is added back. There are over a dozen other nutrients that are not added back, including vitamins E and B_6. Enrichment standards are illustrated in Table 9–4. Observe in Table 9–1 that the protein in one pound of whole wheat bread is 47.6 grams, as compared with enriched or unenriched white bread, which has 39.5 grams. This is one reason informed people think the term "enrich" is misleading and that "fortified" would be a more accurate term.

RESTORED. "Restored" is the word sometimes used to express the addition of lost nutrients back to refined ready–to–eat cereals.

table 9–4   Enrichment Standards Required for 1 Pound of Cereal-Bread Products*

NAME OF FOOD	MINIMUM TO MAXIMUM REQUIREMENTS FOR			
	Thiamine (mg)	Riboflavin (mg)	Niacin (mg)	Iron (mg)
Bread and rolls	1.1–1.8	0.7–1.6	10.0–15.0	8.0–12.5
Flour	2.0–2.5	1.2–1.5	16.0–20.0	13.0–16.5
Cornmeal, grits	2.0–3.0	1.2–1.8	16.0–24.0	13.0–26.0
Macaroni-noodles	4.0–5.0	1.7–2.2	27.0–34.0	13.0–16.5

*SOURCE: U.S. National Archives, Code of Federal Register Title 21, Food and Drugs, 1955, with supplement to 1957.

CONVERTED. This term is applied to rice, and represents a quite different process. The rice is steeped in hot water under pressure in a cylinder containing no air. The result is that a large amount of the nutrients is forced into the starchy part of the grain. Then, when it is polished, these nutrients are not lost. This method has been used in India in a simplified form for many decades and it accounts for the fact that beriberi is not a common disease there, as it has been in other parts of Asia.

Benefits of whole grains

Refined white bread and cereals are not the foods that earned the title of "staff of life." This name applies rather to the many benefits derived from whole grains. However, the "enrichment" program has returned some of the lost benefits to this important group of foods.

In 1970, an experiment conducted by a reputable scientist made glaring headlines—"White Bread Diet Starves Rats." This is an inaccurate interpretation of the data. It simply underscores what we have been discussing in this book, namely that the healthy diet is a balanced one. It is composed of not one or two foods but a balance of those found to meet the nutritional needs of the body—milk, meat, eggs, poultry, fish, organ meats, vegetables (cooked and raw), fruits, some fat, and bread. The experiment further demonstrates that whole grains are more nutritious than the refined or so-called enriched.

Four servings of whole-grain or enriched bread-cereals provide a generous source of energy, low-cost protein, iron, and significant amounts of the three B vitamins likely to be too low in the diet but important in helping the food balance.

Meaningful words

beriberi
complex carbohydrate
converted
energy-heat
enriched
glucose
ketone body
pyruvic acid
simple carbohydrate
vitamin B_6 (pyridoxine)

Thinking and evaluating

1. Explain how the culture and health of people in different lands are affected by the cereal-breads they eat.

2. What is meant by "Bread is the staff of life"?

3. What are the contributions made by cereal grains to the daily diet? Explain why they are so important in a low-cost diet. Why do we need four servings daily?

4. Why is starch the more important carbohydrate? Did you have any mistaken ideas about starch before this study? What were they? What do you think about it now?

5. Since the percentage of protein in cereal grains equals the percentage recommended in a balanced diet, explain why we cannot depend on these foods alone to provide the amount of protein we need.

6. On the basis of our discussion, do you consider bread-cereals "fattening"? Explain your answer.

7. What is meant by the terms enriched, restored, converted, and whole-grain?

8. How do you account for the fact that millions of people kept right on eating white polished rice after it was discovered that "something" present in the unpolished brown rice prevented or cured the dread disease beriberi? In what ways does this relate to our discussion in Chapter 2 of eating habits?

9. What is the nature of thiamine? How does it help our life? What precautions would you use in cooking food to retain the maximum of thiamine? Apply the same questions to vitamin B_6.

10. If you were trying to reduce weight, which carbohydrate-rich foods would you include in your daily diet? Explain your reasons for your choices.

Applying and sharing

1. On the basis of the record of the food you eat daily, what percentage of the total calories is derived from carbohydrates? How does this compare with the percentage for the average American? Do you think you made the wisest choices among these foods? Show how you might improve?

2. From the foods you ate in one day, calculate the amount of protein in total grams provided by cereal-breads. Calculate the amount contributed to your diet by animal foods. Was each meal balanced in the combination of foods needed for a good use of the amino acids? Make similar calculations for thiamine in your day's diet.

3. If you were managing your own home on a low food budget, how would you plan menus for one week, using bread-cereals to help meet the daily recommended allowances in protein, calories, thiamine, riboflavin, niacin, and iron?

4. Plan balanced menus that you would enjoy eating and prepare one of them that includes the following cereal-breads:

> Breakfast: Oatmeal cooked with nonfat dry milk
> Lunch: Corn muffins
> Snack: Pizza
> Dinner: Brown rice

5. Balance this menu: macaroni-and-cheese salad, candied sweet potatoes, hot rolls, steak, carrots, cola drink, chocolate pie.

bread-cereals in meals

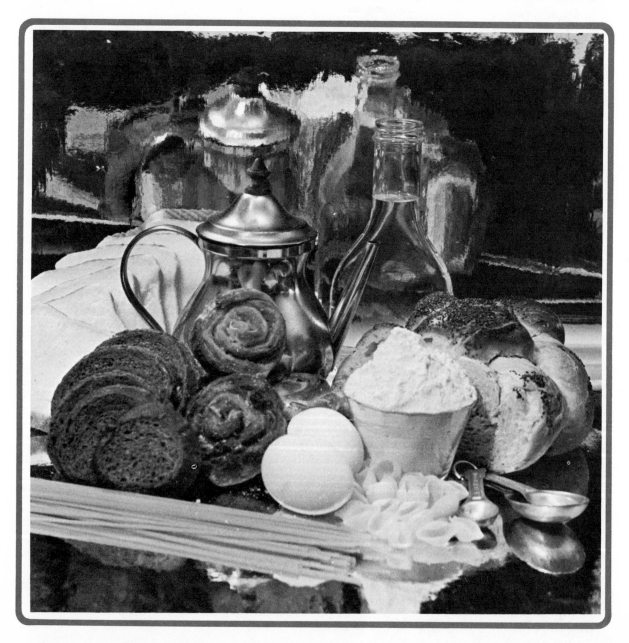

Breadmaking is probably the most basic art of women. For centuries, one of the most important questions a prospective husband asked was: Can she make good bread?

With over 40 million loaves of commercial yeast bread made in the United States daily, there is no need for any homemaker to make bread. But, by doing so, she can put in the ingredients she prefers for flavor, can make a more nourishing food, and can save money. Women often find relaxation and creative fulfillment in making breads. It is a feminine way of expressing love for the family.

Classifications of bread-cereal

Unleavened bread was the first kind man made. He gathered and crushed the grains, mixed the meal thus produced with water and some vegetables, and boiled or baked it on hot rocks. Matzos and tortillas are two modern counterparts of this type.

Leavened breads are basically of two classes, quick breads and yeast breads. We eat about three-fourths of the cereal products in our diets in this form. Quick breads are made with baking powder or soda, or both, and include muffins, biscuits, pancakes, waffles, doughnuts, coffee cakes, sweet rolls, and loaf breads. Yeast breads, leavened with yeast, take longer to make but are rewarding to eat. They are produced in the same forms as quick breads, but most are found in loaves and rolls.

Cereal products are used in many different forms. They may be raw (to be cooked), quick-cooking (that is, partially cooked), ready-to-eat, and in alimentary pastes or macaroni products.

There are hundreds of choices among breads and cereals on the market. Some are quite expensive per serving. Others are among the lowest-cost foods. Some are dependable basic foods that help balance the meals of the day. Others may throw the meals out of balance when they are high in fat, sugar, and calories. Their value to us depends on how wisely we select them, how well we prepare them, and how they fit into the meal and the diet as a whole.

Kinds of flour

Flour is made from grains of wheat, buckwheat, rye, corn, rice, barley, and oats, and from the potato, sweet potato, cottonseed, soybean, peanut, and lima bean. Studies show that soybean or peanut flour, when mixed with wheat flour, provides a more valuable food for those who don't have sufficient animal protein than any cereal eaten alone. Our forebears' habit of eating beans or peanuts with bread as a snack was therefore sound.

Wheat flour

Wheat flour is preferred for all kinds of baking because of the protein *gluten* which it contains. When mixed with liquid, gluten gives elasticity as it swells, to hold air and lighten the bread. Hence the term "light bread."

WHOLE WHEAT FLOUR. Whole wheat (or graham) flour contains all the nutrients of wheat. Bread made from this flour has a nutty flavor and is of a coarser texture and darker color than that made from white flour. It is the most nutritious flour and, since it has less starch and more bran, contains 5 to 8 fewer calories per slice than other types.

WHITE FLOUR. White flour is produced by milling off the bran, aleurone layer, and germ of the grain. The aleurone layer lies beneath the bran and contains the highest-quality protein in wheat —almost as good as animal protein (see Figure 10–1). White flour is composed mostly of the endosperm or starch of the grain. Although this part also contains protein, it is a weaker type of protein. Since vitamins and minerals are lost in milling, white flour is usually enriched. Some is unbleached, but most is bleached with peroxide, chlorine, and other chemicals to produce the desired whiter product.

Hard wheat flour is often labeled "bread flour." Its high gluten content gives the framework for yeast bread.

Cake flour is made from soft wheat and is lowest in gluten. It is used for the finest-textured cakes. Though less nourishing than other flours, it costs more.

All-purpose flour is a blend of hard and soft wheat white flours and is used for any purpose. It absorbs less liquid than bread flour, but more than pastry flour. For cakemaking, less of this flour is required—2 tablespoons less per cup—than of pastry or cake flour.

Self-rising flour is soft wheat or all-purpose flour with added salt and baking powder, and sometimes soda. We buy it in all types of mixes and also simply as self-rising flour.

Read the label to be sure you get the flour you want. Ask for whole wheat if you want it, for consumer demand is heeded.

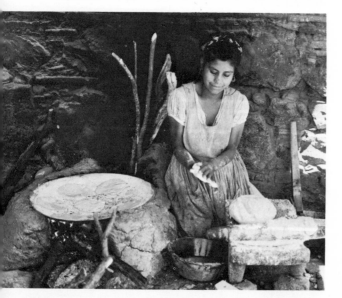

Tortillas, which are a form of unleavened bread, are usually made over an open fire in an ungreased pan or griddle.

Function of Ingredients in breadmaking

Flour

Flour provides gluten and starch, which swell in the presence of liquid to give structure and volume to bread. In yeast bread, the aim is to develop gluten by beating and kneading a stretchy mass of dough. But in quick breads, overbeating develops "tunnels," especially in drop batters, such as muffins and butter cakes.

Liquid

Liquid is essential for the starch to swell and the gluten to develop. The liquid may be water, but milk is more desirable in any form to produce a moist, tender, nourishing bread. The water from macaroni, potatoes, and some vegetables or fruits may also be used.

fig. 10–1 STRUCTURE OF A GRAIN OF WHEAT

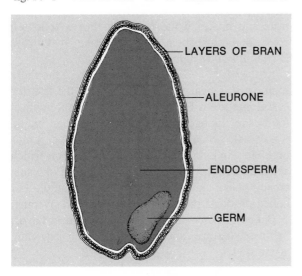

— LAYERS OF BRAN

— ALEURONE

— ENDOSPERM

— GERM

Salt

Salt has two major functions in breadmaking. It is used to enhance flavor and also to delay the growth of yeast plants in yeast bread.

Leavening agents

Leavening agents include yeast, baking powder, soda, egg white, and steam. The purpose of the leavening agent is to produce carbon dioxide gas, which is held in the meshlike structure developed by the gluten or in the beaten egg whites, or both.

YEAST. Unlike soda and baking powder, yeast is a microscopic plant and a good food in its own right. It contains protein and is rich in B vitamins, iron, and probably additional still-unknown nutrients. One tablespoon of dry yeast yields 1.4 milligrams of iron—almost one-third more than a whole egg. Our ancestors called yeast bread healthy bread. Over a long period of time, the contributions of the tiny yeast plants have been substantial factors in keeping a family well.

When yeast is combined with a warm liquid and sugar, an enzyme, zymase, starts fermentation and the yeast plants multiply, producing carbon dioxide gas to leaven breads.

Store dry yeast in a cool pantry and compressed or cake yeast in the refrigerator. Cake yeast works best at temperatures between 80°F and 86°F, or slightly below body temperature; dry yeast granules between 110°F and 115°F.

Bread dough needs a warm place in which to rise, so that the yeast may grow and leaven. Less time is required to make yeast bread when the yeast in the recipe is doubled in quantity.

Sourdough yeast bread is made in a simple way that has been used for thousands of years. A portion of the dough is removed before baking

Bread products achieve tremendous variety through the use of different types of flour and leavening agents. Breads for every taste and need are available in our markets.

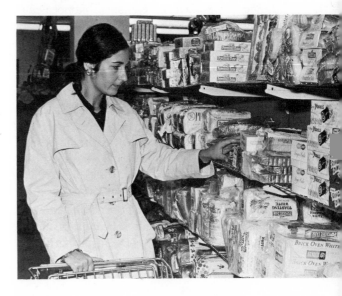

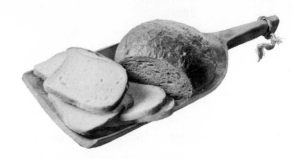

and is used as a source of yeast plants to start the next batch of bread. This is what gives a special flavor to sour rye and some other breads. Lacking refrigerators, many families in developing nations use this method today.

Salt-rising bread, probably the first form of leavened bread, also has a distinctive flavor. Formerly, large amounts of salt were added to prevent an undesirable flavor from the growth of other bacteria, hence the popular name "salt-rising" came to describe it. Today, bakers use selected bacteria cultures (bacteria Clostridium) rather than so much salt to produce fermentation.

BAKING POWDER. Baking powder is the leavening agent used for most quick breads and cakes. All baking powders contain cornstarch and some soda. In addition, they have other ingredients that may be classified as follows:

1/*Tartrate*, in which the leavening agent is tartaric acid. This reacts quickly to contact with liquid and is not popular in our country.

2/*Phosphate*, which contains monocalcium phosphate or monosodium phosphate. About two-thirds of the gas is formed when this type of baking powder meets with the liquid and one-third is formed in the presence of heat in the oven. Too much of it gives food a bitter taste.

3/*S.A.S.* (sodium aluminum sulfate) is a double-acting baking powder and is most preferred. Some carbon dioxide is formed as the liquid and the baking powder combine, but the sulfate is slower to act than other types of baking powder. It leavens in the presence of heat. Less is needed.

SODA. Soda was used before baking powder for quick breads that include sour milk or molasses. Carbon dioxide is produced in proportion to the amount of acid in the liquid and the amount of soda used. Too much soda produces a bitter taste and makes white products turn a yellowish color. Soda darkens a chocolate cake. It destroys B vitamins and vitamin C.

EGG WHITE. Egg white traps air in the fluffy foam as it is beaten. To hold the air, the flour or cereal mixture is folded into the stiff foam in angel food cake, sponge cake, soufflé, and spoon bread.

STEAM. Steam leavens all baked flour products. Heat in baking changes water to vapor, which expands about 1600 times in volume. Popovers, cream puffs, and pound cakes are examples of baked products dependent on steam for leavening.

Baked products are greatly influenced in flavor, lightness, texture, and nutrients by the leavening agent used.

Fat

Fat is added to flour mixtures to give tenderness in texture and to improve the flavor and browning. It does this by shortening the strands of gluten in the flour. The fat coats the gluten strands and prevents their holding together. Hence the term *shortening* is appropriate.

Eggs

Eggs improve the flavor, color, tender texture, lightness, and browning or glaze in baked foods. They are a fine addition to any bread or cereal dish to supplement the weaker protein in these foods.

Sugar

Sugar provides food for the yeast plants, retards the development of the gluten in flour, and improves browning and flavor. You may have noticed that sweet yeast doughs or batters don't rise as high as bread. The sugar is responsible for this. When much sugar is present, a higher temperature is required to coagulate the protein in eggs and flours. Molasses, honey, and brown sugar bring their own distinctive flavor to bread. When the first two are used as alternates for white sugar, the amount of liquid is decreased and the oven baking temperature lowered, lest the food burn. Both sugar and fat delay the development of gluten. This accounts for the fact that cakes are baked in a moderate oven and quick breads in a hot one.

These, then, are the basic ingredients that go into breads and other products made from flour. For variety in flavor, to suit individual tastes, flavoring extracts, spices, herbs, onions, garlic, or cheese may be included. Adding nuts and dried or fresh fruits increases the cost and the calories, but also the nutritive value.

Keys to success in making breads

You may have success in making breads, while your friends' breadmaking is poor. What causes the difference? Here are some points for success:

1/Understand the basic ingredients. This enables you to work with confidence.

2/Use high-quality ingredients suited to the purpose, but not necessarily the most expensive. Grade B or C eggs or dried eggs or milk may be used as effectively as the most expensive kinds. All ingredients should be clean and fresh, with a good odor and taste. Even a small amount of stale nuts, rancid fat or flour, lumpy baking powder that has lost its leavening power, or moldy dried fruit may spoil the flavor and waste the product.

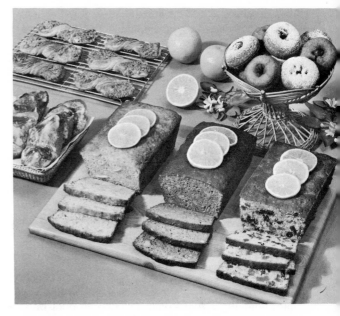

Success in baking depends on good ingredients, tested recipes, correct equipment, and care in following directions.

3/Use only a tested recipe and follow it exactly in all basic ingredients, varying the flavoring to suit your individual taste.

4/Measure each ingredient accurately and combine ingredients according to directions. This is where some beginners fail, while others succeed better than more experienced, but less meticulous, homemakers.

5/Use the correct equipment for making and baking the product. For instance, if the mixing bowl is too small, poor mixing results. If the bread is baked in a pan that is too small, it runs over, may burn, and is less attractive. If the pan is too large, the product is thin, burns quickly, and has a dry crumb.

6/Preheat the oven and be sure that the temperature is accurate. Companies that sell stoves will regulate the oven temperature without charge. If you don't have an accurate thermometer in your oven, get a reliable one to stand on the rack.

7/Bake the bread or cake until it is done, and no longer. The time given in a recipe should be observed, but test to make sure that the product is done. Although the outer edge may look done, the center may be raw and may fall.

8/A baked product is done when
  a. It shrinks from the side of the pan.
  b. A cake tester or toothpick inserted in the center comes out clean.
  c. It springs back after being gently touched in the center.

9/Serve hot breads hot. Most people enjoy rolls and homemade loaf bread hot, though cool bread slices more easily. Hot bread will slice smoothly if you use the bread knife gently as a "saw," rather than vigorously as an "axe."

Quick breads

Quick breads are easily made and homemade baked products are much less expensive than those that are purchased. If freezer space permits, bake extra muffins or loaf breads to freeze and use later for any meal, party, or snack.

Batters are made into a product that will pour or drop from a spoon. Among the products made from batters are popovers, pancakes, waffles, muffins, corn breads, coffee cakes, and loaf breads.

Dough is a flour-and-liquid mixture that can be rolled or kneaded. It produces biscuits, cookies, yeast breads, dumplings, and pastas.

table 10–1 *Standards for Bread and Rolls*

QUALITY	REQUIREMENT
APPEARANCE	Shape evenly rounded, with no humps or large cracks. (Uneven shape indicates it was not shaped and set to rise evenly. Large cracks show that it did not rise enough before baking or rose too much and too quickly while in the oven.)
CRUST	Tender, crisp, and mellow in flavor.
COLOR	Golden brown or darker, according to ingredients.
TEXTURE	Crumb moist, soft, tender. Fine, even holes—not tunnels.
FLAVOR AND AROMA	Fragrant, characteristic for kind, delicate, mellow.

Yeast breads

Batter yeast bread is easy, for it requires no kneading, only mixing and beating. It is baked in a round pan, in a fancy-shaped mold, or in a muffin tin. The outside is rougher and the texture softer than those of standard-type bread. It is moist and keeps well in the refrigerator or in the freezer, when properly wrapped. Most yeast breads, however, are made from kneaded dough.

Shortcuts in making standard yeast bread

Almost no other bread is so appetizing in aroma and flavor as hot yeast bread. Making it is very simple in our modern kitchens, with the superb appliances we have today. With practice, it be-

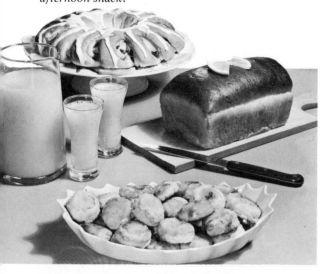

These delicacies, variations of sweet yeast bread, are delightful treats for Sunday brunch or an afternoon snack.

comes an increasing delight. For the method of making yeast bread, and recipes for various types, see pages 432–434.

If you prepare yeast bread in the morning and wish to bake it for dinner, set the loaf in the refrigerator, where it will rise more slowly, and take it directly from there to place in the hot oven. All the bread may be shaped and baked at once. That portion not for immediate use can be wrapped in an airtight package and frozen, to be reheated in a slow oven when needed. Or you may bake one loaf at a time and let the remainder stand in an oiled covered bowl in the refrigerator until you are ready to bake another loaf of fresh, hot bread. Some of the yeast plants will die from the cold and the bread will be less light and of a firmer texture. If it remains as long as a week, it tastes like sourdough bread, but is delicious in its own way. The colder the refrigerator, the sooner the yeast dies.

Basic sweet yeast breads

The basic sweet dough contains, in addition to yeast, more fat, sugar, and eggs than plain bread

and rolls. Delightful in tender texture and mellow flavor, sweet yeast breads are, unfortunately, high in fat, sugar, and calories. The steps in making them are the same as for the plain breads, whether it be a batter sweet dough or a kneaded one. Select a recipe that you like and follow it.

Every country has its special sweet roll. Historians tell us that sweet yeast bread originated in Vienna. The Danes liked it and made it so well that many call this type of sweet roll Danish pastry. Many forms and fillings are used in all countries.

When you have baked bread, judge it critically and give it a score. Note any mistakes you may have made and correct them when you bake again.

Macaroni products

Macaroni, or noodles, originated in China and were brought to Italy by Marco Polo. It is from Italy that the use of this product spread throughout the world. We consider it commonplace today, but it was once a gourmet dish. In the sixteenth century, while traveling in Florence, an Englishman ate and liked this food so well that he later organized a gourmet club called the Macaroni Club, where macaroni was a specialty. Its fame spread even to America, and we have the line "He stuck a feather in his cap and called it macaroni" in our song "Yankee Doodle."

How macaroni products are made

Macaroni products are made from durum hard wheat of high protein content, that holds its shape well and can be formed into many shapes and sizes. Technically called alimentary pastes or pastas, they (like many ready-to-eat cereals) are made from a flour paste. They are alternates for bread and may be used in many different and delightful ways.

Vermicelli is the smallest in diameter of the cord-shaped pastas. Noodles are made from the same flour paste, except that eggs are added. Some are enriched and others are not. Added coloring sometimes makes them look as if they have more egg yolk. You must read the label on all these products. Often a chemical, disodium phosphate, is added to cut down the cooking time. You would not wish to use this type of product if a member of your family is on a low-sodium diet. The weight is on the label, and often the number of servings. Salt does not have to be declared on the label, nor does a gum often used to prevent the product from breaking.

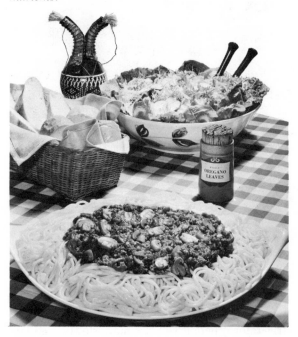

Macaroni products should never be overcooked. Brief cooking in little water preserves the maximum nutrients.

How to cook cereals and macaroni products

Both cereals and macaroni products are boiled in water or other liquid. Select a pan that will hold about three times the volume of the food to be cooked. It should have a firm, heavy bottom and a lid that may be used when desired. If water drips from the sides of the pan, place the lid only slightly ajar to allow steam to escape or reduce the heat further.

Macaroni and cereal are clean and ready to cook. **There is loss of nutrients from pouring off the cooking water of macaroni products or rinsing them after cooking.**

PROPER COOKING TIME. The aim in cooking pasta and other cereal products is to cook them until they are just tender and to use as small an amount of water as can be absorbed by the

food or otherwise used in meal preparation. Experiment until you find the correct time for cooking each macaroni-noodle product and the amount each will absorb. B vitamins and iron are added for enrichment of macaroni.

USES OF COOKING WATER. When some water is left over from cooking, use it in making white sauce or cheese sauce, cook potatoes in it, or use it in soups or in breadmaking. You have paid for the nutrients. Save them and use them. This is good management at the highest level. It comes with understanding foods and the nutrients in them.

Homemakers who run cold water over macaroni products and rice to "firm up" the product after it is cooked make a mistake. When properly cooked, every grain of rice will be separate and macaroni will be firm.

DANGERS OF OVERCOOKING. Overcooking causes macaroni products to lose their shape and all cereal grains to lose thiamine. If they are to be used later in a casserole, cook them until they are barely firm-tender, as they will cook more when baked in the oven.

Remember that directions for cooking, as given on the package, often do not take into consideration what the procedure does to the nutrients. The method given for cooking oriental rice on the brown rice package is an exception.

WAYS OF ADDING NUTRIENTS. Cooking breakfast cereals in milk improves the health values. Nonfat dry milk is excellent for this purpose, as it improves the flavor with only a slight increase in calories per serving and adds all the nutrients of whole milk, except fat and vitamin A. Macaroni and cheese may be used on a low-fat diet with cottage cheese substituted for three-fourths or all of the whole-milk cheese and the white sauce made with nonfat milk.

TIPS ON COOKING CEREALS AND MACARONI PRODUCTS. It is easy to retain the maximum nutrients and obtain a tasty, healthful, and attractive product if you follow three simple steps:

1/Measure about twice as much water (or milk for cereal) as food to be cooked—more, if you like a thin cereal or plan to use the macaroni water in a white sauce or a soup. Bring the water to a boil and add salt.

2/Add the cereal or macaroni, slowly stirring so that each part is kept separate and does not stick or lump. When cereals boil vigorously for two to three minutes, the starch swells and the cereal will not settle to the bottom. This is the time to lower the heat, cover the pot, and just maintain boiling. Do not stir macaroni products or rice while cooking, as this tends to break the

shape. If macaroni sticks together, lift the pan and use a circular motion to shake the mass apart.

3/Cook macaroni products and rice until they are just tender, and no longer. Serve hot.

Good management in buying and storing breads and cereal products

In 1965, American families increased their consumption of bakery foods by 14 percent over the 1955 figure and decreased their consumption of cereals and home-baked foods by 20 percent. This provokes the question: Are homemakers using the cereals and products made from them as wisely as they might?

Buying principles

The place of cereal-breads in our meals is especially important when money is limited. The following principles evolve from our study of cereals and breads.

1/You get more nourishment for your money by buying whole-grain breads and cereals than you do by buying any other kind. The flavor is preferred by gourmets who make an art of cooking. The whole grains are available in fine grind as whole wheat flour and cereals for cooking; in flakes as raw oatmeal or 100 percent whole wheat ready-to-eat cereal; cracked, as bulgur; precooked, as instant whole wheat cereal; or as natural brown rice.

2/Enriched, fortified, restored, and converted breads and cereals are next to whole grains in value and the best choice for those who prefer white cereal-breads.

3/Breads and baked foods made at home from basic ingredients and raw cereals that are completely cooked at home cost less per serving than ready-to-eat, partially cooked, brown-and-serve, thaw-and-heat, separate-and-bake, or mix-and-bake products. But the convenience foods save time. If you have more time than money, it is good management to use your time in preparing most of these foods.

4/The cost of ready-to-eat cereal is higher per serving than any other type.

5/Sweet-fat rolls, breads, and breakfast cakes that are ready to eat cost more than plain breads and rolls per serving. They are higher in fat, sugar, and calories. Use them as special-occasion foods and not as a regular alternate for plain bread. This habit saves money—and the waistline.

Various breads, popovers, and corn sticks may be made from cornmeal. Added cheese, seasonings, and/or hot pepper sauce give greater zest to these foods.

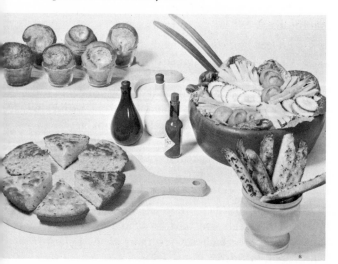

6/Compare the cost of cereals that have added vitamins, minerals, and amino acids with those that do not have them (other than in the standard "enrichment" program). Remember that you can balance the weakness of the amino acid in cereal-breads with milk, cheese, egg, or lean meat in the meal and the deficiency of vitamin C with the fruits and vegetables. When money is limited, spend it for foods that bring nutrients to balance the whole meal, and not for those added to the cereal product, if it is priced much higher per pound.

7/Buy by net weight, not the size of the loaf or the package. Often the small loaf may be heavier than the large one. The weight of the box may be greater than the weight of the cereal in it. A large package may be deceptive in being only partially filled, despite a law that prohibits deceptive packaging. You pay for packaging, as well as for the food.

8/Avoid sugar-coated cereals. You can add the sugar for less and can limit the amount used. It is important not to encourage the "sweet tooth."

9/Read the labels on all bread or cereals carefully. The label tells the kind of cereal; whether it is enriched, fortified, or whole grain; the type of grind; whether it is raw, partially cooked, or ready-to-eat; whether chemicals or coloring are added; whether other ingredients are included, such as sugar, salt, malt flavoring, and so on. Labels help you select the cereal and bread that suits your taste, purse, and needs.

10/Plan the bread and cereals to bring variety to your meals.

11/If storage space permits, shop for bread-cereals for an entire week at the same time that you shop for other foods.

Pancakes, fruit, milk, and sausage add up to a tasty breakfast.

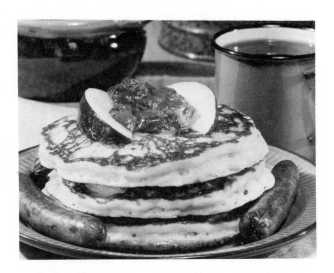

Storage tips

Storage that is adequate is a good part of management in the use of breads and cereals. Commercial baked foods have chemicals added to retard mold and ready-to-eat cereals contain some to help retain freshness.

1/Keep breads that are to be used immediately in a clean, fresh breadbox or in the refrigerator, as you would homemade breads. This latter is especially desirable in hot, humid weather, as it helps retain freshness, prevents rancidity, and deters weevils.

2/Store ready-to-eat cereals in the boxes in which they come. Once opened, tightly close the inner wax container to keep the product moisture-proof. They lose crispness and become tough when they absorb as much as 7 percent moisture from the atmosphere. The large bulk requires large storage space and limits the amount to be bought at one time. Storing cereals in a cabinet over the stove helps keep them crisp. If they become tough, heat them in a low oven to crisp them before serving.

3/Raw cereals and partially cooked cereals may be stored in their original container. Keep the lid on, or close the spout securely when the product is not in use.

Use of bread, cereal, and macaroni products in meals

Since cereal-grain products are made in a wide variety of choices, it is an easy matter to meet the recommendation of four servings in the daily diet. Any of these is counted a serving: 1 slice of bread; 1 roll, biscuit, or muffin; 3 average-size pancakes; 1 ounce of ready-to-eat cereal; ¾ cup of cooked cereal, grits, or macaroni-noodle products.

Breakfast

At breakfast, we usually eat toast or some type of bread. Plain breads low in fat and sugar are the wisest choices for control of weight or of the fat content in the diet. This does not mean an austerity program. Muffins, griddle cakes, waffles, biscuits, and other cereal-bread products are good foods that may be made at home with vegetable oil high in linoleic acid and fortified with nonfat dry milk (see Chapter 11 for discussion of fats). Use sweet rolls as a special treat, not as a habit.

Bread or cereal may be used as alternates at breakfast. Growing young people or those who exercise strenuously may need both. Cereal requiring milk is a better-balanced combination than bread eaten with butter and jam and no milk. When you choose bread instead of cereal, balance its nutrients with a glass of milk.

Cereal may be chosen in a different form for breakfast each day, either hot or ready-to-eat. As a measuring stick on bread-cereal, remember that for the calories in one doughnut you can eat two and one-half slices of bread or have three-fourths of a cup of cooked oatmeal and a glass of skim milk.

Lunch

At lunch bread, cereal, or macaroni is often an important part of the main dish. This may be in the form of bread as:

1/Sandwiches—a teen-age boy might easily eat four slices, or two sandwiches, with his lunch. Variety is obtained through different choices of bread to blend with meat, cheese, eggs, or fish.

Lasagna is an excellent main dish for lunch or supper.

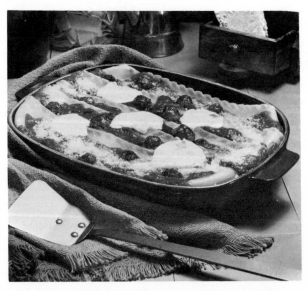

2/Hot breads to accompany a salad as the main dish—for example, hot rolls or corn, bran, wheat, blueberry, or other muffins. Popovers give an elegant, tasty, and special touch when the main dish is a chef's salad or a fruit salad with cottage cheese.

3/A main dish, such as pizza when properly made, English muffins, hot biscuits, or corn bread to serve as a base for creamed chicken, turkey, or fish.

4/Accompaniment to a soup or salad, such as crisp crackers or toast.

5/A main casserole dish, as, for example, macaroni products, spoon bread, rice, or bulgur (cracked wheat), all of which are excellent with tomato sauce, cheese, meat, fish, poultry, or a combination of favorite vegetables and meats.

Dinner

Dinner is a meal in which bread usually does not play such a large part, but it may accompany the meal in the form you like.

1/Hot biscuits, muffins, corn bread or sticks, or homemade yeast breads may act as bread or as dessert, if a jam is served.

2/Dumplings or hush puppies are delicious with poultry.

3/Stuffings in poultry, pork chops, fish, and breasts of veal or lamb are made of rice, bulgur, buckwheat groats (kasha), corn grits, corn bread, stale white bread, or a combination of any of these with (or instead of) white bread.

4/Cereals are used in such desserts as rice or bread pudding, Indian pudding (made of cornmeal), fruit cobblers or deep dish pies (made with low-fat biscuit dough), pies, cakes, cookies, pastries, and sweet breads of all types.

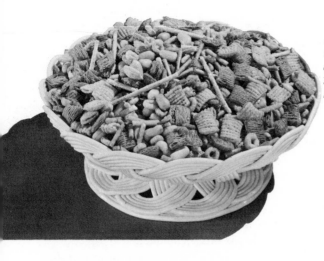

Prepared cereals become tangy, nourishing snacks when mixed with a small amount of vegetable oil, seasoned, and baked for a half-hour in a moderate oven.

Snacks and appetizers

These foods may employ corn, wheat, soy, rye, or a mixture of grains with many types of seasonings. They are served plain, with beverages of various sorts, as a base for canapes or for dips. Watch these, for many are quite high in fat and calories. For instance, only five small pretzel sticks yield 20 calories, and they are much less rich than some other varieties of snack foods.

Popcorn, a whole grain, is one of the best snack foods when you pop it at home and control the amount and kind of fat added. One cup of popcorn with no fat added has about the same number of calories as one slice of bread.

Some bread or cereal has a place in every meal. The exact amount and kind depend on the need of the individual, as well as his income and taste.

Meaningful words

aleurone
alimentary paste (pasta)
batter
disodium phosphate
endosperm
gluten
leavened bread
monocalcium phosphate
monosodium phosphate
quick bread
salt-rising bread
sodium aluminum sulfate
sourdough
tartrate
zymase

Thinking and evaluating

1. What are the advantages of making a part or most of your own bread? Are there any disadvantages? If so, name them. Which is the most economical type of bread to use on a low-cost budget? Which cereal? Which do you enjoy most? Your family? Your friends?

2. What are the functions of the primary ingredients in making bread? What ingredients may be added to give variety? In what way may a homemaker distinguish herself by making bread? How can she help her family? Herself?

3. What principles, once mastered, can enable you to succeed in breadmaking?

4. Referring to the Cookbook section, explain the steps in making yeast bread. How does it differ from the method of making quick breads? What kind of flour would you use for each? Why?

5. Which costs more, ready-to-eat yeast bread or ready-to-eat quick breads? How do you account for this? What do you consider good management in the kinds of bread you buy ready-to-eat? In other convenience forms? Which form of cereal and bread costs least, considering food value?

6. By what standards do you judge a bread? How can evaluation of the breads you make help you become more skillful in the art of making bread? How can keeping a notebook to record your successes and failures help you?

7. Explain the ways in which high calories may "sneak" into breads.

8. What can you learn from reading the labels on breads and cereal products? How can this help you save money? How can it add to the nutrients in your diet?

9. Why is it so important to learn the right technique for cooking cereals? Macaroni products? What is this technique?

10. In what ways may cereal-bread be used in each meal to bring balance and enjoyment to the day's diet?

Applying and sharing

1. With the information you have acquired about the cereal-bread group, make a trip to the market and, with notebook in hand, make a comparative study of the following:
   a. The variety of whole-grain, enriched, and unenriched bread and cereal products in your market, including flours, breads, plain yeast rolls, and those with added ingredients in different forms; cost per pound; cost per serving.
   b. Quick breads, analyzed in the same manner.
   c. Raw cereals, quick-cooking cereals, cereals precooked and ready-to-mix with hot liquid, ready-to-eat cereals—all analyzed as in (a).

2. From the above study, what did you learn about
   a. The price of flour per pound, compared with the price of bread, rolls, and sweet breads made with yeast? Quick breads?
   b. Cereals to be cooked the regular length of time? Quick-cooking? Ready-to-mix with liquid? Ready-to-eat?

3. With the above information, figure out the cost per serving of each type, allowing 1 ounce of flour or cereal per serving or 1 slice of bread or 1 roll. Which is the most nourishing per serving? Do you see any relationship between the cost of bread-cereals and the health values they contribute to the diet? Explain.

4. Discuss what you have learned with your class; with your family at home. Did your discussion clear up any previous false ideas? If so, what were they and how did you disprove them?

5. Experiments in cooking and tasting:
   a. Prepare yeast bread at school. With the class divided into groups, have all make the same basic yeast bread, using one-third whole wheat flour and two-thirds white flour for the first experiment. Mix and set the bread to rise the first day. Cooperate with other classes, so that you may experience handling the dough, baking the bread, and test-tasting it. Judge the bread on the basis of the standards given for bread on page 192. Decide what mistakes, if any, were made and how you can improve.
   b. Repeat this experience at home and make rolls with some of the dough. Which takes less time, bread or rolls? Which did your family enjoy more? How did your work at home compare with that at school? What was the cost per serving? If you can analyze your mistakes, try the bread again until you have a perfect result.

6. Divide the class into groups, each trying a different type of quick bread. Judge the breads and compare results. Decide how each can improve and what mistakes, if any, were made. Share these results with your mother and practice making different kinds of quick breads as part of balanced meals at home.

7. Conduct similar experiments at school and at home by mixing different kinds of cereals and macaroni products. Cook some in water and some with nonfat milk added. Compare the cost per serving and the nutrients for the different kinds.

8. On the basis of your study, plan balanced meals for four days, using different kinds of bread-cereals to meet the recommended amount per person each day. For a young couple on a low food budget, how could you increase the amount of cereal-bread used to give variety without adding excessively to the cost or the calories?

fat in the diet
-ally or foe?

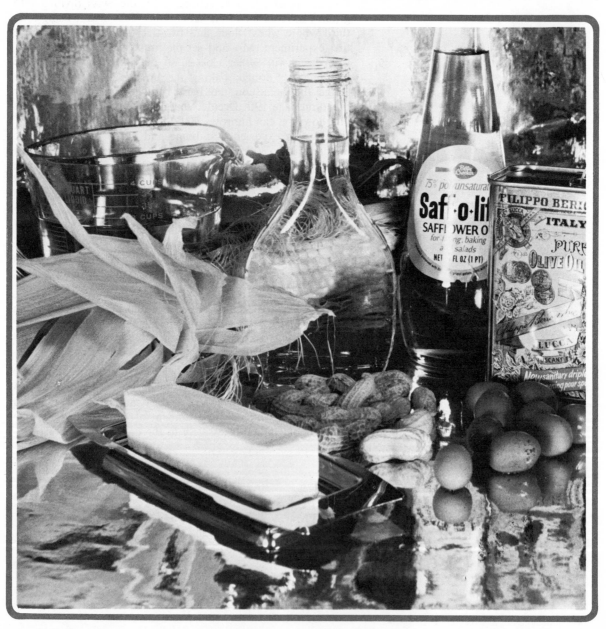

Throughout man's history, fat has been a symbol of the desirable. In the Bible, "live off the fat of the land" symbolized "enjoy the best of everything." To this day, in countries where the contrast between rich and poor is great, the "important" man is often fat. The connotation of the word is now changing as a result of scientific studies on how fat may relate to heart disease and overweight.

Fat in the diet and heart disease

As income has increased in our country, so has the amount of fat in our diets. At the turn of the century, fat constituted 30 to 33 percent of the total calories consumed; it rose to 44 percent in the 1955 survey and remained about the same in 1965. Does this really matter? Yes. So much so that the relationship between fat and heart disease has become headline news.

Focus on fats

Public excitement centers in three major events: first, the release of U.S. Public Health Department statistics that reveal that heart disease is the Number One cause of death in our country; second, the body of knowledge which has built up, showing that the kind and amount of fat we eat are factors contributing to heart-circulatory disease; and, third, the recommendations made to the public in 1965 and again in 1968 by the American Heart Association, and first made to physicians in 1961. The aim, as stated in 1965, was to lower the amount and specify the kind of fat used in the diet, in the hope of lessening the amount of atherosclerosis (ath ə rō sklə rō′ səs), a disease of the arteries in which fatty deposits are laid down inside the artery walls, of the whole American population. In 1968, further studies justified another recommendation confirming and elaborating on the first, stating, "An intake of less than 40 percent of the calories from fat is considered desirable. Of this total, polyunsaturated fats should probably comprise twice the quantity of saturated fats."

Correcting concepts

The concept in the past has been that heart disease is for the "aging." Studies show that the plaques found in older people's arteries, contributing to their hardening, are found in all age groups, even infants. Plaques are irregular streaks of mushy fat and cholesterol that form on the inner walls of the arteries. At the point where they appear, the diameter of the artery is smaller, thus interfering with the normal strong flow of the blood. If large molecules of fat associated with cholesterol pile up in the bloodstream at a partially blocked passage, this is conducive to the formation of clots, with undesirable effects on life and health.

New approaches

These were not only new ideas about food, but also new words to understand, if we are to eat wisely. This is important for all, but you who are young have the most to gain. Young people have time to learn new eating habits and prevent a future date with heart-circulatory disease or control it partially through diet, if it occurs.

Before we examine the meaning of "saturated" and "polyunsaturated" fats and "cholesterol," let us look at some of the other ways in which fat can help or hurt us now and later.

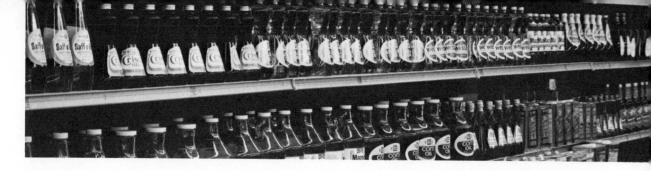

Fat as an ally or foe?

Fat is an ally in the diet when properly used, but it becomes a foe when it is overused or misused.

1/It adds a highly desired flavor to food because of the crisp texture it gives to fried foods, the flakiness to baked products, the juiciness and tenderness to meat, and the delightful seasoning to vegetables and other foods. It becomes a foe when we overeat fatty foods.

2/It gives "staying power" to a meal, for it takes longest to digest of any nutrient, thus delaying hunger. This was a great advantage to our forefathers. Fat sustained them as they burned it up at hard labor. But we are physically less active. Fat becomes a foe when it piles up in the bloodstream. It increases the tendency for the blood to clot, a factor that contributes to heart attacks, strokes, and circulatory ailments.

3/It is our most concentrated source of energy-fuel. (Alcohol is next, with 7.1 calories per gram of alcohol, as compared to 9 per gram of fat. Alcohol contains no nutrients, only calories.) Fat becomes a foe when we eat so much of it that we gain excess weight.

4/Fat is essential for the absorption of the fat-soluble vitamins A, D, E, and K and for their use by the body. Otherwise they are eliminated as waste. One fat, mineral oil, is a foe. It is not absorbed or utilized by the body, but absorbs fat-soluble vitamins and eliminates them as waste, depriving us of nutrients we need.

5/It lubricates the digestive tract. Too much sometimes causes diarrhea in infants and others.

6/A thin fatty sheath helps control body temperature against excessive heat or cold, pads the organs and joints (such as the soles of the feet) to insure greater comfort, rounds out the figure, provides a reserve source of energy, and works on a team of nutrients to make vitamin D with the aid of ultraviolet rays of the sun on the skin. However, when the fatty sheath becomes excessive and the individual becomes obese, the body works less efficiently and its processes are slowed down by the fat.

7/It provides essential fatty acids required for growth, for life itself, and for a good complexion and healthy hair. When "essential" fatty acids are in insufficient supply, eczema develops, together with a rough skin and coarse hair. In lower animals the hair falls out.

Essential fatty acids

Essential fatty acids include linoleic (**lin ə lē′ ik**), linolenic (**lin ə lē nik**), and arachidonic (**ar ə kə dän′ ik**). Linoleic can make arachidonic in the body when the diet includes enough vitamin B_6. Linoleic is by far the most important. It cannot be made in the body, is essential for life, and must be supplied through the food we eat. These three fatty acids are polyunsaturated.

Meaning of saturated and polyunsaturated fats in the diet

The words "saturated fats" and "polyunsaturated fats" are used glibly in advertising foods. Many who use and hear them have only a vague notion of what they mean. Many are confused and some are frightened because of the possible link with heart disease. There is no need for either confusion or fear when we understand what these words mean: that the fat we use in our diet may help our lives now and later.

*The display of fat products in our
supermarkets can be bewildering.
We can protect our health by
choosing polyunsaturated fats.*

Saturated fats

A saturated fat is the largest and heaviest fat molecule (a molecule is a chemical combination of two or more atoms to form a specific substance, such as a fatty acid). Fat molecules are large and complex and contain much more carbon than either protein or carbohydrate. It is the concentration of carbon in fats that makes the calorie count so high.

Let us illustrate with a fragment of a saturated fatty acid and one of a polyunsaturated fatty acid in the simplified diagram (Figure 11–1). You will note that the saturated fatty acid is the larger. Each carbon atom is linked up with hydrogen. To use a baseball term, all bases are loaded. The molecule can hold no more. That is what saturation means.

FOOD SOURCES. Saturated fats comprise 40 to 45 percent of the fat in the average American diet. The most tasty fats are saturated. We eat them in fat of all animal foods—meats, whole milk, cream, butter, cheese, ice cream, egg yolk, lard—and man-made firm fats from vegetable oils, including some margarine and hydrogenated shortening. Saturated fats are also hidden in many convenience foods, and are also found in coconut oil, coconut, and chocolate. Since large amounts of saturated fats in a meal result in a high proportion in the blood serum, we can clearly see the reasons for cutting down on animal fats in the diet, to the degree that it is consistent with an otherwise balanced diet. We need the lean of meat and eggs and the nonfat parts of milk to provide a well-balanced diet.

FATS AND FATTY ACIDS*

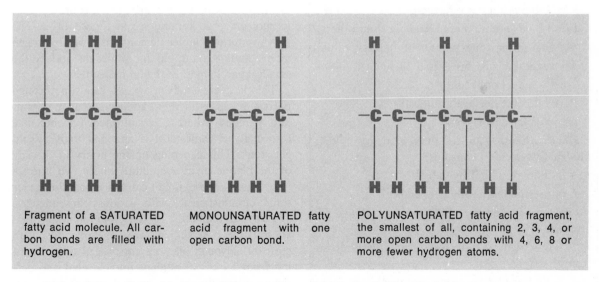

Fragment of a SATURATED fatty acid molecule. All carbon bonds are filled with hydrogen.

MONOUNSATURATED fatty acid fragment with one open carbon bond.

POLYUNSATURATED fatty acid fragment, the smallest of all, containing 2, 3, 4, or more open carbon bonds with 4, 6, 8 or more fewer hydrogen atoms.

*Adapted from Callie M. Coons, "Fats and Fatty Acids," *Food: The Yearbook of Agriculture 1959* (Washington, D.C.: USDA), p. 77.

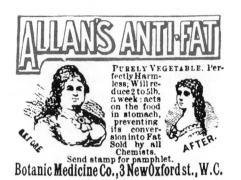

An 1883 magazine ad

Monounsaturated fats

Monounsaturated fats in various foods are illustrated in Tables 11–1 and 11–2. *Mono*, a Greek word meaning *one*, indicates that the fatty acid has only one open carbon bond. It is not so large a molecule as the saturated fat, but not nearly so small as the polyunsaturated ones (*poly*, meaning *many*). Eighty percent of the fat in olive oil is in this class and 44 percent of pork fat.

FOOD SOURCES. Monounsaturated fats constitute a large part of the fat in our diet, as the above-mentioned tables show. Table 11–1 demonstrates that olive oil is the richest source, with hydrogenated shortening, margarine, peanut oil, lard, and butter as next richest sources.

Polyunsaturated fats

Polyunsaturated fatty acids is a term loosely used to imply the "desirable" type of fat. *Unsaturated* means that some of the carbon bonds are open in its molecule, as you can see in Figure 11–1. The polyunsaturated molecule contains fewer hydrogen atoms than a saturated fat molecule and is the smallest and lightest of the fat molecules.

This is a great advantage. It can slip through narrow passages in tiny capillaries that may contain plaques, whereas a saturated fat molecule (especially if cholesterol is attached to it) would get stuck. This can plug up the artery at the site of the plaque or at a juncture where two arteries join. In either case, it can cause a blood clot under some circumstances, with serious consequences.

FOOD SOURCES. In the common foods that we use, the best sources are vegetable oils, with corn oil, soybean oil, and cottonseed oil containing from 51 to 55 percent linoleic acid and safflower oil as the richest source, with 76 percent. Linoleic acid is the key to polyunsaturated fats.

Folklore and superstition

Have you heard that . . .

Heart disease is caused by eating too much dairy fat?

Butter is a more healthful fat than margarine or vegetable oils?

Fat that surrounds meat should be eaten with the lean?

Margarine is harder to digest than butter?

Vegetable oils are not fattening?

Fried foods are no more fattening than others?

All margarines are equal in health value?

All vegetable oils are equal in health value?

Lard is not a healthful fat?

Pork fat is the hardest to digest?

All fat is hard to digest?

Heart disease can be prevented by taking linoleic fatty acid in capsules?

A fat baby is a healthy baby?

A fat person has a jolly personality?

One should become slightly fatter as age increases?

The best way to reduce is to eliminate all fat from the diet?

The best way to prevent heart disease is to eliminate animal fat from the diet?

Don't you believe it!

Linoleic acid: most important of fatty acids

Linoleic acid is the most important fatty acid for good appearance and good health.

1/It is essential for growth.

2/It is essential for normal reproduction.

3/It is essential to provide partial protection against radiation.

4/It helps protect us from excess loss of water.

5/It plays a key role in helping lower the cholesterol level of the blood. This is the focal point in research, because of its link to heart-circulatory disease. It is thought that its beneficial effect may be due to both mechanical reasons—the fact that it is the smallest of the fatty acids—and chemical reasons, which are explained more thoroughly under our discussion of cholesterol later in this chapter.

Food sources

Food sources of linoleic acid are important to learn and use. The richest sources are the seeds of grains and nuts, as illustrated in Table 11–2. Table 11–1 shows the vegetable oils that are excellent sources of linoleic acid. By far the richest known source is safflower oil, which is now on the market at competitive prices. Other good sources are corn, soybean, and cottonseed oils. Sunflower oil is also a good source and may in future be found on your grocery shelves. Peanut oil, another domestic oil, has 31 percent linoleic fatty acid.

Olive oil has been widely favored internationally as a "superior" salad and seasoning oil. Research shows this belief to be inaccurate. It contains only 8 percent linoleic acid. You can save money and improve your diet by using our domestic oils. It is a foolish waste of money, too,

to buy any oil in capsule form to obtain linoleic acid.

"Soft" margarines are our richest source in table spreads. However, there is wide variation among the different brands and types.

Factors influencing use of fat

The way the body uses fat varies a great deal with the age, health, and activity of the individual. It also varies with the kind of fat eaten. Some infants

table 11–1   *Comparison of Saturated and Unsaturated Fatty Acids in Oils and Fats**

(Grams per 100 Grams of Total Fatty Acids)

NAME OF FOOD	POLY-UNSATURATED LINOLEIC FATTY ACID Percent	MONO-UNSATURATED OLEIC FATTY ACID Percent	TOTAL SATURATED FATTY ACIDS Percent
Safflower oil	76	15	8
Sunflower oil	66	21	12
Corn oil	55	30	12
Soybean oil	55	21	18
Cottonseed oil	51	22	26
Peanut oil	31	50	19
Olive oil	8	80	12
Butter	3	35	59
Margarine**	9	60	27
Shortening, hydrogenated	8	68	24
Lard	11	48	40

*Adapted from Callie M. Coons, "Fatty Acids in Some Animal and Plant Foods," *Food: The Yearbook of Agriculture 1959* (Washington, D.C.: USDA), pp. 84–5.
**Margarine varies according to kind.

and people of other ages have difficulty in digesting it. Most people have no trouble at all, especially if they are healthy and physically active. Nature provided that the breast-fed baby has a finely emulsified fat (in fine droplets) three times as high in linoleic acid as cow's milk. Both are good.

Fats in digestion

In digestion, fat is split into a fine emulsion of fatty acids and glycerol (**glis′ ə rol**). This begins in the stomach, but most of it takes place by action of

This Korean child is enjoying a seafood meal that is low in fat.

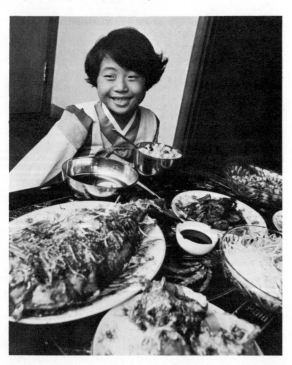

bile and enzyme (lipase) in the small intestines. Tiny fat globules absorb the fat-soluble vitamins and carry them through the intestinal walls and lymph system as they circulate to all tissues. Here the tissues trap the fat and vitamins they need. Excess vitamins are stored in the liver, and fat beyond the body's immediate need is stored as a reserve throughout body tissues.

When the reserve exceeds the need, we become overweight. When the body needs reserve energy and the carbohydrate is all used, it calls on fat, which is now changed back to carbohydrate and burned for energy. This is what happens when we lose weight. In order to be properly oxidized (burned), fat needs some carbohydrate. Hence the saying that "fat is burned in the flame of carbohydrate."

The fats with the lowest melting point are easiest to digest. These include milk fat, egg yolk, and vegetable oil. These are about 97 percent digested, as compared with 93 percent for beef fat and 88 percent for lamb. This is significant for the person who has to plan and prepare meals for people who need help in digesting fat.

The mineral magnesium and vitamins B_6 and E are needed in the diet for the body to use fat well. Since these are lost in highly processed food, we probably eat less of them today than formerly.

Adjusting fat levels

For most young people, the fat level of the blood returns to normal before the next meal—three to six hours. But for older, inactive persons, and especially those with some kinds of disease, the fat piles up in the bloodstream after meals. Studies show that the blood clots more rapidly after a fatty meal and that the fat level may remain high as long as 12 hours—an undesirable condition for anyone, but especially for those with heart disease.

FAT INTAKE. Figure 11–2 represents a summary of the study from which we first learned that Americans are eating about 44 percent of their total calories from fat. Analysis showed that 42 percent of this total was saturated, 43 percent oleic acid (monounsaturated), and only 10 percent linoleic (polyunsaturated) fatty acid. The other 5 percent is in other fatty acids.

Research accumulated since then confirms this study. In the 1965 dietary survey, it was found that we used slightly larger quantities of vegetable oils and slightly smaller quantities of saturated fat. This is encouraging, for we see that those who

know how fat relates to present and future health wish to apply what they learn.

Table 11–2 shows that, weight for weight, chicken, turkey, and fish contain more linoleic acid and less saturated fat than lamb or beef, and that pork contains less saturated fat than other red meats. Scientific evidence explodes the false belief held by many that "pork is a less desirable food than either beef or lamb." On the contrary, it is not only higher in linoleic acid, but also in thiamine, an important point to remember in meal planning. Only two fruits and no vegetables contain enough fat to merit mention. Contrary to popular belief, the avocado is high in total unsaturated fat and low in saturated fat. Olives, on the other hand, contain less than half the linoleic acid of avocado. The whole grains are all high in linoleic acid and low in saturated fat. Here we see the soundness of eating generous amounts of vegetables, fruits, whole grains, and nonfat milk in a meal to balance meat and its fat.

fig. 11–2 **FAT SOURCES IN THE AMERICAN DIET***

Average percent

MILK/DAIRY FOODS	25
PORK/BACON/LARD	24
BEEF/VEAL/LAMB	14
MARGARINE/SHORTENING	13
BAKED GOODS/NUTS	12
OILS/SALAD DRESSINGS	6
POULTRY/FISH/EGGS	6

*Adapted from Callie M. Coons, "Fats and Fatty Acids," *Food: The Yearbook of Agriculture 1959* (Washington, D.C.: USDA), p. 87, and from USDA Household Consumption Survey, 1955.

Relation of cholesterol to heart disease and to fats in the diet

Cholesterol fell under a cloud as being a cause of cardiovascular disease for two reasons, first, because blood serum cholesterol was often high in some types of heart disease, and, second, because in such cases it was a part of fatty plaques inside the arteries. The plaques hardened as the individual grew older, contributing to heart attacks and strokes.

Confusion and fear have been present in the minds of many concerning cholesterol, owing to lack of accurate information which was readily

table 11–2   Comparison of Unsaturated and Saturated Fatty Acids in Some Animal and Plant Foods*

(Grams per 100 Grams of Total Fatty Acids)

NAME OF FOOD	Polyunsaturated Linoleic Fatty Acid	UNSATURATED Monounsaturated Oleic Acid	Other Unsaturated	SATURATED Total Fatty Acids
MILK				
Whole cow's	3	35	3	59
Skim or nonfat	—	—	—	—
Buttermilk	—	—	—	—
Human milk	8	36	8	48
MEATS, FISH, POULTRY				
Beef	2	46	2	50
Pork	9	44	9	38
Lamb	2	37	2	59
Liver, pork	5	28	31	33
Salmon	——together, 27——		55	16
Tuna	——together, 26——		48	26
Chicken	21	40	5	34
Turkey	22	46	4	30
EGG, whole	21	40	11	34
NUTS				
Almond	21	70	—	9
Coconut	1	7	1	91
Peanut	30	46	1	23
Pecan	21	70	1	8
Walnut, English	65	16	12	7
FRUITS AND VEGETABLES				
Avocado	15	50	13	22
Olive	7	80	1	12
WHOLE GRAINS (not oils)				
Corn	47	37	4	12
Oats, rolled	43	33	1	23
Rice	38	42	1	19
Wheat	48	28	6	16

*Adapted from Callie M. Coons, "Fatty Acids in Some Animal and Plant Foods," *Food: The Yearbook of Agriculture 1959* (Washington, D.C.: USDA), pp. 84–85.

understandable to the general public. When we understand the overall picture, which includes the recent research on fat and other factors, we can do something positive about it.

Nature of cholesterol

Cholesterol, a fatlike waxy substance, is part of all human tissue, composing 11 percent of the dry weight of the brain, where it is thought to form a protective sheath, and it is the major component in earwax. It works on a team of nutrients to form vitamin D when the sun shines directly on the skin and also produces good vision, along with vitamin A and other nutrients.

It is part of the liver, spleen, sex glands, and hormones and is essential for the formation of bile salts needed for digestion of fat. Since fat is lighter than water, cholesterol is important in helping transport fat through the liquid bloodstream. It is a rich part of white blood cells. Plasma and liver cholesterol drop sharply, it has been found, during some acute infections. A nutrient that contributes so much to life needs to be understood. Foods containing it should be used intelligently.

New findings

Research is revealing that cholesterol is not the villain once suspected. For one thing, a diet low in it does not always solve the problem of heart disease. Human beings with quite high blood cholesterol have not suffered from heart disease. On the other hand, others with low cholesterol have been found to have heart ailments.

We ingest on the average about 500 to 600 milligrams of cholesterol per day. Since the body

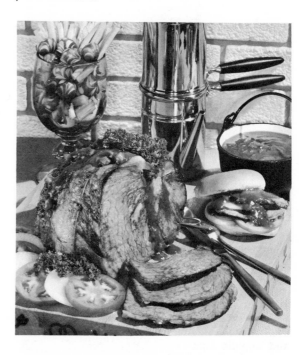

The fat in meat is saturated. The diet should have twice as much unsaturated fat as saturated.

must have it for normal functioning, if we don't eat enough cholesterol-bearing food, the body can manufacture 2000 to 3000 milligrams daily, and does. This occurs mostly in the liver but the skin, intestinal mucosa, and other body tissues can manufacture it. The point to remember is: food alone is not responsible for raising blood cholesterol. If we don't eat it, the body makes it.

Radioactive elements have made it possible to label carbon atoms and follow the cholesterol molecule through the body. From this technique we learn that blood cholesterol may be higher (a) during the normal menstrual cycle; (b) when women reach the age of 55, or during or after menopause; (c) in men from the time they are 25 years old; (d) when there is history of coronary disease in the family; (e) when the thyroid gland is underactive; (f) when a person is putting on weight; (g) when the diet is too high in protein (a high-protein diet is often used by food faddists in crash diets to reduce weight); (h) when too much sweet food is eaten at one time and quickly absorbed; (i) when a person eats large amounts of foods rich in animal fat or other saturated fat; (j) when a person consumes too much alcoholic beverage; (k) when the diet is too high in cholesterol; (l) when a person indulges in overeating in any form; (m) when a person experiences emotional stress in any form; and (n) when the person engages in insufficient regular exercise.

Remember that fruits, vegetables, and cereal grains contain no cholesterol. Table 11–3 indicates the range found in foods. Become familiar with this in planning your day's diet.

Cholesterol and linoleic acid

Exactly why blood cholesterol lowers when linoleic acid constitutes 25 percent or more of the calories is not yet known. But studies show that this occurs even when the total fat in the diet is as high as 40 percent, if linoleic acid is also high and saturated fat low.

The lowering of cholesterol is thought to be due to two things. One is mechanical—that is, the linoleic fatty acid molecule is the smallest one. The other is chemical—linoleic acid tends to have a liquefying effect on cholesterol. We need further research to clarify its role. The fact that now stands out is: We do know that linoleic acid works for us in a balanced diet. Saturated fat can work against us in contributing to heart-circulatory disease when we eat large amounts of it with small amounts of polyunsaturated fats.

table 11–3   Cholesterol Content of Common Foods*

FOOD	CHOLESTEROL CONTENT
(Milligrams per 100 grams—3½ oz.)	
Beef brains	2000
Eggs, fresh whole (2)	550
Liver, raw	300
Butter	250
Oysters, Lobster (meat only)	200
Cheese, cheddar	100
cottage, creamed	15
cream	120
American process	155
Lard and other animal fat	95
Shrimp, Crab (flesh only)	125
Heart, beef, raw	150
Veal	90
Beef, round, medium-fat, raw	70
Chicken, raw, flesh only	60
Fish fillet or steak	70
Lamb, Pork	70
Ice cream	45
Milk, whole	11
skim, liquid	3
Vegetable oils	0
Plant foods	0

*SOURCE: *Composition of Foods*, Agriculture Handbook No. 8, Agriculture Research Service (Washington, D.C.: USDA), Table 4, p. 146.

Ireland-Boston cholesterol-fat study

In this connection, it is interesting to consider the "Ireland-Boston" Heart Study. The Harvard University Department of Nutrition cooperated with the Department of Preventive Medicine of Trinity College in Dublin, Ireland, on this project. A report was made in 1964 of 174 pairs of brothers between 30 and 60 years of age. In each pair, one brother had lived in the Boston area for ten years or more; the other had never left Ireland. Those who remained in Ireland consumed about 300 more calories daily, on the average. Animal fats accounted for 94 percent of their total fat calories, twice as much as those of their American counterparts, and they ate an average of one pound of butter per week. They had less hypertension than their American brothers, and lower blood cholesterol. What other facts were involved?

The brothers in Ireland also (a) weighed less; (b) walked and bicycled more, indicating that they used up the fat in their bloodstream, instead of letting it pile up; and (c) were engaged in agricultural work without the pressures associated with urban living and working, which formed the environment of the Boston brothers.

Harvard medical student study

In another study, made of medical students at Harvard, it was found that young men who had a caloric intake of 5000 a day—enough for a lumberjack—maintained steady weight and steady cholesterol levels, so long as they exercised enough to avoid gaining weight. But when the calories remained at the same level and exercise was reduced, weight rose and blood cholesterol also rose. These experiments have significance for all ages, if we read the message and are guided by it.

Chicken is low in fat content. To balance its saturated fat, the salad dressing should be made with vegetable oil high in linoleic acid.

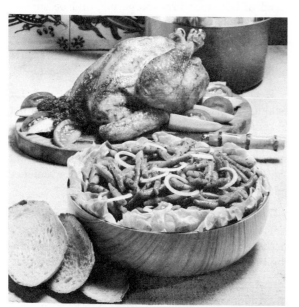

How much fat do we need daily?

The exact amount of fat for best health is not known at present. It is known that a wide variation in fat consumption exists around the world. In the Orient, the mass of people get about 10 percent of their calories from fat and heart disease is low there. But among the rich in India and Guatemala, who eat a high saturated fat diet, studies show that the incidence of heart disease is comparable to that of Western countries, where 40 percent or more of the caloric intake is derived from fat.

The National Research Council's Food and Nutrition Board recommended in 1948 that the average diet should derive 20 to 25 percent of its calories from fat. These figures were supported by the American Medical Association's Council on Foods and Nutrition.

Studies show that for some—the diabetic and others—when fat is lowered and carbohydrates increased, there is a rise in blood triglycerides (trī glis′ ə rīds) or fat, which may also correlate to coronary heart disease in a manner similar to that of cholesterol. When excess carbohydrate, protein, or fat is eaten, it is changed into triglycerides and stored in the form of adipose tissue, or body fat. Then, when we need immediate energy and have to call upon reserve fat, it is changed back into glucose, the form of energy used by the blood. But, in the case of diabetics and some heart patients, this change is not efficient and triglycerides may rise in the blood serum. On the other hand, the large population in the world who derive 65 to 85 percent of their calories from carbohydrate also have a low incidence of coronary heart disease.

Dr. Jean Mayer, Professor of Nutrition at Harvard, expresses the view of many in nutrition in recommending a balanced diet containing no more than 30 percent of fat in the total calories for the day.

How to lower saturated fat and increase polyunsaturated fat in our diets

Both saturated and unsaturated fats are important to us, for we need meats, dairy foods, eggs, fruits, and green leafy vegetables, as well as other vegetables, in a balanced diet. It is thought that a good proportion is one part saturated fats to two parts unsaturated.

We should know our foods. It is essential that we realize, for instance, that 3 ounces of beef roast has 16 grams or 144 calories of saturated fat to 1 gram or 9 calories of linoleic acid. Beef is our favorite meat. We frequently select foods on the

basis of convenience. For example, consider frankfurters—a food eaten by the millions in our country. One hot dog (8 to a pound) has 170 calories, 135 of which were formerly from fat, mostly saturated. Two ounces of tuna has 113 calories, with 41 from fats, most of which are not saturated. It is encouraging to learn that our newer knowledge of fat has caused the government to require a lowering in the fat content of hot dogs to 30 percent, or about 94 calories each. These are important things to know.

Tips on planning the diet

The following are suggestions for planning and preparing meals that contain more polyunsaturated fat and less saturated.

1/Use special soft margarine as a spread, instead of butter or firm margarine, and be sure to read the label when you buy, to see that the first ingredient listed is liquid safflower or corn, soybean, cottonseed, or sunflower oil, as this indicates a high percentage of linoleic acid (see Table 11–1).

2/Use vegetable oil high in linoleic acid for baking quick breads, cakes, pastries, and other baked products, when possible. To improve the flavor in cakes and cookies, use more extract, spices, or lemon or orange peel, as oil brings out the flavors in herbs and spices. Most convenience mixes contain saturated fat.

3/Use vegetable oil to season vegetables, white sauce, casseroles, salads, and other foods and use herbs, onions, garlic, and other seasonings, including brown meat drippings, to bring out the flavor.

4/Use vegetable oil to fry, sauté, or brush meat in broiling or baking, if the meat is lean.

Both saturated and unsaturated fats are essential for health. We need foods from each group to give us the variety of nutrients the body requires.

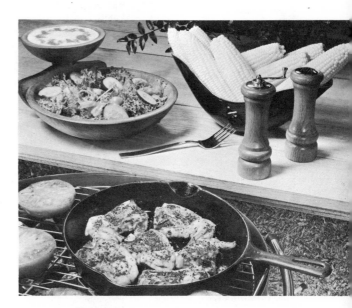

5/Cook cereals in skim milk and add 1 teaspoon of safflower or other oil per serving, and cook your egg in a teaspoon of this oil to provide a share of linoleic acid at breakfast.

6/Use more low-fat chicken, turkey, fish, shellfish, veal, and baby beef in the diet and season dry beans with vegetable oil and herbs, onions, and garlic for good flavor as a meat alternate.

7/Trim all visible fat from red meat before cooking as it is saturated, and trim the marbled fat away as you eat red meat. Enough remains in the fine marbling that you can't trim out, to provide more than the amount of saturated fat you need. Skin poultry and remove all visible fat before cooking, if you need to keep the saturated fat low.

8/Divide the amount of fat used in the day about equally among the three meals, rather than eating little or none at breakfast and overloading at dinner. Remember that when the day is before you, there is time to be active and burn up fat, but a high-fat meal in the evening with no activity and then bed can pile up the fat level in the bloodstream for as much as 12 hours, as studies show.

9/Keep a sharp eye out for "hidden" saturated fats in many premade foods and meals and in snacks and appetizers. Formerly, if the label said, "Made with butter," the product was considered superior. We now shun such products if we wish to keep the saturated fat low.

10/Study each recipe for the kind and amount of fat it contains before using it. Some, but not all, food editors of magazines and newspapers and authors of cookbooks are most interested in flavor and appearance and seem to care little about applying in their recipes the modern knowledge of nutrition on fat. You can prepare tasty foods that have the correct kind and amount of fat by studying the tables in this book, and thus make an intelligent choice that will serve your needs.

11/In shopping, take time to read labels to find the kind and amount of fat used in processed foods. Remember that the visible fats in meals amount to about two-fifths of the total, leaving the lion's share—three-fifths—to fat we can't see. This is usually highly saturated.

12/In eating out, learn to analyze dishes for fat content. For instance, knowing that French fries are usually fried in oil, you would naturally conclude that, though high in calories from fat, the oil is polyunsaturated. But by spot-checking it has been found that coconut, which is almost completely saturated, is the oil most often used for deep-fat frying in public eating places. It is cheaper. In such a case, you might wish to order a baked potato instead.

table 11–4   "Hidden" Calories from Fat in Common Foods*

FOOD		MEASURE	CALORIES FROM FAT	TOTAL CALORIES
MEAT	Sirloin steak, broiled	6 oz.	486	660
	Bacon, fried	2 slices	72	90
	Hamburger, regular	3 oz.	153	245
	Lamb, roast leg	3 oz.	144	235
	Pork, roast fresh (lean only)	2.4 oz.	90	175
	Ham, cured, roast	3 oz.	171	245
	Chicken, half breast (with bone and fried)	3.3 oz.	45	155
	Drumstick, fried	2.1 oz.	36	90
	Chicken, canned boneless	3 oz.	90	170
	Crabmeat, canned	3 oz.	18	85
MILK AND MILK PRODUCTS	Heavy cream	1 T.	54	55
	Cream cheese	3 oz.	288	320
	Ice cream	3-oz. cup	45	95
	Malted milk	1 cup	90	245
NUTS	Peanut butter	1 T.	72	95
	Peanut halves, roasted	½ cup	324	420
	Almonds, shelled	½ cup	347	425
	Pecan halves	½ cup	347	370
	Walnut halves	½ cup	338	345
LUNCHEON MEATS	Bologna	2 slices	63	80
	Frankfurter	1	94	170
DESSERTS	Devil's food cake	1/16 of 9-in. cake	81	235
	Fruit cake, dark	1/30 of 8-in. loaf	18	55
	Plain cake, no icing	1 slice	108	315
	with boiled white icing	1 slice	108	400
	Angel food cake, no icing	1 slice	trace	135
	Brownie	1	54	95
	Apple pie	1/7 of 9-in. pie	135	350
	Mince pie	1/7 of 9-in. pie	144	365
	Lemon meringue pie	1/7 of 9-in. pie	108	305
	Pumpkin pie	1/7 of 9-in. pie	135	275
SALAD DRESSING	Mayonnaise	1 T.	99	100
	French	1 T.	54	65
	Home-cooked	1 T.	18	25
	Thousand Island	1 T.	72	80
SNACKS AND APPETIZERS	Potato chips	10 chips	72	115
	Pizza	⅛ of 14-in. pie	54	185
	Olives, ripe black	2 large	trace	73
	green	3 large	trace	78

*Adapted from *Nutritive Value of Foods*, Bulletin No. 72 (Washington, D.C.: USDA, revised 1970).

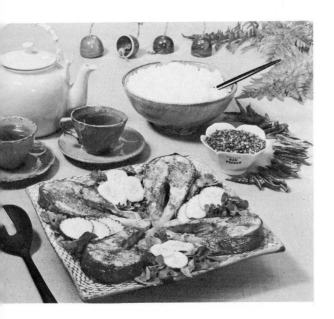

Fish is a valuable food that is high in essential nutrients and low in saturated fat.

—foods which contain little or no saturated fat—you are holding down on total fat and cholesterol. Prepare your menus accordingly.

13/In planning meals, see that the kind and amount of fat are balanced among the three repasts of the day. When you have a sirloin steak, use fresh fruit for dessert and season the salad and vegetables with an oil high in linoleic acid. When fish, liver, broiled chicken, or beans are used as the main protein dish, you may have your favorite dessert that is high in fat (preferably polyunsaturated).

14/Though the percentage of fat is lower in the imitation ice milks than in standard ice cream, the fat used in the ice milk is often coconut oil and/or hydrogenated vegetable oils. The same is true of imitation coffee cream. This might be changed by consumer demand, and the demand that the kind and percentage of each fat used in preprocessed foods be stated on the label.

15/Remember that when the meal contains vegetables, fruits, cereal-breads, and non-fat milk

Kinds of fats in our markets

Oils

Oils are fats that stay liquid at room temperature or when refrigerated. They come from the seeds of plants, with the exception of olive and coconut oil. These two are derived from the fruit.

CHARACTERISTICS OF OIL. Oils are similar to other fats in that they taste and feel greasy, provide a concentrated source of energy, absorb strong odors and flavors from foods, become rancid when exposed to the air, and make food more tender, crisp, and tasty. All become undesirable for eating if heated to the point of burning.

Oils and fats differ in flavor, melting point, smoking point, congealing point, the rate at which they become rancid, and their ability to "shorten" a baked food. The practical approach to the study of oils and fats is to consider their values in terms of what they do for your health, as well as making food tasty.

LINOLEIC CONTENT. Remember that corn, soybean, and cottonseed oils have about two-fifths more linoleic acid than peanut oil and six-sevenths more than olive oil. On the other hand, if you are in a grocery store (not a health food store) and can find pure safflower oil competitively priced, it is your best buy, as it is highest in linoleic acid.

BLENDED OILS. Blends of oils afford opportunity to the unscrupulous processor to add low-cost coconut oil that is highly saturated. It is wise to buy a straight oil of corn, soybean, cottonseed, or safflower. Buy processed foods that state the kinds of fat used. Watch this on convenience foods and meals.

Read the fine print on the label to see what you are getting. If the label does not provide this information, write to the company about it.

Butter

Butter, a highly saturated, firm fat, was considered the best table spread among Europeans and Americans until an alternate was found in the form of margarine. Butter and margarine look alike and have similar flavor and food value, except that the vitamin A content in a pound of margarine is always 15,000 I.U. (International Units). The amount in butter may be more or less, depending on the feed of the cow. Butter costs more to produce and sells for more per pound.

CONTENT. There are no federal restrictions to prevent the addition of color and flavoring to butter and most butter has both added, though many people do not know this, for it is not stated on the label. It contains about 80 percent fat and may have 3 percent added salt. Some is unsalted. It is made from both sour and sweet cream. The remainder of butter is milk solids and water.

GRADES. The highest grade is AA, which is rated 93 points. U.S. Grade A is rated 92 points. The higher the grade, the higher the cost. Store butter well-covered, in the coldest part of the refrigerator, as it becomes rancid quickly when warm and exposed to air.

Margarine

Margarine, a man-made alternate for butter, is made by a process of hydrogenation (hī dräj ə nā′

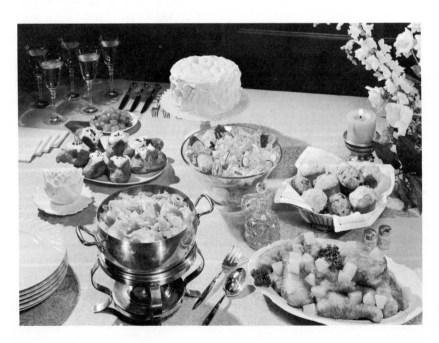

All these tempting dishes were made with safflower oil, which is highest in linoleic acid content.

shən). Margarine and hydrogenated shortening are made by heating vegetable oils under pressure in the presence of a metal catalyst (a catalyst, you recall, is an element that stimulates a reaction without becoming a part of it). As hydrogen gas bubbles through the vegetable oils, the double carbon bonds are forced open. Each takes on hydrogen. Thus a polyunsaturated oil becomes partially or completely saturated. In general, the firmer the margarine, the higher the degree of saturated fat in it.

SPECIAL MARGARINES. Research on fat and its relationship to heart-circulatory disease has prompted the manufacture of special margarines, called soft. In these, only a portion of the oil is hydrogenated. Then the firm fat is blended with pure vegetable oil. It is too soft to form into sticks, and is sold in tubs. The softer it is, the more liquid oil. Therefore, the word "soft" in the name of margarines has come to mean in the minds of many consumers "high in polyunsaturated fat."

One manufacturer produces three forms of margarine—regular, "soft," and "diet"—all with approximately the same percentages of the various fatty acids. This illustrates why the consumer must read the label and understand it, and not buy by a descriptive name alone.

The word "soft" appears in the name of five of the ten margarines recently studied by Peter Miljanich and Rosemarie Ostwald,* yet they vary in the amount of linoleic acid from 22 to 48 percent. One so-called soft margarine lists as its first ingredient "Partially hydrogenated vegetable oils," which means that there is more saturated fat in it

---

*Peter Miljanich and Rosemarie Ostwald, "Fatty Acids in Newer Brands of Margarine," *Journal of the American Dietetics Association*, Vol 56, No. 1, January 1970, p. 30.

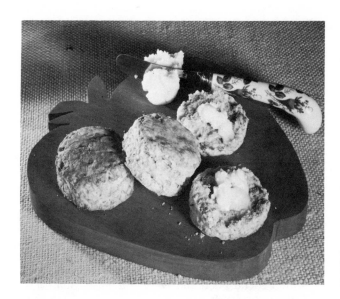

Soft margarine as a table spread is higher in polyunsaturated fat than butter. There is little difference in flavor.

than any other ingredient. Nevertheless, its label also says, "Low in saturated fat, ideal for low saturated fat diets." The names and the advertising, therefore, can be confusing to the purchaser.

One margarine in this study lists on its label "Made with liquid safflower oil, hardened safflower and cottonseed oils . . . Polyunsaturated." For the informed shopper, this means that the chief ingredient is liquid safflower oil, as it is listed first. Hence it is highest in linoleic acid. Since it takes about 2 tablespoons of safflower oil to provide the linoleic acid of 3 tablespoons of corn, soy, or cottonseed oil, for example, you can use one tablespoon less of safflower oil and save 125 calories from fat. Such information is significant for those who wish to increase their intake of linoleic acid and hold down their total calories from fat.

The shopper can decide which to buy on the basis of facts, not the advertiser's claims. The study reemphasizes the fact that we need to have a clear understanding of foods before we go to the markets.

"IMITATION" MARGARINES. Two margarines in the study were "imitation" margarines, meaning that they contain less than 80 percent fat. Both contain 56 percent water, and water is the first ingredient on the label. But these margarines are a boon for those who wish to restrict their intake of total fat and calories and at the same time enjoy a spread with a high ratio of linoleic acid in it. They should cost less.

MARGARINE STANDARDS. Margarine must contain at least 80 percent fat, a standard set by the Federal Food and Drug Administration. Most margarines also contain whole or nonfat dry milk, salt, and the required 15,000 I.U. of vitamin A per pound. Unlike butter, all ingredients are listed on the label with the largest amount first, and the others in descending order. This helps you acquire accurate information about the range of linoleic acid in margarines and to use that information to promote better health.

Hydrogenated shortening

Shortening, also made by hydrogenating vegetable oils, usually contains no color, vitamin A, or butter flavoring. It is spoken of as a plastic fat, being precreamed by whipping air in during hydrogenation. It is easy to mix with flour and sugar for baking. Chemicals are added to prevent oxidation and rancidity, to give moistness, and to increase volume. These are monoglycerides (män, ə glis′ ə rīds) and diglycerides—the same chemicals added to commercial bread as "softeners."

Lard

Lard, the fat from hogs, is about 40 percent monounsaturated and has almost four times as much linoleic acid as butter. It is also high in the essential fatty acid arachidonic, which hydrogenated fats do not have. It is the choice fat among chefs for the finest pastries and was the primary fat used in early America. It is soft at room temperature, but firm when refrigerated.

Lard and vegetable oils yield 125 calories per tablespoon, as compared with butter, margarine, and shortenings, which have 100 calories. About ⅞ cup of lard and vegetable oils equals a cup of butter or hydrogenated fats in baking, or about 2 tablespoons less per cup.

Cooking with fats

Acquiring skill in cooking with the type of fat you wish to use is the test of what you know. Look critically at the fat in your recipes. Experiment, using less fat than many recipes suggest. You can obtain excellent flavor in seasoning vegetables with less saturated fat and more imagination in the use of herbs. Since we all enjoy some foods that use high fat in preparation, let us consider cooking with fat and put into practice what we have learned.

Pastry

Pastries are highly desired by people around the world and involve the most complicated technique in cooking with fat. Pastries are a mixture of fat with flour, cold or hot water or cold milk, salt, and in some instances baking powder. These are discussed in Chapter 10. It is easy to learn to make delicate, tender pastry that melts in your

table 11–5 *Comparison of Fatty Acids and Calories in Common Foods**

	FOOD	MEASURE	SATURATED FATTY ACID		LINOLEIC (POLYUNSAT-URATED) FATTY ACID		OLEIC (MONOUNSAT-URATED) FATTY ACID	
			Grams	Calories	Grams	Calories	Grams	Calories
FATS	Margarine, soft	1 T.	2	18	4	36	4	36
	Butter	1 T.	6	54	trace		4	36
	Margarine, firm	1 T.	2	18	3	27	6	54
	Lard	1 T.	5	45	1	9	6	54
	Corn oil	1 T.	1	9	7	63	4	36
	Cottonseed oil	1 T.	4	36	7	63	3	27
	Soybean oil	1 T.	2	18	7	63	3	27
	Olive oil	1 T.	2	18	1	9	11	99
MEATS	Pork							
	bacon	2 slices	3	27	1	9	4	36
	roast, fresh	3 oz.	9	81	2	18	10	90
	Roast beef	3 oz.	16	144	1	9	15	135
	Hamburger, regular	3 oz.	8	72	trace		8	72
	lean		5	45	trace		4	36
	Steak, broiled	3 oz.	13	117	1	9	12	108
	Lamb roast, leg	3 oz.	9	81	trace		6	54
	Chicken, flesh only							
	(broiled)	3 oz.	1	9	1	9	1	9
	Veal breast	3 oz.	7	63	trace		6	54
	Salmon, pink, canned	3 oz.	1	9	trace		1	9
NUTS	Almonds, shelled	⅓ c.	2	18	5	45	17	153
	Peanuts, halved	⅓ c.	5	45	7	63	10	90
	Peanut butter	1 T.	2	18	2	18	4	36
	Walnuts, shelled	⅓ c.	1.3	12	12	108	9	81
OTHER	Milk, whole	1 c.	5	45	trace		3	27
	Milk, nonfat or skim	1 c.	0	0	0		0	0
	Egg, large	1	2	18	trace		3	27
	Avocado	1	7	63	5	45	17	153
	Bread	1 slice						
	white enriched		trace		trace		trace	
	whole wheat		trace		trace		trace	
	Corn muffin	1	2	18	trace		2	18

*Adapted from *Nutritive Value of Foods*, Bulletin No. 72 (Washington, D.C.: USDA, revised 1970).

Pastry made with vegetable oil is crisp, tender, and flaky.

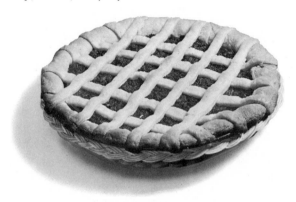

mouth, if you select a tested recipe and follow it accurately.

PASTRY WITH VEGETABLE OIL. Practically all the pastry you buy ready-made in convenient forms is made by the standard method with saturated fat. However, increasing numbers of homemakers want less saturated fat in the diet and use oil when they cook. A recipe for oil pastry is given in the Cookbook, page 437.

CRUMB CRUST. Crumb crust may be made to suit your taste and calorie need. This type of crust can eliminate most of the fat and calories, if you wish. Recipes for various crumb crusts appear in the Cookbook, pages 438–439.

Remember that if you use a tablespoon of soft margarine for one crust this yields 100 calories, as compared with 590 in the hydrogenated shortening used in the standard one-crust pie recipe.

HOMEMADE PASTRY MIXES. These may be made in dry form and stored in the refrigerator, with nothing to add but the liquid. Compare what it costs you to make a piecrust at home in the form you like, with what it costs to use the ready-to-make pastry mix. It is simple to make good pastry,

standard or puff. The basic method of mixing pastry and a recipe for a basic homemade pastry mix are given on pages 435 and 437 in the Cookbook section. Standard pie crust is also given in the Cookbook (page 437).

Deep-fat frying

Deep-fat frying is a world-favorite way of cooking some types of foods. When properly fried, such foods are highly satisfying. They are crisp and crunchy on the outside and, since hot fat seals in the juices, they are tender and delicate in flavor and retain vitamins and minerals. However, when

Foods fried in deep fat are tasty and satisfying. Southern fried chicken is one of the most popular dishes in America.

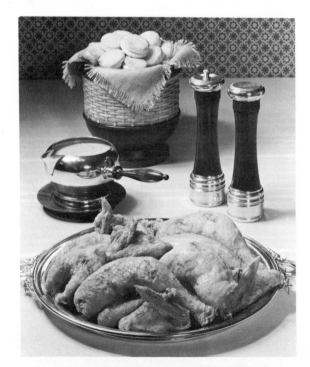

foods are sliced thin, as for potato chips, they lose vitamins. If blanched first or held in water in pieces, they lose vitamins, minerals, amino acids, and sugars.

However, fried foods taste so good that this method will continue to be used, at least on occasion. Therefore, if it is done at all, let us learn to do it well.

SMOKING TEMPERATURE. The smoking temperature of fats is important to learn. Butter and margarine have the lowest smoking temperature, and are not suited to more than sautéing. The smoking temperature of hydrogenated vegetable shortenings is 350° to 370°; lard is 360° to 378°; and oils, such as corn, 440° to 450°F. When a fat smokes, the molecule is breaking down and the food will have an unpleasant flavor. This is also irritating to the lining of the digestive tract. Discard fat that turns brown or smokes on being heated. The safe way to cook with fat in frying is to use a thermometer.

FATS IN SALAD DRESSINGS. These fats were discussed in Chapter 8 in connection with salads.

Storage of fats

All animal fats should be stored in the refrigerator. Hydrogenated fats have chemical additives to prevent oxidation and hence rancidity, but it is well to store margarines in the refrigerator, and also oils that are not promptly used.

Meaningful words

arachidonic
atherosclerosis
diglycerides
emulsion
glycerol
"hidden" calories
hydrogenation
linolenic
lipase
monoglycerides
monounsaturated fat
oleic acid
palmitic acid
"plastic" fats
polyglycerides
polyunsaturated fat
saturated fat
stearic acid

Thinking and evaluating

1. Which foods do you like best? Write down the foods you ate yesterday and today at meals and between meals.
   a. From these menus, classify the foods rich in saturated fats, then foods high in linoleic acid.
   b. Consult Table 11–4 on page 216 and make a list of "hidden" calories from fat in the foods you ate yesterday and today.
   c. Multiplying the number of grams in each food by 9, calculate the total calories you ate from saturated fat and those from linoleic acid (polyunsaturated fat). What did you learn that can help you?

2. What contributions does fat make to a well-balanced diet? What are its weaknesses?

3. What is the difference between a saturated and a polyunsaturated fat? Give examples.

4. Why is linoleic fatty acid so important in the diet? Give examples of how you would use it in each meal to increase its amount and decrease the amount of saturated fat.

5. Do you think it really matters to select one kind of fat over another? Why?

6. Explain what is meant by cholesterol. How does it function to help your life? When may it become an enemy? What foods are rich in it? Why does the body make cholesterol if it is cut too low in the diet? On the basis of what you have learned here and in Chapter 3, explain why an egg is desirable in the daily diet for a normal person. Why include some fat high in linoleic acid in the meal? Why might a person with heart disease need only three to four eggs per week?

7. How much fat do you need daily? On the basis of the record you made, how much fat do you eat? How many calories of fat were saturated? How many were from linoleic acid? Make a plan to improve, if necessary.

8. Explain how a girl can influence her own life and those of her future husband and children by knowing how to prepare and serve balanced meals using the best knowledge of fat we have.

Applying and sharing

1. Visit the market where you shop and in a notebook list the different kinds of fat and the price per pound of oils (usually sold by the quart, which is 2 pounds or 32 ounces), shortenings, firm margarines, soft or "special" margarines, and lard (usually sold by the pound).

    a. Using Table 11–1, list the percentage of saturated fat in each one; the linoleic acid; the cost per pound. Share with your family what you have learned.

    b. Do you need to change your habits as regards the kind of fat used in cooking? The amount? Your table spread? Why? Is your family agreeable to a change? Would it be wise for them to read this chapter?

2. Plan balanced menus for four days, lowering the total fat intake to below 40 percent of the total calories and using at least 50 percent of your fat calories in the form of linoleic acid.

    a. What meats would you use in meals? Which meat alternates? Why would you trim the visible fat from meats? Would you use all the meat for one day at one meal or divide it among all three? Why?

    b. How would you season vegetables? What type of spread would you use? Why?

3. **Cooking**—Make the following dishes and use them as part of a balanced meal:

    a. A one-crust pie using the type of crust and the kind of fat you consider best suited to your need.

    b. A two-crust pie made according to what you have learned about the use of fats in the preparation of pastry.

    c. One cup of French dressing for salads, using a vegetable oil high in linoleic acid; also variations from your favorite basic dressing.

4. Prepare at school at different times a balanced breakfast, dinner, and party refreshments, using the principles and procedures you have learned. Repeat this experience at home.

5. Using Table 11–2 on page 210, calculate the total calories, the calories from saturated fat, and the calories from linoleic acid in each of the following foods:

    a. Milk—3 glasses whole, 3 glasses nonfat, or buttermilk

    b. Vegetables and fruits—1 serving citrus, 1 serving green leafy, 1 serving yellow, 1 potato, 1 serving dried beans, 1 serving other fruit or vegetable

    c. Bread-cereal—enriched or whole-grain, 4 servings in desired form

    d. Meat, poultry, fish, eggs—2 servings of meat or 1 alternate, 1 serving of egg or alternate.

    Evaluate what you have learned by these calculations and explain how you would use this information.

sugar in a balanced diet

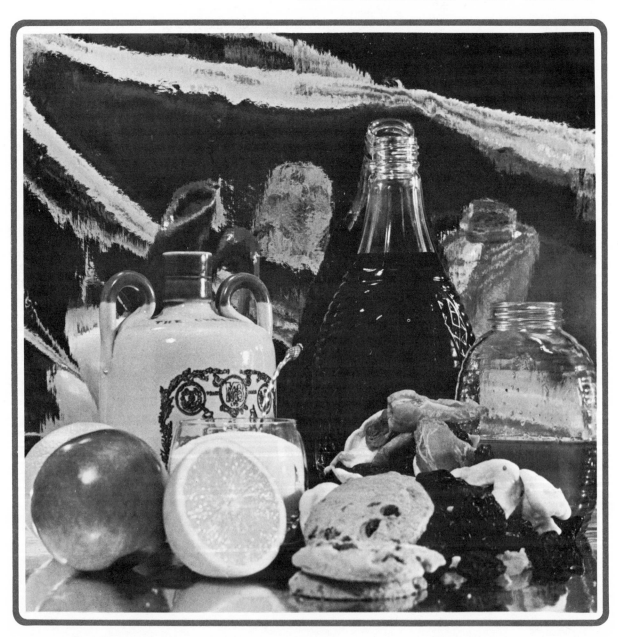

The use of sugar has increased during this century, until now the average American consumes about 225 cups annually. This amounts to approximately 420 calories a day from sugar.

Like fat, sugar is not grouped among the recommended foods in the Daily Food Guide. This does not mean that it is to be ignored. On the contrary, we need to understand its advantages and disadvantages, so that we may know its place in the diet.

Advantages of sugar

Taste

Sugar has a delectable taste. We enjoy and eat many fruits, some vegetables, and sweet milk for the appealing taste the sugar adds. With the exception of honey, it does not appear in concentrated form in nature. Thus the sugar we eat as it appears in foods naturally is in better balance for us. Primitive man chewed the canes for sweet juice. Sophisticated man boils the juice from cane, beets, and maple trees to make sugar, molasses, and syrups. These sweetening agents are added to foods to make them more tasty and emotionally satisfying.

We associate sugar (in sweet foods) with happy events—birthdays, weddings, Christmas, and other occasions. So do people in other lands. The Turks enjoy its flavor so much that they named their most sacred holiday Seker Byram (shā′ kär bī′ rəm), meaning Sugar Holiday. This takes place at the end of Ramadan, the month of religious fasting. Children are given candy. Families and friends visit one another and are served favorite cakes, candies, and other sweets, along with Turkish coffee or tea.

Energy source

Sugar is a quick and inexpensive source of energy. Along with starch, it helps the body build tissues and utilize fat. There are two types: single sugars, known as monosaccharides (män ə sak′ ə rīds)— glucose, fructose, and galactose—and double sugars, known as disaccharides (dī sak′ ə rīds)— sucrose, maltose, and lactose.

In digestion, starch and sugars are changed to glucose. Glucose is maintained at a constant level in the blood, though there is only a 10- to 15-minute supply in the bloodstream at any one time, and only about a 24-hour reserve stored in body tissues as glycogen (glī′ kə jən). When we eat more sugar than the body requires for immediate use as energy and for glycogen reserves, the excess is stored in the body as surplus fat. When the blood sugar is lowered, the glycogen is changed back to glucose. This was dealt with more thoroughly in Chapter 9.

Food sources

GLUCOSE. Glucose, also called dextrose, is widely distributed in foods. It is about 20 percent of the weight of grapes. Mediterranean people boil down the juice of grapes for sugar, in the form of syrup. It is abundantly present in fruits, plant juices, sweet corn, unripe potatoes, onions, and the blood of animals.

FRUCTOSE. Fructose, also called levulose, constitutes about one-half of the solid matter in honey and is widely found in fruits and plant juices. Glucose and fructose are the only sugars absorbed directly into the bloodstream.

SUCROSE. Sucrose is the sugar we get from cane, beets, sorghum, maple, and many root vegetables, such as carrots. Pineapple is rich in it. Sucrose is our table sugar and the one we use most in cooking. During digestion, sucrose yields one molecule each of fructose and glucose. This is expressed chemically as

$$\text{sucrose} \longrightarrow \text{fructose} + \text{glucose}$$

MALTOSE.   Maltose is found in cereal grains and malt products. It is rarely used in its pure form.

LACTOSE.   Lactose is found in milk, constituting 6 to 7 percent of mother's milk and 4.5 to 5 percent of cow's and goat's milk. It has the least taste of sweetness and is a healthful sugar for babies. It may be bought in pure form for formula-fed infants. In digestion, it yields three molecules of galactose and one of glucose:

Children and grown-ups alike prefer sweet snacks. Why should we avoid eating too many sweets?

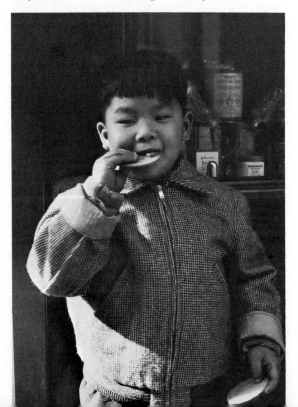

$$\text{lactose} \longrightarrow 1 \text{ glucose molecule} + 3 \text{ galactose molecules}$$

Most people think candy is the quickest source of energy. This is a mistake. The same steps are required in digestion for cane sugar as for milk sugar. Only fruit and vegetable sugars are immediately absorbed into the bloodstream as glucose and fructose.

GALACTOSE.   Galactose does not occur in natural food, but is an end product in the digestion of some sugars, such as lactose.

It is important to understand that the "quick lift" can be provided by foods such as fruits and vegetables, their juices, and milk, all of which also carry protein, vitamins, and minerals. By understanding the nature of sugar, we can see that it cannot substitute for other foods that contain protein, minerals, and other essential nutrients.

Disadvantages of sugar

"Empty" calories

Unfortunately, the calories in sugar are empty. They yield 100 percent energy, and nothing more. It follows that, if you derive a large share of your calories from sugar, you are likely to be poorly nourished. Young people should recognize this before they marry, for their own sakes and also for the sake of the children they may have.

The table of Nutritive Value of Foods in the Appendix shows that, while sweets in the daily diet give good flavor and high calories, they lack nutrients, and are thus empty.

Overweight is encouraged by a sweet tooth, which not only provides empty calories but also accumulates body fat that we don't want or need. Sugar then also becomes a foe, like fat.

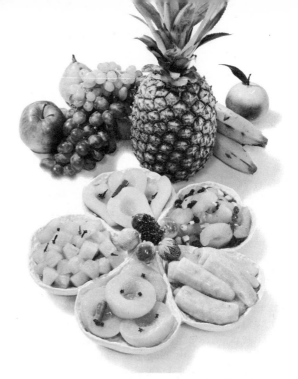

The amount of sugar we eat that is "invisible" is staggering. Who would believe that by our own choice we eat on the average over a half-cup of sugar a day? Many of these 420 calories are hidden in foods. The point to remember is that this is over a fifth of your total calories, if your daily need is around 2000.

What makes the high sugar content of the diet so serious is that:

1/You can add almost a pound of weight per week with 420 calories per day from sugar.

2/If overconsumption of sweets means being deprived of foods carrying nutrients you require, your good looks and good health are being undermined, causing you to "age" prematurely.

The same 420 calories now devoted to sugars could give you a balanced breakfast consisting of a whole orange, a slice of toast, a teaspoon of margarine, an egg, and a glass of whole milk—with about 17 calories left over.

Sugar and disease

DIABETES. Sugar contributes directly and indirectly to some diseases. Among these is diabetes. Hippocrates, the physician of ancient Greece, who is known as the father of medicine, noted the "sweet urine" of the diabetic in the fifth to fourth century B.C. Through modern physiology, we now understand the meaning of what he observed. The hormone *insulin*, secreted by the pancreas, enables individual cells in tissues to oxidize glucose and release energy from food. When there is not enough insulin in the bloodstream, glucose is not normally burned and blood sugar rises.

This is what happens in diabetes. So much blood sugar piles up in the blood that the kidneys are unable to pass it back into the bloodstream, and sugar is excreted into the urine. High blood sugar causes frequent urination, dehydration of body fluids and tissues, and deep thirst.

When diabetes is severe or long-standing, complications may appear, such as increased hunger because of the body's inability to utilize food normally; decreased resistance to infection and healing of wounds; and the accumulation of fatty acids in the blood, known as ketosis, which may result in coma or unconsciousness, cataracts on the eyes, or heart disease. Once fatal, diabetes can now be medically controlled. Major factors in this control are maintaining normal weight and regulating the diet. There are over two million diabetics in the United States, with 2500 deaths annually. It has been found that 75 percent of the diabetics treated were above the normal weight range. Diabetes occurs in all age groups.

TOOTH DECAY. Sugar contributes to tooth decay. The condition of the teeth of Americans is unbelievably poor. While there are many factors that lead to dental caries, poor choice of foods is a basic cause from conception on. It affects tooth decay directly through fermentation of sugar and formation of acids in the mouth, especially when sweets stick on the teeth.

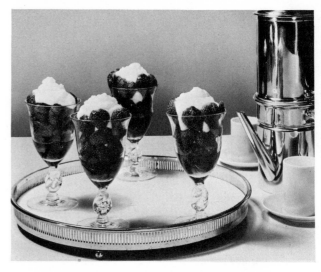

Fruits are the natural and desirable way to include sugar in the diet. Yogurt with berries is a satisfying dessert.

Studies show that about one-half of the two-year-olds in our country have at least one decayed tooth and that this reflects poor natural diet; 90 percent of the children up to six years of age have one or more decayed teeth. In 15-year-olds, the figure rises to 95 percent. It is unnecessary and undesirable that we "eat ourselves right out of our teeth."

Dr. J. H. Shaw of the Harvard School of Dental Medicine points out that the most successful way to achieve teeth with high resistance to decay is "by close adherence to a diet throughout tooth development that is ideal for the formation of caries-resistant teeth." Since the period of tooth development is prolonged, this objective cannot be realized overnight, but requires the same high standard of nutrition for years. We can't get good teeth by taking a vitamin pill. In preceding chapters we saw that a team of foods in balance is needed to do this job.

GASTRIC DISTRESS. Sugar eaten in large amounts at one time produces a feeling of over-fullness in the stomach. What is happening? Water is drawn from our body tissues into the stomach to dilute the sugar concentration. You recall from your courses in science the principle of osmotic pressure: a concentrated solution draws fluid into it from outside and tends to equalize the concentration on opposite sides of the semipermeable membrane (the stomach wall, in this case).

Sweets between meals raise the blood sugar on the one hand, and on the other, large amounts give a feeling of "fullness," thus dulling the appetite. This is what may happen to the meal skippers who snack on sweets between meals. Hence they deny themselves nutrients they require to build and maintain life on a high level.

Coronary heart disease is related to the type of carbohydrate in the diet, as was discussed in Chapter 9. Some research is showing that high sucrose in the diet may be one factor contributing to it.

It is possible that the change in American food habits to eating more fat, sugar, and protein with smaller quantities of vegetables, fruits, cereal, and milk results in a weaker diet, and poor nutrition.

Place of sugar in the diet

With this background, we can see that:

1/The desirable way to eat most of the sugar in the diet is as it occurs naturally in fruits, fruit juices, vegetables, cereal-breads, and milk and milk products that carry other nutrients we need.

2/The amount of sugar eaten in the day should be distributed among the three meals, rather than consumed in a large amount at one meal or as a snack.

3/We should learn to like cereal and fresh fruits with little or no sugar added and avoid presweetened cereals.

4/We should learn to enjoy dried fruits as an alternate for candy, because they carry valuable nutrients along with the fruit sugar.

5/A little sugar should be added to some vegetables to improve the flavor—for example, salads, carrots, peas, turnips, cabbage, coleslaw, collards, and summer squash (if a little sugar added makes the food taste better and makes you eat more vegetables, this is all to the good).

6/The time and place to eat a concentrated sweet is as dessert, after a good balanced meal. But remember to save a place for it, lest you add unneeded calories that end up as body fat.

We might return to the early American habit of reserving sweets for special days.

In breakfast

At breakfast, sugar is often used visibly on cereal or fruit or as syrup on pancakes and waffles, or as sweet spreads. Less visibly, it is used in coffee

Helping Mommy make cookies is a favorite "chore" for children. Why are homemade cookies better for them than the bought variety?

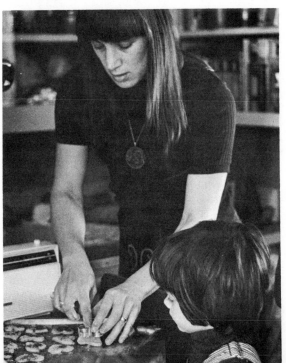

cakes, sweet breads, doughnuts, and the like. When overweight is your problem, you need not give up these sweets completely, but use them sparingly. A teaspoon of marmalade spread thinly over bread is tasty and adds only 18 calories.

Learn to analyze the calories in the sweets you eat. To find out how many calories are in a serving of a sweet bread for breakfast, set down the ingredients in the recipe. This you can do if you make it. Figure out the calories per serving by the method suggested in Chapter 2.

Here is an example of how much sugar you may use on pancakes, French toast, or waffles through syrup, a tablespoon of which has 60 calories from sugar. Pour the syrup into a measuring cup, use as much as you usually do, then record the amount you ate. This can add up to over 300 calories—all empty (unless you use dark molasses, a tablespoon of which has 45 calories and a few nutrients). Pancakes, waffles, and French toast are good foods. It is the large amount of fat and sugar syrup added that is undesirable.

In lunch or dinner

At lunch or dinner, have a sweet in the form of fruit, rather than concentrated sugar. If you have a sweet tooth, try a few dried dates. Dried fruit is a ready-to-eat sweet that teams up calories with nutrients. Fresh fruit is low in calories and a gourmet delight with cheese. Use light syrup or water-packed canned fruits and cut down calories from sugar by 125 percent. Custards and milk puddings have little sugar and are desserts containing essential nutrients. Angel food, sponge, and plain cake and gingerbread are all sweets with health values, as are deep-dish fruit pies.

At dinner, many people eat their big meal of the day, topped off with a sweet-fat dessert. The modern concept is to divide the nutrients and

At lunch or dinner, have fresh fruit for dessert. Or, for a low-calorie variation, make it into a pudding or pie using little sugar or fat.

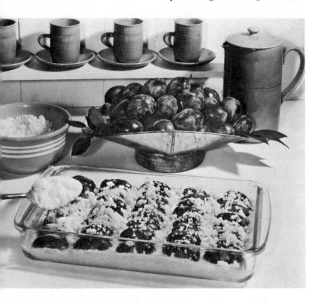

calories more evenly among the three meals and any snacks that may be eaten.

Have your favorite pie or cake when you have a low-fat, low-sweet dinner, such as baked beans, fish, or liver as the main protein, or a fish, meat, or poultry vegetable chowder. Thus we need not give up any food we enjoy eating, but can eat smaller amounts of it in balance for the meal and the day.

Table 12–1 illustrates how easy it is for one-half cup to one cup of sugar to "sneak" in hidden forms into the day's diet. By giving the daily diet informed thought, the consumer can control this intake, as Menu 2 indicates. Such thought prevents a gain of about one pound per week from sugar alone.

Cake and spaghetti are favorite foods of many, but they should not be served in the same meal. If you have one food high in sugar in the meal, such as candied sweet potatoes, serve a fresh fruit

or a low-calorie dessert. Sherbet, which is high in sugar, is usually thought of as low-calorie, but it has 130 calories in a half-cup serving, as compared with ice milk, which has 93 for the same amount.

Buying sugar

The table of Nutritive Value of Foods in the Appendix can help you see the different forms in which you may buy visible sugar.

Molasses

Molasses is 60 percent sugar, but dark molasses is a good source of iron and some B vitamins. The young homemaker today might return to the gingerbread or molasses cake of her grandmother for a satisfying, simple dessert.

Syrups

Syrups are available in many flavors and forms. If you like special flavors and are imaginative, make your own syrups and save money. For instance, boil one pound of brown sugar with a cup of water, adding maple flavoring at the end to provide a tasty substitute for much more expensive maple syrup. It takes little time to measure sugar and water and boil it. Syrups with "butter added" can also be made at home at lower cost, using the amount of soft margarine you need. Store the surplus in the refrigerator.

Read the labels on bottles marked "Maple syrup," to avoid paying a high price for a small amount of maple syrup mixed with sugar, water, flavoring, and coloring. The shape of some bottles is deceptive, but the weights give the accurate standards for determining the actual cost of the product.

Table 12–1 *Comparison of Added Sugar in Two Basic Menus*

1 tsp. Cane Sugar = 13 Calories

MENU 1 Food	Added Sugar (tsp.)	MENU 2 Food	Added Sugar (tsp.)
BREAKFAST		**BREAKFAST**	
Grapefruit, ½	2	Grapefruit, ½	0
Cereal, milk, sugar	3	Egg, soft boiled	0
Toast, spread, 1T jam	3	Toast, spread	1
Coffee, milk, sugar	2	Milk, 1 glass	0
		Coffee, black	0
Total	10	Total	1
LUNCH		**LUNCH**	
Baked ham sandwich	0	Baked ham sandwich	0
Sweet pickle	1	2 leaves lettuce	0
2 leaves lettuce	0	Milk, plain, 1 glass	0
Chocolate milk, 1 glass	3	1 banana, eaten from peel	0
1 sliced banana, cream, sugar	2	Cookie, med.	3
Cookies, 2 med.	5⅓	Total	3
Total	11⅓		
		SNACK	
SNACK		Lemonade, 1 glass	2
Cola-type drink, 1 glass	6		
		DINNER	
DINNER		Fried chicken	0
Fried chicken	0	Baked sweet potato	0
Candied yams	3	Frozen peas	⅓
Frozen peas	⅓	Green salad, dressing	⅓
Green salad, dressing	⅓	Raw apple	0
Apple pie	10	Milk, 1 glass	0
Coffee, sugar	2	Coffee, black	0
Total	15⅔	Total	⅔
Grand total	43	Grand total	6⅔
TV SNACK BEFORE BED		**TV SNACK BEFORE BED**	
Candy, 1 piece	7	Tangerine	0
Day's total (incl. snacks)	50	Day's total (incl. snacks)	6⅔
Total calories 50 × 13 = 650		Total calories 6⅔ × 13 = 86⅔	

Fruits retain their shape better when cooked in syrup. Syrups and molasses may also be used as a glaze for meats.

Cost of sugar

Granulated white sugar costs least per pound and maple sugar most, when compared with brown, lump, or confectioners' sugar, and also less than molasses, syrups, and honey. Lactose, the most expensive form of sugar, is purchased at drug stores for infant milk formulas.

Storing sugar

White sugar should be stored in a canister or jar with a tight lid. Brown sugar usually becomes hard

The Sally Lunn, a tea cake made in America since earliest Colonial days, uses very little sugar and is light and delicious.

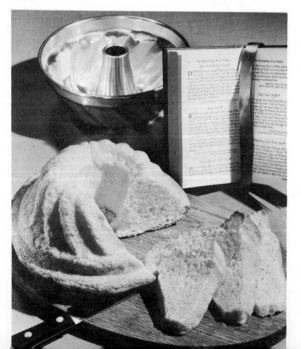

and dry when left in its box in a dry climate, unless it is kept in the refrigerator. It should be stored in a closed metal or glass container or with half a fresh apple added to retain moisture.

Commercial syrups may be stored on a cool pantry shelf. If a mold tends to form on top, the syrup should be stored in the refrigerator. Once opened, natural maple syrup should be stored in the refrigerator. Molasses and honey keep well on a cool shelf.

Use of preserved fruits in meals

Preserved fruit—jelly, jam, conserve, marmalade, and apple butter—is a popular spread on breads at breakfast or to accompany hot breads at any meal. It yields about 55 calories per tablespoon. It may be used as dessert with a hot bread. Here we have the pleasure of a sweet without weighting the day's diet with sugar and calories.

These products are also used to top a pastry tart, on breakfast sweet breads, in a jelly roll, as icing on a cake, as a spread on pancakes or waffles, or over pudding, yogurt, or ice cream.

Role of cakes

No one knows when the first cake was baked— probably back in history when the first crude earthen oven was invented and woman gave vent to her creative impulse to please those she loved by making a sweet treat. We still celebrate with a cake as our expression of love at a birth or a wedding, for an honored guest, or to express love and sympathy when sorrow comes to a family.

Cakes may be purchased in all sizes and in many varieties, including sponge, butter, and chiffon. The cake mix is one of the most popular

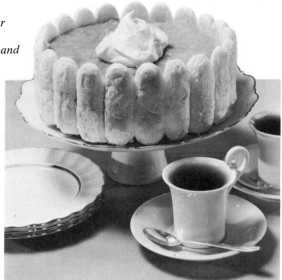

In this beautiful dessert, low-sugar ladyfingers form a crown around a mold made of vanilla ice cream and spiced canned applesauce.

of all mixes. The volume sold is so great that such a mix is not expensive. The mix is used by many homemakers who wish a cake to be warm and home-made in effect, but can't or don't wish to make one. But the hostess who can make a good cake from basic ingredients, without a mix, gets a loud round of applause from guests and family. When properly made, a cake is an artistic gem and a culinary delight. It is the symbol of the finest in cooking.

Sponge cake

Considered by some to be the most difficult, sponge cake is really quite simple and quick to make, once you understand the principles of

The basic butter cake recipe can be varied to produce many types of cakes. Cupcakes, frosted and topped with fruit and nuts, are especially appealing as holiday treats.

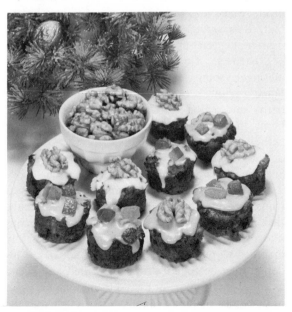

baking this type of cake and follow them. Sponge cake contains flour and sugar, but no fat and no liquid, except that of eggs and flavoring. Leavening is accomplished by incorporating air in the egg whites and producing steam by heat.

Angel food cake

This cake is just what its name suggests. It is made with only the white of egg, flour, sugar, salt, cream of tartar, and flavoring. One slice has a third more protein than a slice of bread, no fat, and only 110 calories. It is the ideal cake for weight watchers and those who need a low-calorie, low-fat diet to help prevent or control weight problems or cardiovascular disease.

A serving of sponge cake—one-twelfth of a cake eight inches in diameter—has 120 calories, 18 of which come from the fat in egg yolks. The egg yolk also adds iron, vitamin A, and thiamine, and the white carries the same amount of protein and riboflavin as does angel food cake.

With electric mixers and other excellent cooking equipment in our modern kitchens, you can successfully make a good cake, provided you have a good recipe and follow it accurately in every detail.

Butter cakes

Butter-type cakes differ from sponge cakes in ingredients and technique of mixing. Cakes using fat are usually layer, loaf, pound, or fruitcakes. Variety of flavor and appearance is achieved by using different types of pan, flavoring, fat, and sweetening or by adding fruits or nuts. The cakes typical of different countries are dissimilar because of the many possible combinations of these factors.

Ingredients for basic butter cakes include sugar, fat, flour, eggs, liquid, leavening agent, and flavoring. The flour may be cake, pastry, or all-purpose. The first gives a finer grain and smoother texture, but all-purpose flour works well when two tablespoons of the sifted and measured flour are removed from each cup specified in the recipe and it is more nourishing, as it is enriched, higher in protein, and less refined. The functions of each ingredient are described on pages 188–191 (Chapter 10).

Types of butter cakes

POUND CAKE.   This cake was popular before modern refrigeration, as it is simple to make, is tasty, and keeps moist a long time. It was originally made with one pound each of butter, flour, and sugar, with eggs and flavoring to taste. The eggs, heat, air, and steam leaven it and the texture is compact and smooth. Fruits and nuts added to this cake produce fruitcake. Pound cakes and fruitcakes are usually baked in oblong deep pans or round ones or any fancy shape that might express the esthetic tastes of the homemaker.

CHIFFON CAKE.   Chiffon cake is a combination of the butter cake and the sponge type and merges the fine quality of both in volume, lightness, texture, and flavor. Higher in calories and fat than the true sponge, it also has a wider variety of nutrients. When made with wisely chosen oil, it can contribute desirable linoleic fatty acid. Orange chiffon is the most popular and the flavor mellows when the cake is made a day or two before it is needed. It requires no frosting, only a simple dusting with confectioners' sugar, but an orange frosting gives it a festive appearance. It is delicious plain or with fresh fruit, ice cream, or ice milk.

TORTE.   Tortes, which are rich in eggs and nutmeats, are special cakes in middle-European countries. A torte has five to seven thin layers and looks like a cake. A filling of chocolate, lemon custard, fruit preserves, sour or whipped cream, or confectioners' sugar icing is spread between the layers. Since it is very rich, it is cut in small servings. It is served at teas and receptions, and as dessert at special meals.

COOKIES.   Cookies are miniature cakes— meringue, sponge-type, butter-type, or fruitcakes. Some are low in fat and sugar. Others are high in both—and calories. When you make them at home, they can carry a fair share of nutrients along with the sugar and fat.

Each country has its own specialty in cookies. Scandinavians have many tasty filled or bar cookies, as do the Swiss and Germans. Honey, dried fruits, and nuts are used in these. The Scots have their shortbread, a rich, sweet tea cake. Americans like a basic cookie dough that may be only slightly modified to produce many kinds of cookies. This dough may be rolled, dropped, chilled and sliced as an ice-box cookie, or forced from a cookie press in a variety of fancy shapes. The dough may be

Every country has its own cookie favorites, especially for Christmas.

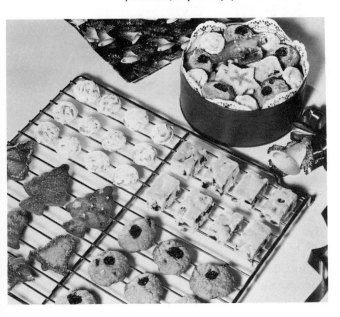

kept in the refrigerator and cookies baked fresh as needed, or they may be baked all at one time and stored in a tightly covered container.

Standards for cakes

The standards for judging a good butter cake are
Appearance: Rounded, smooth top
Color: Golden brown, unless a dark cake
Grain: Moist
Texture: Fine, with a velvety crumb
Flavor: Mellow and characteristic for its kind

Use of vegetable oil in cakes

The quick, or one-step method of making a butter-type cake saves time. Oils high in linoleic acid may be used as all or part of the fat. This is a modified muffin technique, but it requires more sugar than the standard cake. See the Cookbook for the basic recipe.

Storing cake

Cake designed for use the same day should be stored in a covered cake unit, but not in the refrigerator. Cake may be made and frozen several days ahead of time, if desired. This is good management for a party, for it helps the hostess avoid making all her preparations in one day. On the day of the party, the cake may be removed from the freezer and brought to room temperature. It may also be warmed in a low oven just before serving. A hot frosting may be added to give the flavor and appearance of a cake fresh from the oven.

Fruitcakes and chiffon, applesauce, banana, and all sponge-type cakes may be stored in the refrigerator and kept for more than a week. Fruitcakes "ripen" by standing in storage. If you warm this type of cake in a slow oven before serving, it tastes just like a fresh one.

Serving cakes

To serve a cake is an art in itself. An attractive cake on a pretty plate or cake stand may be used as a centerpiece. Think ahead and put on your bride's list for gifts a pretty cake stand, a cake knife, and a server. The cake plate may be the same pattern as your dinner service or a different, more elaborate one. Serve cake on a five- or seven-inch plate. A cake with frosting cuts smoothly if the knife is dipped in hot water and wiped before each serving is cut.

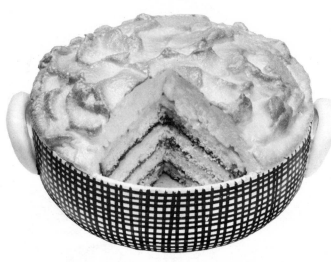

How to use leftover cake

1. **Fruit Melba:** Slice and place the cake on a serving plate, centering on it a half-peach, a slice of pineapple, and/or two apricot halves. Spread it with applesauce and top with ice cream or serve it with yogurt, sour cream, or milk.

2. **Ruth White's Quick Fruit Pudding:** Use applesauce, stewed rhubarb, or any drained cooked or canned fruit. Place one-inch cubes of cake—or slices—in the bottom of a pie pan or an oblong pan and cover them with the fruit topping. Add brown sugar lightly over the fruit and sprinkle with nutmeg and cinnamon. Heat under the broiler (being careful not to burn it) about three to five minutes, or until it is lightly browned.

3. **English Trifle:** Place fresh or canned fruit over pieces of cake in a fruit dish or parfait glass and top it with thin "boiled" custard. Add one teaspoon of sherry or rum over the top, if desired.

4. Toast slices of cake and top them with ice cream or fruit preserves.

5. Use the cake in puddings or mix it with dried, fresh, frozen, or drained canned fruit and top with yogurt, then more fruit, as a "yogurt short-cake."

6. Use the leftover cake as crumbs for Apple Brown Betty or other such puddings.

7. Use it as a crumb crust for a cream-type pie, laying the cake in slices or strips.

8. Reheat the cake in a pan. Sprinkle it with a small amount of cold water. Cover it tightly with foil and heat it in a low oven until it is moist, hot, and delicious. Serve it plain or topped with ice cream, fruit, and/or yogurt.

Candies and frostings

Crystaline candies and frostings

Well-made candy and cooked cake frostings are made by the same principles and are examples of the art of sugar cookery. The basic aim is to produce a fine, smooth crystal when liquid is cooked with sugar. Both need the same precautions and care in making. The major difference between fudge frosting and fudge candy is that the candy is cooked longer to a thickness that will cut and the frosting must be soft enough to spread before it firms. Penuche, pralines, and fondants are other examples of crystal-forming candy.

Noncrystaline Candies

Noncrystaline (amorphous, shapeless) candies are brittle, sticky, or both. They include caramels, taffies, toffees, caramel popcorn, and all types of brittles. They are made by melting all or part of the dry sugar until it is golden brown, but not burnt. Caramelizing changes the chemistry of the sugar and prevents the formation of crystals. Soda is added to increase the speed of caramelizing. Nuts or raisins may be added with the soda. Brittles should be spread quickly, for they harden rapidly.

In view of the recent research concerning sugar, showing it to be a less desirable type of carbohydrate than the starches found in vegetables, fruits, and cereal grains, many modern homemakers use unfrosted cakes. Therefore, the making of candies and frostings is given less emphasis than formerly.

Artificial sweeteners

During the '60's, sugar substitutes were being increasingly used by the manufacturers of beverages and various processed foods for persons desiring sweet flavor without calories. Many foods appeared on the market, aimed at diabetics and dieters. In 1968, for example, Americans consumed 500 million cases of low-calorie soft drinks. These drinks, and most of the other low-calorie foods, contained sodium cyclamate, a sugar substitute. The soft drinks alone used 17 million pounds of cyclamate!

For a time, it seemed that this artificial sweetener was the perfect answer to the sugar problem. However, tests on animals began to show undesirable results. The Food and Drug Administration became increasingly concerned because of the possibility of serious dangers to human beings from widespread and prolonged use of this substance, and in 1970 banned the use of cyclamates. Products containing these sugar substitutes were ordered removed from store shelves. The low-calorie foods appeared with the notation on the label "Sugar added." Exactly how much lower they were in calorie content than the regular product was not indicated on the labels.

Tests on saccharin, another sugar substitute, have indicated undesirable effects on the test animals and have led to a re-evaluation of its safety for human beings. At present, intensive research is going on concerning the entire question of sugar substitutes and their relative safety for human consumption. Probably new sugar substitutes will be developed that are acceptable for human use.

Meaningful words

artificial sweeteners
cyclamates
dental caries
diabetes
disaccharides
empty calories
fructose
galactose
glycogen
insulin
"invisible" sugars
ketosis

Thinking and evaluating

1. What contributions do sugars make to the diet? What are the disadvantages of too much? What is too much?

2. How does sugar differ from meat? Vegetables and fruits? Milk? Eggs? Cereal-bread? Fat? Which sweets do you like best? Least?

3. What is the most useful place of sugar in meals? What form of sweets do you consider best for snacks? Why? How would you try to train a child in regard to the eating of sweets?

4. Give 12 examples of "hidden calories" in foods. Why must one understand each?

5. Explain how sugar is used by the body. How is it stored in the body? In what form is all carbohydrate food circulated in the blood and used by the cells? Which is the only food that is 100 percent carbohydrate? Is this an advantage or disadvantage? Why?

Meaningful words

levulose
maltose
monosaccharides
osmotic pressure
polysaccharides
sucrose

6. Recalling the chapter on cereal-breads, what is the difference between starch and sugar? Complex carbohydrates and simple carbohydrates? Which are more valuable to you now? To a growing child? To a middle-aged or older person? Why?

7. Do you think Americans in general eat too much sugar? Do you? How do you account for this?

8. In terms of energy yielded, is sugar an economical food? In terms of nutrients, is it a dependable food? Explain your answer.

9. In what ways could beverages with sugar substitutes work to your advantage? Disadvantage? How would you use them in a day's diet?

Applying and sharing

1. Discuss with your family and friends what you have learned about sugar in relation to other foods.

2. Record all the food you ate yesterday and today and all the beverages you drank. Using Table 12–1, figure out:
   a. How many calories you got from concentrated sweets.
   b. How many of these calories were "hidden." How many were visible.
   c. The total number of calories; calories from complex carbohydrate foods and from sugars; protein in grams and calories; fat in grams and calories; milligrams of calcium and iron; milligrams of vitamin C, riboflavin, thiamine, and niacin; and I.U. of vitamin A you derived from each meal and snack, giving the hour of the day for each.

3. How did your diet compare with the one you kept for seven consecutive days at the beginning of this study? How did it compare with the recommended daily diet? Have you improved? Make a plan to improve your diet, if necessary.

4. Plan balanced menus for one week for a young couple on a low food budget to include enough sweets to satisfy your emotional needs but not so much as to unbalance the diet.

5. With a tested recipe, make one in each category of the following:
   a. Cakes—butter-type, sponge
   b. Cookies—roll, icebox, drop, bar
   c. Icing or candy
Show how you would use each as part of a balanced meal.

part ii

nutrition
and the
beginning of life

13

food-as life begins

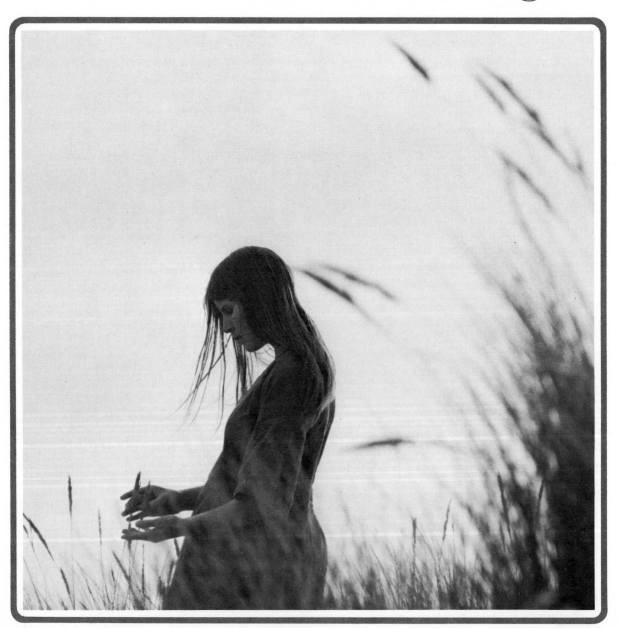

Most young people dream of the day when they will be the parents of a perfectly formed, healthy baby. We have long known the important role that heredity plays in making this dream come true. Only within the last few decades have we discovered that next to heredity, food plays the major role in the development of a healthy, well-formed infant.

The microscope was developed toward the end of the seventeenth century. But not until the 1960's was it possible to photograph the development of cells during the first six days of life and understand more fully, therefore, our biological beginnings.

How life begins

Life begins as two cells, the ovum (or egg) from the mother and a sperm cell from the father, unite to become one. Life is made possible through the food carried in the tiny egg cell of the mother—protein, vitamins, minerals, carbohydrates, and fats. That is why the egg is 85,000 times as large as the sperm which fertilizes it, though it is as tiny as the "fine point of a needle."

The ovum

From the time the menstrual period begins in a girl until it ceases at menopause, each month one ovum ripens in one of her two ovaries and is emitted. This occurs for some every 28 days and for others every 35 days or more. At birth, a girl's body contains approximately one-quarter million immature egg cells, some of which will mature and be released throughout her life.

The ovum has no locomotion, and for this reason nature provided the ovarian tubes (also called Fallopian tubes) with spongy, hairlike cells around the area where the ovum is emitted. These are in constant motion, drawing toward the Fallopian tubes, and there is fluid here and in the tubes. The egg is moved by means of this motion and fluid, so that 90 to 100 percent of the ripened eggs move into the tube toward the uterus. The ripened egg lives only 24 hours unless fertilized by the male sperm cell.

The sperm

The enlarged sperm cells (also called spermatozoa) are made in the testicles of the father. Nature so provided for the survival of the species that between 20 and 500 million sperm cells are available to fertilize the ripened ovum in one emission.

Unlike the egg, they can, by force of their large head and long tail, propel themselves like tadpoles, which they resemble when magnified some two thousand times. They move toward the egg at the rate of three inches per hour, A. C. Guyton reports. Though many sperm may enter the egg, only one—the first to reach the nucleus—can fertilize it. A sperm can live in the female genital tract from 24 to 72 hours but, like the egg, its span of life for fertilization is only 24 hours. The nucleus of the sperm is in the head, while that of the egg is in the center. If fertilization does not take place, these cells become as "grains of dust." But if the sperm reaches the egg, it burrows its head into it with the aid of a built-in enzyme. The content of the sperm is then thoroughly intermixed with the yolk or nucleus of the egg. When the fusion is completed, the two cells become one living cell. This cell now divides to form the nuclei of two new cells, and this is the remarkable beginning of life. Dr. Geraldine L. Flanagan, a noted embryologist, has described this moment as "zero hour of day one."

The genes

The hereditary traits from all ancestors on both sides of the family are carried in the genes which are in the nucleus of each cell. Sperm and ovum each contribute exactly one half of the hereditary traits. It is the genes that carry the architectural plan for the development of the baby and the "time clock," so that each different part develops at exactly the right moment, unless it is interfered with. Development is so precisely timed that, on seeing an embryo, an embryologist can estimate its age within one day.

It is remarkable that hereditary characteristics are set in the first half-hour of the new life: the color of hair, eyes, and skin; the potential height, shape of the face, and size of the head. Indeed, the potential intelligence, temperament, and a tendency to some kinds of disease come through the genes, though these qualities are also affected by environment.

Cell division

In 10 hours after the first cell divides, there are 4 cells, and 100 by the end of the first week, all held together in the original egg sac. As the new life grows, the content of the egg sac is used up as food. In about four days the cluster of cells, if viewed under a microscope, looks something like a berry. At about this time, the cluster arrives from the ovarian tube and attaches itself to the cozy inner lining of the uterus (also called womb). Here it will remain for the first nine months of nurturing and extraordinary growth. Usually the physician dates the prenatal age of the baby from the first day of the mother's last menstrual period. He adds nine months and seven days for the estimated time of delivery. The baby is now dependent on the mother's blood supply for its food and normal growth.

The father's contribution

Once the egg is fertilized, the father has made his biological contribution. In recent years, scientists have learned that it is the father who contributes the sex determination of the child. Incidentally,

Food plays an important part in the development of a healthy, normal baby.

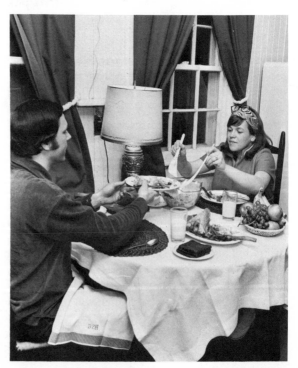

there are 106 male children born to every 100 females.

However, the father's contribution is not only biological. He has much more to give. We are learning that the emotions influence the ability of the mother to produce the balance of hormones needed for successful pregnancy. Her emotional condition influences her ability to absorb and properly utilize the nutrients from the food she eats. By providing his wife with love and security, the father contributes to a happy and emotionally well-balanced mother, and indirectly to the child they are expecting.

Another responsibility of the father is to provide a suitable home, necessary medical care, and the kind and amount of food required by the mother and the baby. At a recent Nutrition and Pregnancy Symposium of the Council on Foods and Nutrition of the American Medical Association, it was emphasized that the father should eat the same good diet as the mother. This helps her manage family meals more easily and helps both of them develop good eating habits for their own benefit and for the example they will thereby be setting for their children.

The mother's contribution

It is the mother's direct responsibility to supply nourishment for the normal development of the baby before birth. The ovum that the mother initially supplies is the largest human cell, mainly because it is stocked with microscopic bits of food for the first nourishment of life.

The embryo (the baby in its first eight weeks of life within the mother) cannot go far without the amount and kind of food and liquid it needs, for the genes cannot reach their full potential without good nutrition. Dr. Genevieve Stearns, Research Professor Emeritus in the Department of Orthopedic Surgery (former Research Professor of Pediatrics) at the University of Iowa, put it this way:

> The well-nourished mother can nourish her fetus well; therefore, the best insurance for a healthy infant is a mother who is healthy and well-nourished throughout her entire life, as well as during the period of pregnancy itself.

What happens if the mother fails to provide adequate nutrition?

At the Nutrition and Pregnancy Symposium referred to on this page, it was stated that "loss of human life in the newborn period is the third leading medical cause of death in the United States." This is a startling revelation. The symposium further disclosed that "Human and animal studies suggest that all defects enumerated here can arise from nutritional deficiencies." The defects referred to include problems of production (sterility, spontaneous abortion, premature or immature birth, stillbirth, toxemia, labor problems, and anemia of the mother during pregnancy and of the baby during the first year) and also "some neurological defects in children, the convulsive, mentally deficient, and so-called cerebral palsied may be related to nutritional factors."

Although there are other causes of these conditions besides nutritional deficiencies, the lack of any particular nutrient may produce different harmful effects at different stages of pregnancy. The time clock for the development of each organ and part of the body is set at the time of conception. Hence the expectant mother and her baby have an enormous advantage if she is continuously well-nourished.

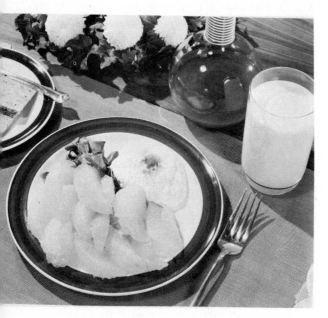

Cottage cheese, citrus fruit, wafers, and milk make a nourishing, simple lunch for an expectant mother.

Young mothers who begin with good eating habits and maintain them throughout the entire childbearing period of life have the best chance of producing healthy, strong, full-term babies. There is less chance of illness during pregnancy or after the baby is born, less loss of maternal tissues during and after birth. There is reduced trauma in the mother (shock from labor and delivery) and the baby will be stronger and better nourished as he begins life as a separate person.

The importance of a balanced diet for the expectant mother will stand out more clearly if we trace briefly the biological development of the baby and the rapid changes for baby and mother during gestation (the period of pregnancy).

Meaning of the first two months

The first two months of pregnancy are extraordinary. Usually a girl or woman does not know she is an expectant mother until she misses at least one menstrual period. By this time the embryo has already become firmly attached to the lining of the uterus, and is formed into a miniature of what the baby will one day be. This lining, called the endometrium, has soft, spongy cells, rich in blood and nutrients, to receive the new baby.

If no fertilized egg attaches itself to the endometrium, the lining separates from the uterus and is discharged in menstruation. After each menstrual period, the body sets to work to make a new lining. When the fertilized egg is implanted in the uterus, the menstrual cycle in a normal pregnancy ceases until after the birth of the baby. The "spotting" which may occur in the early part of pregnancy is a part of the body's effort to dispose of broken cells in the debris resulting from the establishment of the new life within the uterus.

Earliest development

As early as the ninth day, the embryo starts to take shape. A balloonlike capsule is built, forming a kind of shield around the cell-cluster which provides the "preliminary tissues for the whole body." The largest part of this shield is to become the brain.

In the third week of pregnancy, the baby's heart begins to beat. The brain divides into two lobes; future vertebrae and muscle tissue begin to border the spinal cord. The baby is now only one-tenth of an inch long.

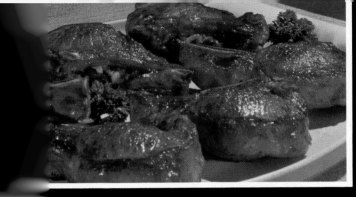

(left) Pork, properly coo[...]
succulent treat. (below)[...]
cottage cheese and fruit m[...]
refreshing and nutritious [...]
an expectant mother—lo[...]
calories, too.

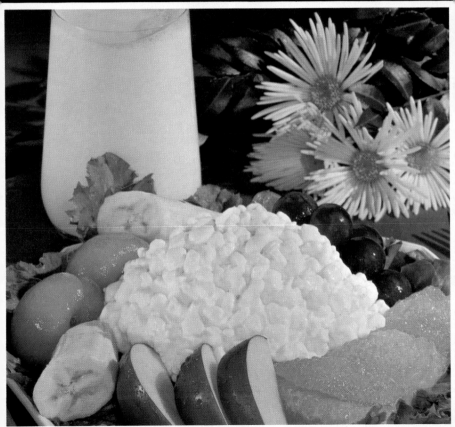

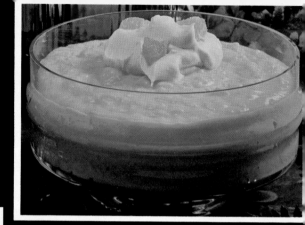

(right) *Rice is the base for many luxurious and delectable desserts.* (below, left) *Meat is one of the most valuable foods, particularly for an expectant mother and her developing child.* (below, right) *There is nothing "dated" about old-fashioned pot roast and noodles. It is a perennial favorite.*

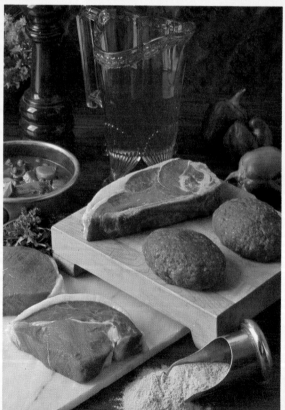

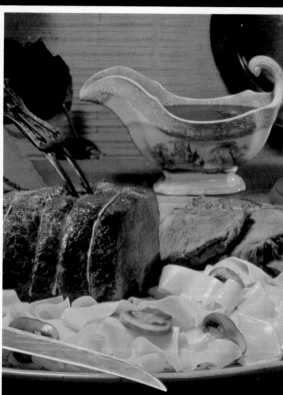

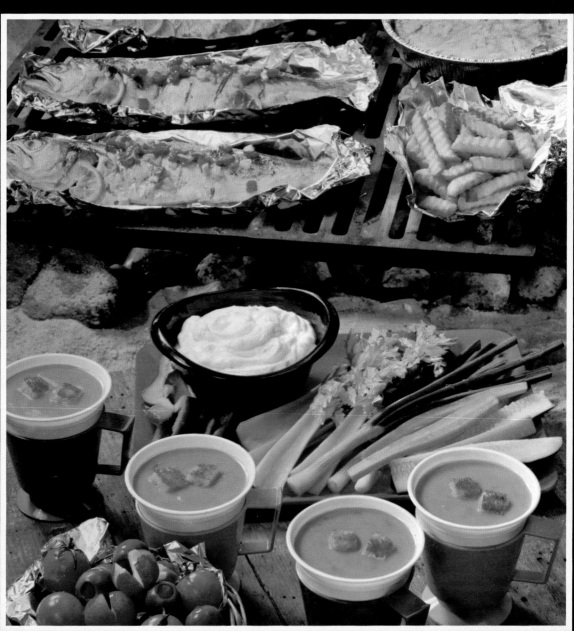

Baked or broiled fish is a piquant main dish of special value to a mother-to-be.

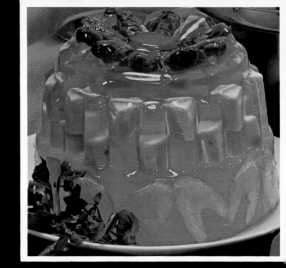

(right) *Molded gelatin salads are light, nourishing, and low in calories. They are useful in helping an expectant mother control her weight.*
(below) *A delightful change from the everyday menu is this shrimp and rice salad—crisp, eye-catching, and totally delicious.*

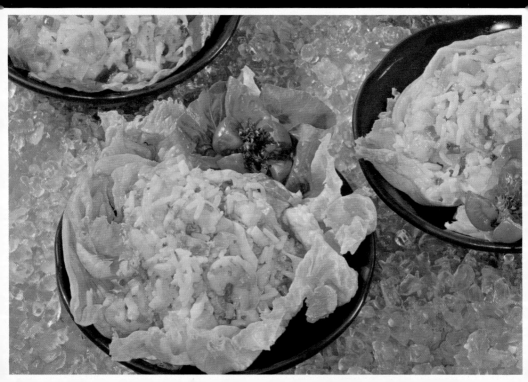

By the end of the first month, the baby is rapidly taking form, with a head, arm buds, simple mouth, eyes, ears, kidneys, digestive tract, brain, heart, bloodstream, and a crude umbilical cord through which food is brought from the mass of spongy, rootlike tissue covering the capsule. What is more, the heart beats about 65 times a minute!

It is now only one-fourth of an inch long, but ten thousand times larger than the fertilized egg. The thin, elastic membrane enclosing the developing baby is filled with a watery fluid. This has been called "the bag of waters," but is technically known as the amnion (am′ nē än), a Greek word meaning "little lamb." Lambs are often born enclosed in this membrane. There is a folk belief that a child born enclosed in the membrane (spoken of as *caul* or *veil*) is destined for a great life.

The seventh week

In the seventh week of life, the embryo becomes a small-scale baby, although it weighs only one-thirtieth of an ounce and is less than one inch long. It has skin that covers a rounded body. Baby teeth are set in the gums, fingers and thumbs have appeared, and the tiny body functions. The brain sends out impulses. The embryonic liver makes blood cells. The stomach produces some digestive juices. The kidneys take uric acid from the baby's blood to eliminate as waste via the mother's bloodstream. The muscles of the arms and body can move, but the mother cannot feel them.

Of this rapid growth, the embryologist G. L. Flanagan says, "When the embryo reaches such completion safely and without impairment, it has a good start in life. It is perhaps unfortunate that the existence of the incipient individual is still largely unnoticed and often unappreciated during the crucial weeks of the formation of the body."*

It is quite important that young people understand that the baby is formed in miniature before most women even know they are pregnant.

Between the forty-sixth and forty-eighth day of life, the first true bone cells appear in the upper arms to replace the cartilage. The embryo now becomes a fetus, which in Latin means "young one." Thus, in less than two months, the original two cells have grown into a living baby.

Why infections in the mother are to be avoided

In addition to poor nutrition, disease in the mother during the first two months may upset the gene pattern for normal development. For example, the virus of German measles can cause gross deformity in the particular part that is growing fastest at the time of the infection. Recent research has found a solution to this problem. Gamma globulin is being administered to young girls by injection, to give them immunity to this disease.

Radiation from X rays can reach the embryo and also cause injury. This is why many physicians avoid taking X rays of an expectant mother.

Maternal transfer system

The baby receives not only nutrients but also other substances that enter the mother's bloodstream, within an hour or two after she takes them. If she takes a drink of alcohol, he gets some. If she smokes a cigarette, he gets some nicotine. Large substances, such as protein and whole red blood, as well as most bacteria, are filtered out by the walls of the umbilical blood vessels. But smaller

---

*Geraldine L. Flanagan, *The First Nine Months of Life* (New York: Simon & Schuster, Inc., 1962).

substances, including the anesthesia used at child-birth, pass into the baby's bloodstream.

The mother's use of drugs may interfere with the normal formation of new life. This was illustrated dramatically during the early 1960's, when a tranquilizer called thalidomide became widely used in several countries. Many babies born to mothers who had used it in the early stages of pregnancy were found to have imperfectly developed arms and legs. The mother's drug had stopped the normal development of the fetus.

The filter-transfer system that created this situation has, however, some benefits for the baby. A major one is the transmission of the mother's immunity to certain diseases.

Function of the placenta

The placenta, so important to the life of a baby before it is born, is a powerful organ made of spongy tissue and a network of large and small blood vessels. You may have seen it presented in modern paintings as the "Tree of Life." The placenta is attached to the mother at the wall of the uterus and to the baby by the umbilical cord.

The mother's blood never directly enters the baby's body, nor does the baby's blood enter the mother's body. The placenta is the magnificent intermediary. It functions as adult lungs do, supplying oxygen from the mother's blood and removing carbon dioxide from the baby's blood. Through it the baby's waste is picked up and eliminated by the mother's blood. The placenta acts like an adult liver in that the mother's blood cells are processed and iron from them is made available to the baby. It also acts as adult intestines do: nutrients from the mother's blood are absorbed through the placenta into the baby's blood. And, like the intestines, it can process food molecules with the aid of digestive enzymes when the baby's own blood vessels pick up the nutrients. It even produces hormones.

To summarize, the placenta serves as (1) a storehouse from the mother's diet to meet the wide nutrient needs of the baby, but it can store only the food it receives; (2) a superb transport system between mother and baby, but able to transport only those nutrients that the mother provides; and (3) the medium for disposing of the baby's wastes.

The placenta expands from three inches in diameter at one month to eight at birth, at which time it weighs about one pound. Studies show that if the mother permanently lives at a high altitude, the placenta grows larger than normal to provide more oxygen. Although the prenatal baby uses very little, it can suffer from lack of oxygen even at lower altitudes if the mother for some reason is denied an adequate supply.

Function of the umbilical cord

During gestation

The umbilical cord is the baby's lifeline to the mother by way of the placenta. In the first stage of life, it is a short, stemlike connection; by birth it varies in length from five inches to four feet. The average length of the cord is two feet. It is a masterpiece of engineering. It has a closed blood system in which blood travels at the rate of four miles an hour. The force of blood is so great that the cord rarely becomes knotted or tangled. It takes only 30 seconds for the blood to make a round trip through the baby and the cord. Inside

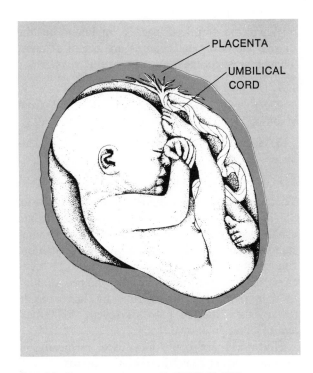

PLACENTA

UMBILICAL CORD

fig. 13–1 **HOW THE HUMAN FETUS IS FED**

the cord are two arteries which carry the used blood from the baby to the placenta. Dr. Flanagan points out that in the placenta "wastes are traded for sustenance" (nutrients and oxygen). Fresh nutrients and oxygen are carried back to the baby through a large blood vessel which enters his body at the navel, where the umbilical cord is connected. From this point, the baby's blood vessels take over, supplying each expanding tissue with fresh supplies of food and oxygen. At four months, the baby's heart pumps blood through his body—the equivalent of about 25 quarts a day. This amount increases to the equivalent of 300 quarts a day by the end of nine months.

At birth

At birth, the umbilical cord has completed its task of supplying vitamins, minerals, fat, proteins, and carbohydrates from the mother's diet or from her body reserves. Nature provides an automatic transition so that the baby's circulatory system becomes completely independent. This is done by a jellylike substance which for the months of intrauterine life has held the blood vessels in place in the cord. At birth, this jelly swells and closes off the connection between the child and the placenta.

After birth

Soon after birth, the umbilical cord is cut, leaving the greater length attached to the placenta. Cord and placenta are discharged together and are known as the "afterbirth." In parts of rural Nigeria, the cord and placenta are given ceremonial burial. Such a religious rite indicates that simple folk perceive the "almost holy" function of these two organs by paying special honor to that which sustained and promoted life in the child before birth.

Function of hormones

Hormones, themselves made from food, are closely related to every stage of successful pregnancy. They work as a team with enzymes, nutrients, and one another. Hormone secretions are stimulated by progesterone (**prō jes′ tə rōn**), which comes from the adrenal cortex and, during pregnancy, from the placenta. Progesterone signals other glands to get busy as a new life starts. One of the observable effects is the change that begins to take place in the breasts of the expectant mother.

A girl is made aware of the physiological and emotional effects of hormones by her monthly period. Estrogen from the ovaries signals the body to build a new endometrium each month after the menstrual period has discharged the old one from the uterus. The hormones especially concerned with reproduction are progesterone, gonadotropin (gō nad ə trōp′ in), and estrogen (es′ trō jən). Among other things, they regulate the nutrition of developing tissues. Today, an early test for pregnancy is the presence of gonadotropins in the urine.

The father helps both mother and baby by providing a secure and happy atmosphere during the gestation period.

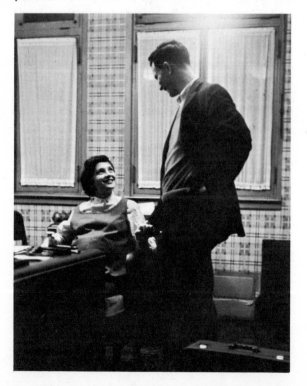

When the fertilized egg is implanted in the uterus, the hormonal changes are begun at once. These may affect the mother in several ways:

1/She may lose her appetite.

2/She may feel nausea and lose food from vomiting.

3/Her digestive system may seem out of balance.

4/She may lose weight.

There are also definite changes in her metabolism. She may retain more nutrients from her food than usual or she may lose more, according to circumstances and according to her health and nutrition. Emotions also have a great influence on this delicate balance. The mother can be helped or hurt by her psychological outlook, by her attitude toward the expected baby or toward its father, and by other emotional factors.

Hormones are sometimes used medically to maintain the endometrium in the uterus instead of having it slough off in menstruation; thus they aid in preventing a miscarriage in the early stage of pregnancy. In the first three months of pregnancy, hormonal secretions are key factors in helping each part of the baby's body assume its distinct form.

The thyroid gland, which regulates the rate of oxidation in cell tissues, increases thyroxin during pregnancy because of accelerated metabolism. The adrenal glands and ovaries also increase their secretions. It is the pituitary gland at the base of the brain that "masterminds" and coordinates glandular secretions.

During the fourth month, the placenta becomes the main source of hormones essential to the pregnancy and to prepare the mother for the production of milk. At the end of pregnancy, some hormones are decreased and others increased to help start labor and birth.

Growth of the fetus from three to nine months

The third month

As the third month begins the baby can easily fit into a cup. He weighs only one ounce, but he can turn his head, kick, frown, curl his toes, make a fist, move his thumb, press his lips together, open his mouth, and swallow amniotic fluid. Though he practices inhaling and exhaling, he doesn't drown in his "bag of water," because oxygen is supplied to him through his mother's blood via the umbilical cord.

In the third month, a period of refinement begins that continues until birth. The eyes come closer to the bridge of the nose. By the ninth week, the eyelids close over the eyes. He does not open his eyes till the sixth month. The baby now has working digestive glands, taste buds, and saliva-producing glands. He can urinate sterile urine, which is carried away through the placenta; he can digest the nutrients in the fluid he swallows from the amniotic sac; and his first teeth begin to form. The ribs and vertebrae start turning to hard bone, requiring more calcium and vitamins A, D, and C from the mother's diet. Sex differences are more clearly defined. The mouth fills out and the face is prettier. The bony plate dividing the mouth from the nose is now fused together. If the fusion fails at this time, the baby has a cleft palate and sometimes harelip. You recall in your study of riboflavin in Chapter 5 that riboflavin deficiency in lower animals causes these conditions. Unfortunately, they are frequently found in people in developing nations where the diet is inadequate and to a lesser degree in our own country.

The second trimester

THE FOURTH MONTH. In the fourth month, rapid growth begins. Length increases to about eight to ten inches and the baby weighs about six ounces, which is a big gain over the third month. The baby needs more food, water, and oxygen. With the aid of digestive enzymes, the placenta processes more food from the mother's blood. It begins to synthesize immunity substances (globulins) to protect the baby from infection. In the fourth month, the heart functions. The fetus is a self-contained functioning system, but dependent on his mother and not ready to live in our world outside.

THE FIFTH MONTH. In the fifth month, the baby is a foot long and weighs one pound. He begins to grow eyelashes and fringe of hair. His bones harden. Nails form on the fingers, then the toes. Muscles grow stronger. The latter part of the fourth month or beginning of the fifth, the mother feels the first flutter of life. The heartbeat is strong enough now to be detected with a stethoscope—two heartbeats, if the mother is to have twins. The baby moves when awake and follows a sleep pattern from which he can be aroused by vibrations of the mother's body or by loud sounds.

THE SIXTH MONTH. This is a month for further refinement of the body. The baby grows about two inches and gains 26 ounces in weight. His grip is strong enough to support his weight. He can maintain breathing and, if born prematurely, has a chance of living as an incubator baby, but he would not live well. His digestive and respiratory systems are not mature enough at this time to perform normal functions. Many expectant mothers do not realize that the food they eat determines the quality of the "baby teeth," and that during the sixth month the buds for the permanent teeth are already set in the jaws behind the "milk teeth."

The third trimester

The third trimester—the seventh, eighth, and ninth months—is the period of greatest growth. The baby gains most of his prebirth weight, usually five pounds or more. His organs are sufficiently formed to permit him to live if born prematurely. He is quite lively inside the amniotic sac, where he has lived much like a spaceman in weightlessness. The fluid reduces now, giving him more space in which to grow. If he is born at this stage, it is more difficult for him to carry on his normal development than in the sheltered body of his mother. He grows hair, gets the hiccoughs, and perfects his sucking ability. Some babies suck their thumb so much before birth that they have a callus on it!

TOWARD THE END OF THE EIGHTH MONTH. At this point he snugly fills up his space, having only enough room to turn from side to side, and he settles into the head-down position for normal birth. His body takes on a padding of fat just beneath the skin to ease his birth and to insulate him from the harsh temperature change he will experience then.

IN THE NINTH MONTH. During the first three weeks, the baby adds more weight and lays down a reserve of iron in his body. All twenty of his baby teeth are formed just as they will be when they erupt, and they are almost completely enameled. He acquires additional antibodies which give him immunity to the diseases his mother has had or for which she has been effectively vaccinated (such as measles, mumps, whooping cough, chicken pox, scarlet fever, poliomyelitis, some strains of streptococci, influenza, and even the common cold). The *gamma globulin* made by the placenta helps protect both baby and mother from contagious diseases during the last three months. These antibodies are not perfect protection, but a full-term baby is better protected than a premature one. At birth, he gains added protection from the mother's milk, even the first watery colostrum.

Regular exercise is important during pregnancy.

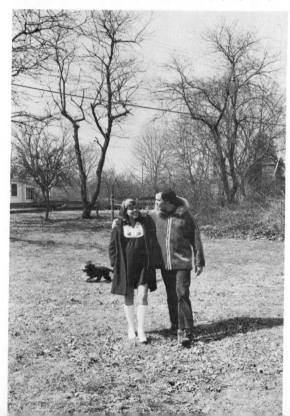

The entire family can enjoy a barbecue meal like this one, which is especially good for a mother-to-be.

The Rh factor, so named for the rhesus monkeys that were used in the study of this problem, is one kind of antibody that can cause trouble. When a girl with Rh-negative factors marries a man with Rh-positive blood and becomes pregnant, their baby may have Rh-positive blood. The mother's body may then manufacture antibodies to combat these Rh-positive factors. This problem usually does not develop with the first child and may not arise with others. Should trouble occur, new drugs are now on the market, enabling the physician to take measures to help both mother and baby. In some cases, a complete transfer of blood may be performed on the baby at birth.

THE END OF THE NINTH MONTH. The baby and mother are now ready for his entrance into the world. The placenta is now old and ending its usefulness. It is said that the placenta goes through all the changes of a human lifetime in nine months. The aging placenta is one signal to the body for birth. Hormones secreted into the blood produce a more elastic, pliable uterus and birth canal that help start labor and birth. It is thought that progesterone, which inhibits uterine contractions, decreases toward the end of pregnancy and that estrogen, which increases contractions, is produced in much larger amounts at the end of term.

The word "labor" is well-chosen, for birth uses energy. In the first part of labor, studies show that the muscles in the upper part of the uterus exert pressure equal to 55 pounds on the baby each time they contract. The pressure usually breaks the amniotic sac. With the rhythmical uterine contractions, the water is released at once or gradually, according to where the rupture is located. The pressure pushes the baby, building up to a "force equal to the weight of nearly one hundred pounds" when the baby's head emerges.

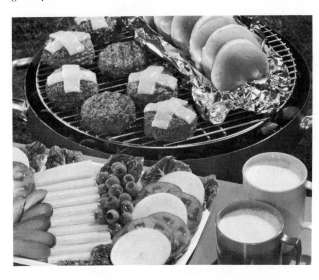

How eating habits can help the expectant mother and her baby

To form a perfect baby from two tiny cells to a strong, healthy infant ready to live and function well after birth requires good eating habits on the part of an expectant mother. Here are some of the reasons:

1/A balance of food is needed to enlarge the uterus from about the size of a finger until it is big enough to hold a 6- to 9-pound baby 19 to 21 inches long. Dr. Ray Hepner has found that the length of the baby is a better measurement of true growth and good nutrition than weight, which has been our yardstick in the past. An "average" baby is 20 inches long and weighs slightly over 7 pounds.

2/A balance of high-quality nutrients is needed to build and maintain the constantly changing placenta.

3/The mother must provide sufficient iron to (a) build a complete blood supply for her baby so that he can live an independent life; and (b) lay down reserves of iron in the baby's body to last about four months after birth because milk, his first food, is low in iron; then (c) supply enough additional iron in the diet to avoid becoming anemic either during pregnancy or afterwards, and (d) build up a reserve to protect her from any undue loss of blood at delivery.

4/She must provide the nutrients required to build the "bag of waters" and maintain fresh fluid in the amniotic sac as the baby grows. The umbilical cord that connects the baby to the mother by way of the placenta must be made and maintained.

5/An adequate diet is essential for enlargement of the breasts and ability to breast-feed the baby.

6/It is the nutrients from the mother's food that build the entire structure of the baby, including the heart, muscles, brains, bones, baby teeth, buds for permanent teeth, hair, skin, muscle tissue, and all the organs, glands, and blood supply at birth.

Thus, from the one-cell life at the beginning, the baby grows to two hundred million cells and from a microscopic fertilized ovum to weigh six billion times more—and all from the food his mother supplies. If she doesn't eat what he needs, he takes nutrients from her body reserves. If they are not available in either her food or her own body tissues, the baby suffers the consequences before birth and afterwards.

Preparing for motherhood

"When," you ask, "is the time for a girl to start preparing for motherhood?" The answer, as you have seen in this chapter, is that, if you are a girl, you have started already.

Indeed, a girl starts preparing for motherhood when she is born. Some of the things that happen in our lifetime cannot be changed, but there is much that we can do for ourselves and our children by managing our food needs intelligently from this point on. This makes it especially important for a young girl to understand why she needs good eating habits at the earliest age possible, long before she starts her family, and why she should learn to eat the right kinds and amounts of required foods each day. One who does this is rewarded twice, in her own good health and that of her child. Indeed, it is both a responsibility she owes her child and an endowment that only she can give.

Meaningful words

abortion (miscarriage)

afterbirth

amnion

cell nucleus

colostrum

embryo

embryology

Thinking and evaluating

1. In what ways are prospective mothers handicapped by the "secrecy" surrounding discussion of the growth of life before birth?

2. What is the basic concept to remember about taking care of the prenatal baby's nutritional needs?

3. What responsibilities can and should the expectant father take in looking after the needs of the expectant mother and their baby?

4. What happens if the expectant mother fails to provide in her diet adequate nutrition for herself and the baby? Do you consider

Meaningful words

endometrium
estrogen
Fallopian tube
fetus
gestation
gonadotropin
heredity
immature birth
intrauterine life
labor and delivery
ovaries
ovum
pituitary
placenta
premature birth
progesterone
Rh factor
sperm, spermatozoa
"time clock"
umbilical cord
uterus (womb)

it important for an expectant mother to have good nutritional reserves? Explain.

5. Describe the first two months of pregnancy.

6. In what way or ways do the substances that enter the mother's bloodstream affect the baby? Give examples.

7. What is the function of (a) the placenta, (b) the umbilical cord, (c) hormones?

8. Describe the growth of the fetus from three to nine months.

9. How would you summarize the role of nutrition in the beginning of life?

Applying and sharing

1. Discuss with your teacher the possibility of inviting an outstanding Doctor of Medicine in your community to speak to your class (or Department) on the subject "The Expectant Mother and Her Baby."

2. Discuss with your teacher the possibility of having a simple Mother and Daughter Tea. For the occasion, ask an outstanding woman in your community to talk to you on a topic of your choosing, such as "The Art of Preparation for Motherhood."

3. As a class project, you might prepare an exhibit of pamphlets and other readable material on prenatal care to share at a P.T.A. meeting.

14
a balanced diet
for the expectant
and lactating mother

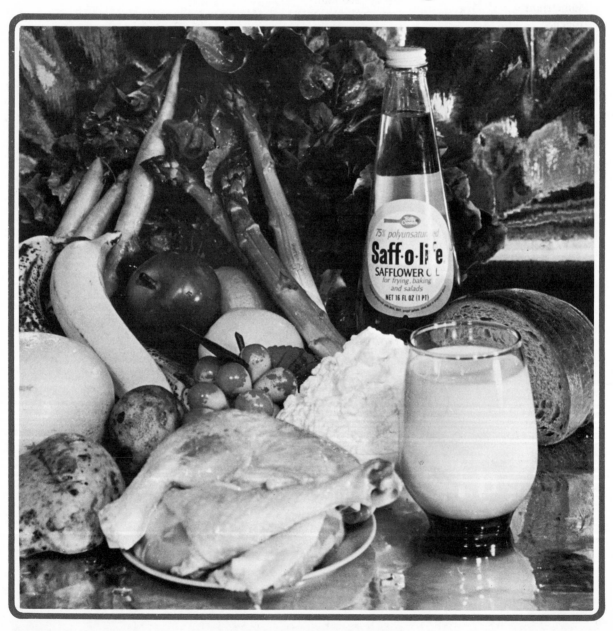

Healthy, well-nourished girls and women sail through pregnancy with no complications. It is natural for a healthy woman to produce full-term, healthy babies. The growth in our knowledge of the important role of good nutrition and the advances in medicine and prenatal care all increase our ability to prevent possible complications of pregnancy that may occur and to cope with those that do occur.

Importance of teen-age diet

In 1967, of all babies born in the United States, 605,038 had teen-age mothers. This figure[*] underscores the need for each school girl and boy to understand not only how life begins, but also the importance of a balanced diet for young people.

Before marriage, three major factors contribute to the poor eating habits of many young people: (1) the desire on the part of the girl to be slender, (2) the tendency to eat the foods that others in the same age group make popular, and (3) the general lack of understanding or disregard of nutritional information. All too frequently, the wife has a poor background and preparation for the responsibility of providing the nutritional needs of a family. In addition, the husband often comes to marriage with strong food prejudices and poor eating habits. These are the major stumbling blocks to the improvement of the mother's diet or that of her family. They can seriously affect the future health of the entire family group.

---

[*]*Vital Statistics Report*, Vol. 17, No. 9, December 1968, p. 4, and *Statistical Abstract of the U.S.*, 1969, p. 50.

How emotional climate affects nutrition of the expectant mother and her baby

An environment in which the young mother-to-be can have peace of mind must be created. Long experience has demonstrated what goes into a healthy "climate" for motherhood. The affection of those we love—a major need we each feel throughout life—is much more important for the girl during pregnancy. She particularly needs the affection of the man she has chosen as her companion in this greatest of all adventures, parenthood.

Illegitimacy

Illegitimacy is a subject discussed among close friends, but generally veiled from the public and often from parents. Of the births in 1967, it is estimated that 151,300 of the babies born to girls 19 years of age or under were illegitimate. This is about one in four. Statistics give us a cold and disturbing picture of this large and gradually increasing number of illegitimate births to teen-age girls. They do not show us the psychological, economic, and social stresses of the girl who is left to bear the child outside of marriage.

EFFECTS OF EMOTIONAL STRESS. At the University of Iowa College of Medicine, Dr. Genevieve Stearns and her associates made extensive studies which show that emotional stress in an expectant mother affects the nutritional state of mother and child adversely. They studied one group of girls and women 13 to 30 years of age who were illegitimately pregnant. It was found that those who were emotionally stable and who ate a well-balanced diet could absorb and retain "more nutrients than were needed by the fetus.

Girls from the poorest nutritional backgrounds were able to retain as much as girls whose nutritional background had always been good."

On the other hand, emotionally disturbed expectant mothers showed loss of nutrients with each disturbing influence. The girl who was most emotionally disturbed over her condition continually lost calcium from the diet, instead of absorbing it. The loss doubled the amount needed by the fetus. And she lost other nutrients that "left her body with a serious deficit."

Remember that it is the emotional disturbance, not the pregnancy, that causes an expectant mother to fail to absorb and retain nutrients. A girl who is emotionally disturbed is in a poor condition to have a strong, healthy baby or to come through well herself.

Longstanding good eating habits help an expectant mother. She feels well and transmits the needed nutrients to her baby.

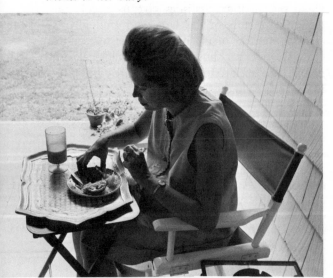

Two other groups of pregnant girls were studied. These studies show how good eating habits of long standing help an expectant mother. The first group had been eating an excellent diet for at least the previous four years. The second group had only a fair diet, but each did have three glasses of milk daily. Both groups were then given a series of increasingly good diets. What were the results? It took five months for the girls with previously poor diets to utilize the nutrients as well as those who had previously had good eating habits. "We had expected the opposite," Dr. Stearns comments, adding, "Adolescent girls greatly need to study nutrition."

Effect of diet on the expectant mother

Russian World War II study

How important the diet of the mother-to-be is for the baby was made abundantly clear during the siege of Leningrad, from August, 1941 to January, 1943. A. N. Antonov reports that in 1942 the birthrate fell strikingly and stillbirths (babies born dead) doubled during the last half of 1942. Premature births increased to 41.2 percent of the total live births; 9 percent of the full-term infants and 31 percent of the premature ones died as newborn babies. The full-term babies that did live "had conspicuously low vitality, suckled poorly, and had low resistance to infection," he observed. The mothers of these babies had had poor nutrition for a long time prior to the siege and there was a serious food shortage during the siege. A mother living under these conditions could not provide for the needs of the growing baby before birth, either from food or from her own body reserves.

fig. 14–1 **PERCENT OF IMMATURE BABIES BORN TO MOTHERS*** (to age 29, New Jersey, 1963)

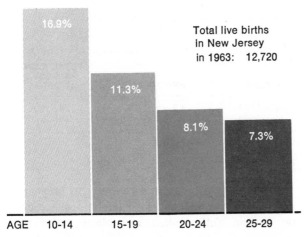

Total live births in New Jersey in 1963: 12,720

| AGE | 10-14 | 15-19 | 20-24 | 25-29 |

16.9% — 11.3% — 8.1% — 7.3%

*SOURCE: Unpublished figures from the Department of Health, Public Health Statistics Program, Trenton, N. J.

British World War II study

By contrast, there was a great drop in the number of stillbirths in the British Isles. This was ascribed wholly to improvement in the diet of pregnant women. During World War II, the British eliminated white bread and only whole-grain bread was available. They rationed sugar, allowing only one pound per person per month. The previous consumption of sugar had been about 10 pounds per person per month. Nutritionists were placed in charge of the whole nation's diet and never has the country had such a healthy crop of babies, despite the emotional stress it was undergoing. "After 1942, the rates for prematurity, congenital debility (malformations at birth) and birth injury (such as spastic condition) fell markedly," the study revealed.

While all pregnant women in Great Britain at that time showed improved nutritional status, those who had had the poorest diets for a long period before the war made the least improvement.

Diet and heredity

In a study in Aberdeen, Scotland, Dr. A. M. Thomson found that girls who are well-nourished grow to the full height that their heredity permits. But girls poorly nourished in childhood tend to be stunted and do not have as good health. This study covered 3500 women who gave birth to their first babies. Thomson found that there were fewer premature births and fewer deaths of newborn babies among those born to mothers 5 feet 4 inches tall or taller than to mothers who were 5 feet 1 inch tall or shorter.

Some U. S. studies

In a similar study in the United States, B. S. Burke found that "all of the stillborn infants, all of the neonatal deaths but one, all of the premature infants but one (and it died as a newborn baby), all of the functionally immature infants, and most of the congenital defects were found in the group of infants born to mothers with 'poor' or 'very poor' prenatal diets. Since no major effort was made to change the dietary habits of these women, it is probable that in the majority of cases the prenatal dietary rating was representative of long-time food habits." In follow-up studies, covering second pregnancies of the same group, it was revealed that, if the mother's diet had improved, so had the condition of this baby. But if her diet was worse than it had been during her first pregnancy, the condition of the second baby was also worse, indicating a relationship between the mother's diet and the health of the unborn baby.

The National Institute of Neurological Diseases has made a study of 55,000 mothers who gave birth to about 60,000 babies over a period of six years. One general conclusion arrived at was that

When a young mother-to-be is emotionally secure and happy, and eats a nutritionally sound diet, she is less susceptible to various complications of pregnancy.

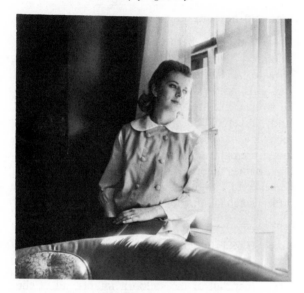

a poor diet on the part of the mother was the single most important cause of many birth defects and a lower predisposed intelligence.

Complications of pregnancy related to diet

Anemia

Anemia, a common condition during the whole or the latter part of pregnancy, is often due to iron deficiency. It is very unlikely that anemia will occur in girls and women who enter pregnancy in a good state of nutrition and who continue eating a well-balanced diet with a good supply of iron-rich foods. On the other hand, babies born to anemic mothers often lack sufficient iron reserves. This results in infant anemia. A full-term infant has about double the amount of iron in his body as a premature one. (See Table 14–1).

table 14–1   Iron in Premature and Full-Term Infants*

INFANT	WEIGHT AT BIRTH	TOTAL IRON IN BODY AT BIRTH
FULL-TERM	3.3 kg (7.25 lbs.)	242 mg
PREMATURE	1.5 kg (4.95 lbs.)	122 mg

*Irving Schulman, "Iron Requirements in Infancy," Infant Nutrition Symposium 7, Council on Foods and Nutrition, American Medical Association, 1959 (adapted from table p. 51).

Another form of anemia common to pregnant and lactating women and their infants is macrocytic anemia (also called megablastic anemia), which is due to a deficiency in folacin (folic acid), a vitamin in the B family. (See Chapter 7, pages 137–138, for a discussion of the role of folacin in the diet.) In this form of anemia, the red blood cells are too few in number and much too large. They also contain too little hemoglobin. Treatment with folic acid can cure this condition.

Toxemia

Toxemia is a condition that sometimes develops in pregnancy. While the cause is not known, it is associated with (1) high blood pressure, (2) a rapid gain in weight, (3) edema (the retention of water in tissues, which accounts for a large part of the gain in weight), and (4) albumin, a protein in the urine, which is not normal. The advanced stage is spoken of as eclampsia (e klam(p)' sē ə). This is marked by convulsions and possibly coma.

B. S. Burke and his associates found that, among the pregnant women in their studies, not one who ate a good or an excellent diet had toxemia. On the other hand, 44 percent of those on poor and very poor diets and 8 percent on fair diets developed it.

It has been noted that this condition is prevalent among excessively overweight women, especially those whose weight has been gained during pregnancy. When a poor diet was supplemented by good-quality protein and increased vitamins, less toxemia resulted.

More recently, research indicates that salt restriction may not be as important in treating toxemia as was formerly supposed. W. F. Mengert found no difference in the progress of the disease when 48 patients who definitely had toxemia were on a high salt diet or on a low one. M. Robinson, in a study of more than 2000 pregnant women, half of whom had a lower salt intake and half a high salt intake, found less toxemia in those who had the higher salt intake. There are other factors to consider, however. These include a detailed study of the patients' nutritional condition prior to pregnancy and the diet during it.

Morning sickness

Morning sickness is the name often given to nausea or vomiting that sometimes occurs in pregnant women on getting up in the morning. It is often among the earliest symptoms of pregnancy. When it occurs, it is during the period when the baby is attaching itself to the mother's body and the first adjustments are taking place. There are great hormonal and tissue changes in the mother's body at this time. If nausea or vomiting persists, medical guidance is needed.

One theory is that the carbohydrate stored in the liver (glycogen) is used up during the night by the embryo, leaving the mother with a shortage of carbohydrate. If she refuses to eat breakfast because of fear of nausea or vomiting, the shortage becomes more acute. A better regimen is to be quiet, instead of moving vigorously, and to eat a

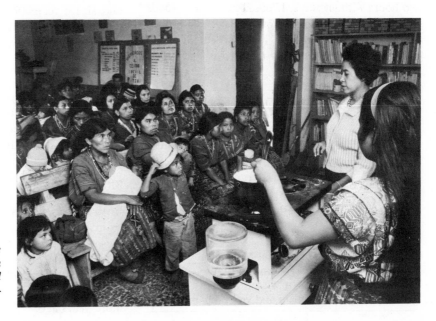

Nutrition classes teach these Guatemalan Indian women how to improve their lives and ensure healthy, normal children.

simple breakfast of cereal, fruit or fruit juice, and milk. Frequent small meals are preferable to three large ones during this period. Tests show that even dry toast taken before arising helps prevent nausea. Juices and milk may be drunk at intervals, rather than at mealtime. Rich fatty or fried foods, pastries, rich desserts, and highly seasoned foods should be avoided.

Pernicious vomiting

Pernicious vomiting—the type that is severe and persistent—can lead to serious nutritional disturbance and requires medical attention. Vitamin B_6 is effective in relieving the symptoms for some and, in a few cases, intravenous feeding of glucose with a mixture of vitamins and other nutrients is prescribed.

The high carbohydrate-low fat diet is fed every two hours without skips. If possible, favorite foods should be included and those disliked should be avoided during this period. The food eaten should be of the type that is easily digested.

EXAMPLES OF MEALS FOR
PERNICIOUS VOMITING

1.

CEREAL WITH MILK AND SUGAR
DRY TOAST WITH JELLY
CRACKERS WITH JELLY
TOMATO JUICE

2.

MEAT BROTH (all fat removed)
BAKED POTATO (without fat)
PLAIN RICE WITH MILK AND SUGAR
PLAIN GELATIN (or fruit and vegetable purée)

If the expectant mother is vomiting severely, she needs liquids and vitamin therapy, at the doctor's direction. Other foods should be added gradually, until a balanced diet is resumed. Small amounts of liquid taken frequently are usually tolerated. Dehydration must be avoided. All food, solid and liquid, is given cautiously under competent medical supervision.

Constipation

Constipation is frequently found, especially during the latter stage of pregnancy, among those who have not established good eating habits. This can be controlled in most cases without the aid of laxatives, provided one eats a well-balanced diet with plenty of bulky vegetables and fruits and whole-grain bread-cereal. Also recommended are regular exercise, such as walking; sufficient rest and sleep; recreation; adequate amounts of fluid daily; and freedom from unusual stress or tensions.

Edema

Edema is one symptom that can be partially or completely controlled by diet, if there is no toxemia. Such a diet, often referred to as salt-free, is actually a low-sodium one.

Birth defects

Birth defects have for centuries been surrounded by mystery. Anthropologists have unearthed drawings on clay rocks in the Middle East showing dwarfism and other birth defects, including those affecting the mouth, nose, ears, hands, feet, shoulders, and sex organs dating from 4000 or more years ago.

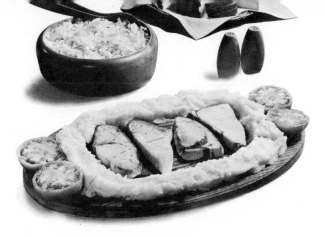

What would you add to make this a sound, nourishing meal for an expectant mother?

Dr. Lucille S. Hurley of the University of California at Davis* reported that "Most of the malformations recorded in these tablets appear to have been based on careful observation, and (the same defects) can be seen today in nurseries or children's hospitals. . . . Today . . . birth defects loom as one of the major health problems. For example, the percent of infant deaths due to congenital malformations has shown a steady increase . . . since 1910. But not all congenital malformations are fatal; they often produce a living but handicapped child. . . . In the infants' ward of a large children's hospital, it was found that over a period of five months, more than one-third of the children were in the ward because of structural congenital malformations. . . . Today it is recognized that congenital malformations can be caused by genetic factors, by radiation, by viruses . . . by drugs and **by other environmental factors such as nutrition.**"

Weight control and normal gain

Some girls and women fear retaining fat after pregnancy. This causes no anxiety for those who understand the meaning of a balanced diet and know how to manage their meals and snacks. Many a well-nourished, emotionally happy girl or woman "blooms" into a more beautiful person when she is expecting a baby. This is a time when she takes especially good care of herself.

---

*Speech at the meeting of The American Home Economics Association at San Francisco in 1966 on "Nutrition and Birth Defects."

Caloric intake

The calorie allowance per day is increased by only 200 during pregnancy, and only from the beginning of the fourth month on. The calorie intake is increased by 1000 per day during lactation; the baby, in turn, uses up these calories for rapid growth.

The normal weight gain during pregnancy is from 16 to 24 pounds. These extra pounds gained consist mainly of the increased size of the uterus; the breasts (about double in size), which prepare the mother for breast-feeding the baby; the placenta; the extra fluid in which the baby floats; the extra blood for mother and baby; and the weight of the baby.

Rate of weight gain

Research has shown that it is best for the gain in weight to be gradual during the first six months, for there is less likelihood of premature births or toxemia under these conditions. A greater frequency of premature births was found when there was severe loss of weight during the first three months. It is extremely valuable for a girl to be aware of this before pregnancy and this is an incentive to establish good eating habits while young.

The concept to remember is this: an expectant mother should gain weight gradually and not lose weight unless she is advised to do so by her physician. The mother can return to her normal weight after the baby's birth, provided she eats wisely during pregnancy and afterwards.

table 14–2 Daily Balanced Diets for Pregnancy and Lactation

| FOOD | | PREGNANCY (Depends on Age) | | LACTATION* (Depends on Age) |
		NORMAL +200 2200 Calories	LOW-CALORIE* 1800 Calories**	NORMAL +1000 3000 Calories
		MEASURE	MEASURE	MEASURE
MILK		1 qt. whole, vitamin D-fortified	1 qt. whole, vitamin D-fortified	1½–2 qts. whole, vitamin D-fortified
MEAT, FISH, POULTRY	(Liver and sea-food at least once per week)	4-6 oz., lean	4 oz., lean	6 oz., lean
EGG		1 whole	1 whole	1 whole
VEGETABLES	(Include dark green leafy or deep yellow, potato, others— 1 raw)	At least 4 servings	At least 4 servings, succulent	At least 4–5 servings
FRUIT	(2 or more serv-ings citrus, 1 other)	3 servings	3 servings	3 servings
BREAD-CEREALS	(Whole-grain or enriched)	4 servings	4 servings	4–6 servings
BUTTER OR MARGARINE	As spread	3 teaspoons	3 teaspoons	1–3 tablespoons
OTHER FOODS	To meet calorie need	Desserts, vegetable oil to season, fruit juices		Other foods desired from recommended group and desserts. Avoid fats, rich and concentrated sweets, highly seasoned foods

*Low-calorie and lactation diets should be supervised by a physician.
**Can be reduced by 300 calories by substituting 1 qt. skim milk for whole milk and taking vitamin A supplement under physician's directions.

Underweight

Underweight, when severe at the beginning of pregnancy and when it continues during pregnancy, is as serious as overweight, for it hurts both the mother and the baby. A physician can determine whether the cause is disease and, if so, can treat it. Sometimes it is due to a false concept of what is beautiful in a figure. If excess slenderness is achieved at the price of malnutrition, it can be corrected by a balanced diet with a larger calorie intake, which will help the expectant mother to attain normal weight.

Underweight may be caused by psychological factors, such as depression and inability or unwillingness to eat a balanced diet. Foods rich in protein of good quality, high in vitamins and minerals, as well as higher caloric content, are needed when the expectant mother is excessively underweight.

All expectant and lactating mothers, regardless of their weight, should be sure to provide balanced and nutritious food for themselves and their babies. The recommended daily dietary allowances for expectant and lactating mothers is given in the Appendix, pages 446–447, and shows optimum quantities of the various important nutrients.

Nutrients required during pregnancy and lactation

Protein

The protein allowance is increased by 10 grams daily for pregnancy and 20 grams during lactation. The mother is building a baby, every cell of which contains some protein and constantly demands more. While she is pregnant, she is not only constructing cells of the fetus, but must also develop new tissues in her own body to take care of the baby and to serve her during pregnancy, delivery, and lactation. The rapidly growing infant requires protein, which he obtains from the mother's milk if she breast-feeds him.

The main point to remember is this: the expectant mother should have a generous amount of animal protein divided about equally among her meals, and some between meals, if she eats snacks. The latter should be foods that she needs for building and for balancing the diet, if she wishes to control her weight at a normal level. How can this be done with regard to protein? Let us analyze the protein content of the 2200-calorie diet pattern given in Table 14–2.

FOOD	PROTEIN (Grams)
1 quart of milk	36
1 egg at breakfast or lunch	6
1½ oz. tuna fish or	
3 T. peanut butter at lunch	12
4 servings of bread-cereal	8
4 servings of vegetables	8
3 servings of fruit or juice	3
3 oz. lean cooked meat, fish, or poultry	16–20
Total daily protein	89–93

This generously meets the need for protein during pregnancy and lactation.

Fortunately, by taking some protein from the different food groups, one can at the same time meet one's need for other nutrients and for the bulk needed to keep elimination normal. By using the tables in this book which present foods rich in the different vitamins and minerals, it is an easy matter to plan menus with variety at any cost level and at the same time please the taste of the mother-to-be and that of her family. In addition, she and her family will be getting an excellent diet.

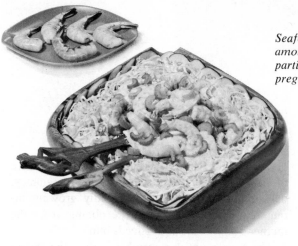

Seafood supplies generous amounts of iodine, which is particularly important during pregnancy and lactation.

Minerals

Minerals are quite important for the expectant mother and her baby. When one gives thought to the minerals that are likely to be low in the diet—calcium, iron, and iodine—it is now simple to devise delicious menus to provide them and others.

CALCIUM. Deficiency of calcium depletes the mother's reserves and starts premature aging. In severe deficiency, the bones may soften and become misshapen. It can affect the length of the fetus. You recall that body length is now considered a more important yardstick for measuring the new baby's status of nutrition than weight. Milk in any form supplies plenty of calcium and phosphorus, but must be teamed with vitamins D, C, and A, amino acids, and other substances to build the bony structure of the baby.

IODINE. If the diet is deficient in iodine, simple goiter sometimes results because of the extra demand on the mother during pregnancy, and even more during lactation. Iodine is easily available in seafoods of all kinds and in iodized salt.

IRON. The menu on page 267 (Table 14–3) shows one day's meals that provide a low-calorie balanced diet with the recommended amount of iron daily during pregnancy and lactation. Such meals help prevent anemia in the mother and the baby.

The total iron for the three meals adds up to 20.2 milligrams. With a total calorie count of 1480, this leaves a margin of 320 calories on the low-calorie diet and 720 on the normal diet for pregnancy, to be filled in with selected foods, such as snacks of fruit or fruit juice between meals and fresh fruit and milk at bedtime. By exercising ingenuity and an understanding of foods, the expectant mother can plan many types of appetizing meals which will provide a similar balance of nutrients and exciting flavors.

Vitamins

VITAMIN D. The vitamin D requirement is 400 I.U. daily during pregnancy and lactation. It is important for the absorption of calcium and phosphorus from the digestive tract and for the laying down of these minerals to build the skeletal frame and the future teeth of the baby.

VITAMIN A. Vitamin A is essential for life and for the formation of the epithelial cells that line every organ, gland, and membrane inside the body of the baby and maintain those in the mother. When we realize the many body processes in which vitamin A is involved, the importance of having the mother's diet provide the extra 1000 to 3000 I.U. daily is obvious.

VITAMIN C. The intake of water-soluble vitamins should be increased. Vitamin C is involved in the life processes of every tissue and 10 to 20 grams more is needed during pregnancy and lactation.

THE B VITAMINS. It is not difficult to provide the many B vitamins for their interrelated roles. They are increased when the recommended variety of foods is eaten.

The balance in each meal means the combination of minerals, vitamins, protein, and other nutrients to provide for normal development of the baby and to maintain the expectant mother's

table 14–3   *Balanced Menu for One Day Providing 20.2 Milligrams of Iron and Low Calories* *

BREAKFAST			LUNCH			DINNER		
Food	Iron mg	Cal- ories	Food	Iron mg	Cal- ories	Food	Iron mg	Cal- ories
1 egg	1.1	80	2 oz. ham	1.6	135	3 oz. pot roast, beef	2.9	245
1 slice whole-grain			½ c. cooked spinach	2.0	20	1 potato	0.7	90
bread	0.8	65	1 raw tomato*	0.9	40	½ c. peas	1.5	58
½ grapefruit	0.5	45	¼ head Boston			½ head Boston		
1 t. soft margarine	0.0	33	lettuce	1.1	8	lettuce*	2.2	15
1 glass skimmed milk	0.1	90	1 slice enriched bread	0.6	65	1 slice enriched bread	0.6	65
			1 t. soft margarine	0.0	33	1 t. soft margarine	0.0	33
			½ c. dried apricots,			½ cantaloupe	0.8	60
			cooked	2.6	120	1 glass skimmed milk	0.1	90
			1 glass skimmed milk	0.1	90			
	2.5	313		8.9	511		8.8	656
Day's total calories: 1480**								

*Add 2 tablespoons of safflower oil or 3 tablespoons of corn, soybean, or cottonseed oil as salad dressing or seasoning during the whole day to provide linoleic fatty acid. This will add 250 calories from safflower oil or 375 from the others.
**Add foods desired to meet the day's total calorie need.

health on a high level. Two other vitamins, E and K, should be mentioned, for they have an especially important role in pregnancy.

VITAMIN K. Vitamin K is not found in the list of nutrients essential for life and likely to be too low in the diet. Further research may disclose new roles for this vitamin, which has been called the coagulation vitamin, for it is indispensable for the normal clotting of blood. It is therefore essential for a normal pregnancy and delivery, as well as for recovery afterwards.

Human babies are born with no vitamin K reserve. That is why many hospitals give vitamin K to the mother just before delivery or to the infant just after birth. Mothers who eat a balanced diet will have enough of this vitamin, as it is widely distributed in foods, especially liver, leafy green vegetables, tomatoes, cauliflower, soybean oil, and egg yolk. Under proper conditions, a small amount is synthesized in the intestinal tract.

In some types of liver disease, when bile salts are not formed, vitamin K is not absorbed from the intestinal tract into the bloodstream, for bile salts must be present to aid this vitamin in absorption—another example of teamwork in the body's use of food. Vitamin K may be deficient when diarrhea or other intestinal diseases are present.

VITAMIN E. Sufficient research has been done on vitamin E to warrant its inclusion in the 1968 Recommended Daily Dietary Allowances (see pages 446–447). While more research is needed, we already know that it is helpful in producing a normal pregnancy.

It is worth noting what research has revealed about this vitamin in studies of animals. The white rat was used for the first experimental studies. When the pregnant animal did not have enough vitamin E in her diet, the placenta failed to function properly, the fetus died, and spontaneous abortion occurred. When vitamin E was provided in the diet, the same mother completed a successful pregnancy with normal, healthy young.

Another experiment showed that male rats with insufficient vitamin E became sterile in 75 to 100 days, owing to injury of the sperm-forming structure. It was not possible to restore male fertility once this injury had occurred.

Then an experiment was performed on the young. Newly weaned animals were placed on a diet deficient in vitamin E. In three to four months on such a diet, their hind legs became paralyzed. The feeding of vitamin E at this time could stop further injury, but could not repair the harm already done.

When sheep, goats, calves, and other large animals ate a diet deficient in vitamin E, their skeletal muscles degenerated. Cattle died of a heart ailment.

In human beings, vitamin E unites with oxygen inside the body to prevent blood-destroying elements from attacking red blood cells, studies reveal. It is also known that vitamin E combines with oxygen to spare the oxidation and hence the destruction of vitamin A, and also to prevent oxidation and rancidity in fats.

What is being learned in these and other scientific studies brings home to us the fact that **many human ailments are nutritional at base.** More knowledge is needed of vitamin E. However, enough is known to show its value in preventing and treating various ailments and some use has already been made of it in treating spontaneous abortion, cardiovascular disease, and muscular degeneration.

In food, vitamin E is found in the germ of whole wheat and also in wheat-germ oil, corn oil, cottonseed oil, milk fat, butter, eggs, liver, and green leaves of plants. If you eat these and other foods recommended for a balanced diet, you are likely to have enough vitamin E.

Meaningful words

congenital debility
congenital defects
eclampsia
edema
neonatal deaths
pernicious vomiting
stillborn
toxemia

Thinking and evaluating

1. What are the advantages and disadvantages of having teen-agers take on the responsibility of parenthood? In your judgment, is it a help to understand and practice good eating habits before getting married and starting a family? Give reasons for your answer.

2. In discussing the young mother's nutritional needs, why is it desirable to consider her emotional needs? Name some of these needs. On what is your answer based?

3. What would you consider the ideal conditions for having your first baby? Which of these conditions could you give up without emotional stress? Which could you not give up?

4. It has been said that illegitimacy puts the burden of both parents on the girl. Is this statement too severe? If so, in what way? How may illegitimate parenthood have adverse effects on the mother or the child? How may it hurt the father, now and later?

5. Which nutrients are required in larger amounts for the expectant mother? The lactating mother? How much of an increase in these nutrients is needed for each?

6. What has research revealed about weight gain during pregnancy?

7. Why is vitamin K sometimes given to mothers or babies at the time of birth? Why is a diet adequate in vitamin E important?

8. What complications of pregnancy are related to diet? How can they be avoided?

9. If you were explaining to a young person who had not read this book why a balanced diet during pregnancy pays dividends to the developing baby and its parents, what would you say?

10. What superstitions, prejudices, and fads about foods are held concerning pregnancy by persons you know? How can these be disproved?

11. There are 12 nations in the world that have a lower infant mortality rate than the United States. How would you account for this in the world's richest nation, with the best food supply?

Applying and sharing

1. Obtain the following information from your public library or by writing to your county and state health department:
   a. In your state, how many children were born to mothers 19 years of age or younger during each of the last two years?
   b. How many of these teen-age mothers were married? How many unmarried?

2. Inquire whether your mother knows of women in your family or community who had an increased number of dental cavities during or shortly after pregnancy. Why might this occur? Share your findings with the class.

3. Make a checklist of five or more points that you have learned from this chapter, which girls and boys should know before they are married. Show your list to six girl friends outside this class. Which points are they finding out for the first time from you? Share your findings with the class.

4. Plan balanced menus for one week, including snacks, for an expectant mother whose husband is just out of school and has his first job. Would you enjoy preparing and eating the meals you have planned?

feeding the baby
and small child

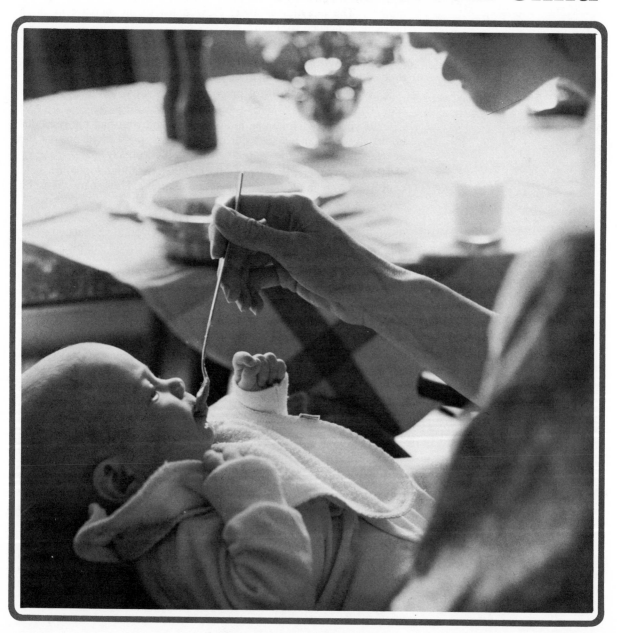

Challenge of starting good eating habits

Early influences

When we are born, our taste for food is remarkably adaptive. A young child can be taught to like any food. Food likes are not determined by flavor alone. They are shaped by what those we love and respect make desirable. They are influenced by the emotional climate of the home, especially at mealtime. The twig is bent the first year of life and a child's eating habits are set long before he enters school. The way a child is taught to like new foods is quite as important as the foods he is taught to eat.

Young couples today have a better opportunity to help their children establish good eating habits than their parents had with them. We know so much more about good nutrition. Our standard of living is higher. There are more foods on the market from which to choose our diet.

Then, too, we know much more about the psychology of eating. Mealtime can be one of life's most satisfying moments when people enjoy well-prepared food and companionship. Some children develop dislikes for foods for psychological reasons which hurt them all their lives. Young parents today can set their children a better example than perhaps they saw in their parents' home as children.

Father's role

The father is a powerful force in helping the child establish good eating habits, psychologists report. He can help, first, by supporting his wife in word and deed and, second, by eating the foods that the child needs and showing his appreciation for them.

The father's role was vividly illustrated by an incident in Buckingham Palace in 1966. Opening the door to the nursery, Prince Philip narrowly missed a flying spoonful of cereal thrown by his young son, Prince Andrew. The father said nothing. He walked across the room to the nursery table, sat down astride a chair, picked up the child's spoon, and quickly ate all the cereal with obvious enjoyment. Wiping his lips and expressing pleasure on his face, he turned to the governess and said, "This stuff's too good for babies. Give it to me instead in the morning." Prince Andrew clamored for his cereal again! His father had made it desirable by eating the food promptly and with enjoyment. How much more effective than saying, "Eat your cereal. It's good for you!" or "I never liked cereal, either."

What is a full-term, normal baby like?

Size

A full-term baby averages 20 inches in length and a little over 7 pounds in weight. He is overweight if heavier than 10 pounds and is probably premature if under 5½ pounds. As we have learned, today it is thought that height is more significant than weight in indicating good nutrition. The baby will double his birth weight in five months and triple it in about one year. But this depends on the type of feeding and the individual baby.

Body functions

A newborn full-term healthy baby can cry vigorously, suckles well, can digest and absorb his food well, has a good color, is lively, responds to stimuli, and sleeps well. He has a good reserve of iron. Up to 75 percent of his weight is water. This de-

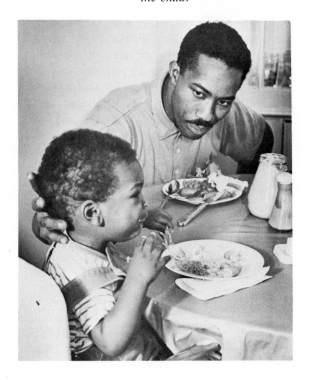

The father plays a vital role in helping a child develop good eating habits. If Daddy eats a food with enjoyment, it becomes attractive to the child.

creases until at age 10 the average amount of water is 47 to 54 percent, as in an average man or woman. His bony structure, most of which is cartilage, is one-fifth his weight. His head is large, his trunk long, and his arms and legs short, as compared with those of an older child.

The seven-month baby

A seven-month baby is not only premature, but also immature, and this makes it much harder for him and his parents. He has a softer skull than a full-term baby, because of inadequate bone mineralization. Such a baby is more likely to have hemorrhage and brain injury at birth because of

pressure on the soft skull. He has less iron reserve and is likely to be anemic, with weak muscles and little fat. His digestion and absorption of food are poor, for the enzymes do not function well and the stomach is small. He may not be able to suckle well, and while eating may become fatigued quickly or his underdeveloped respiratory system may present breathing problems. Since his sweat glands are immature, it is hard for them to regulate his body temperature. All this reemphasizes the importance of good eating habits on the part of the expectant mother, to help produce a normal full-term baby.

Breast-feeding

Man has not yet devised a formula that has all the advantages of breast-feeding. Although a baby may be well-nourished by properly managed formula-feeding, it is generally agreed that there are many advantages for the baby and some for the mother if she can breast-feed even one to three months.

Advantages

Advantages begin with the **colostrum**, which is the first thin, yellowish fluid that appears the day the child is born. It is not milk, but it is rich in protein and minerals and probably contains a variety of vitamins. It is lower in sugar and fat than milk. While there is only one-half ounce of it in 24 hours, this seems to be the food nature meant for the baby to take in his first hours of life.

By the third to fourth day, the breasts enlarge with milk and by the end of two weeks the mother's milk is normal in content. Then the baby begins to grow.

Human milk was meant for human babies and cow's milk for calves. Human milk has twice as much iron, measure for measure, as cow's milk and more vitamins A and C and niacin. Human milk has more milk sugar, the best kind for a baby, and contains about seven times as much linoleic fatty acid. H. H. Williams of Cornell University suggests that nutrients in the undiluted milk of the mother may fit the need of the human baby because of its particular balance of chemicals and nutrients and that of the cow may fit the exact needs of the calf in ways we do not yet know.

Remember that in a formula cow's milk is diluted with boiled water and has sugar added, in an effort to arrive at a food similar to natural breast milk. The baby digests and absorbs human milk excellently and thus helps the digestive tract

A breast-fed baby at one year.

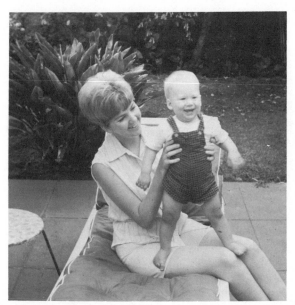

get off to a good start. This makes a few months of breast-feeding worth while.

Another advantage is that mother's milk is clean, fresh, pure, and the correct temperature, and there are few or no problems of constipation. There is less thumbsucking, less illness, and lower mortality among breast-fed babies than others.

Studies prove that the baby derives definite psychological benefits from breast-feeding because of the feeling of security and comfort he experiences in being held snugly in his mother's arms. He begins to communicate with her, and this emotional satisfaction has long-range effects even into adolescence and adulthood.

There are physical advantages for the mother, too. The early stage of nursing causes the uterus walls to contract and return to normal size and position earlier than when the baby is formula-fed.

It is good management (saving time, money, and equipment) to breast-feed, and it eliminates errors in calculating and making formulas.

With the addition of water in a formula, the proportion of vitamins and other nutrients decreases. A new baby needs a food such as orange juice early in life to supply vitamin C, and additional vitamins, especially vitamin D, are recommended to supplement the milk in its diet. The RDA for a baby from birth to one year is given in the table on pages 446–447.

The need for calories and protein is highest in the young baby, but the need for minerals and vitamins increases as the child grows. The intake of B vitamins increases in relation to the total increase in the number of calories daily. Studies show that a full-term infant weighing seven and one-half pounds at birth contains in its body more than twice the amount of iron as a premature baby weighing about five pounds.

The mother who breast-feeds is much more aware of being a major force in providing the food on which her baby grows and develops than she was during the period of pregnancy. Nursing is an expression of love for her child that only she can give. In his content, cozy position, the baby develops a bond with his mother that is richly rewarding to both.

Fears about breast-feeding

Many girls fear that they cannot breast-feed their baby. It has been found that about 87 percent of all mothers can successfully breast-feed, but that less than 50 percent of American mothers do so. Why?

The reasons that some girls do not nurse their babies are based on fear, old wives' tales, superstition, and ignorance. For instance, some think that nursing causes the breasts to sag or get smaller. This is false. The potential size of the breasts is determined by the genes in heredity, and by the girl's hormones and weight. Hormones and weight change with age and they are greatly influenced by good or poor nutrition. On this point Dr. Benjamin Spock says, "I know from my own medical experience that many women breast-feed several babies with no deleterious [damaging] effect on their figure. Others end up with better figures." He adds that overweight in any woman can cause the breasts to sag.

Fear of getting fat is another reason women give for not nursing their babies. This, too, is baseless. A mother will gain weight only if she gorges herself on food and drink, eating more than she and her baby need. A girl who understands and follows a well-planned lactation diet will provide the balance of nutrients her baby needs plus those her own body needs. She will not "lose a tooth for every baby." Nor will she gain excessive weight. If she does gain weight, it is a signal for her to examine what she is eating and drinking, and the amount. Either her diet is not well-balanced or she is overeating. Table 15–1 gives a day's menus for a lactating mother. Such a diet will help correct both factors in overweight.

Many mothers wonder whether smoking on their part will hurt their baby. This question has been investigated and nicotine was found in the milk of all mothers who smoked and in the blood of their babies. There was no evidence that the baby was hurt by the amount of nicotine it ingested, but it was concluded that, while there is no demonstrable effect, the mother's smoking cannot do the child any good. More research on this question is needed.

Breast-feeding aids

Some girls with small breasts fear that they cannot adequately feed the baby. Just the opposite is true. There is no excess fat to interfere with the manufacture of milk. All of the milk the baby gets is not there when he begins. It is manufactured as he nurses. That is why a mother needs to drink a glass of milk about 20 minutes before nursing. This helps her supply the amount of milk immediately required by her baby. Some of the most successful breast-feeding is done by women with small breasts.

During pregnancy, the physician guides the mother of a first baby in the care of her breasts, especially the nipples. This is to toughen them for feeding the baby and to enable the baby to take his food easily. During the first week or two, the breasts are filled with milk and may be tender, but soon they are quite comfortable.

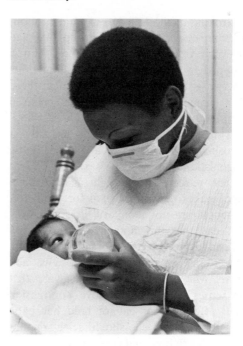

Whether breast-fed or bottle-fed, a baby should be held in his mother's arms. This gives him a feeling of warmth and security.

Technique of feeding the baby

The same techniques apply, whether a baby is breast-fed or formula-fed.

1/The baby should be held in his mother's arms. She should select a comfortable chair and prepare to sit for 15 to 20 minutes. Psychiatrists and psychologists have reported that the way a baby is fed has immediate and long-term influence on his emotional development. When babies are fed with a propped-up bottle of formula, without the closeness and human warmth he experiences when held during nursing, he may not develop well emotionally. This was noted in babies cared for in institutions. A dramatic example of this was found in a study of monkeys from birth to maturity, reported by H. F. Harlow in *The American Psychologist.* You may have noted in the zoo that mother monkeys hold their babies in their arms and caress them as they nurse, smoothing their

table 15–1 **Menu for One Day for a Lactating Mother***
(Normal Weight)

BREAKFAST	10 A.M. SNACK	LUNCH OR SUPPER	AFTERNOON SNACK	DINNER	10 P.M. SNACK
Grapefruit, ½ Ham and scrambled eggs Toast, whole wheat or enriched Soft margarine Marmalade Milk, 8 oz. Coffee, if desired	Milk, 8 oz.	Tomato juice, 6 oz. Liverwurst sandwich on rye bread Salad: green tossed, with cottage cheese mound Canned peaches Cookie Milk, 8 oz. Tea or coffee, if desired	Orange juice or alternate	Pot roast Potatoes Carrots Salad: cab- bage and orange Gingerbread Applesauce Milk, 8 oz. Coffee, if desired	Milk, 8 oz.

*Irving Shulman, "Iron Requirements in Infancy," Infant Nutrition Symposium 7, Council on Foods and Nutrition, American Medical Association, 1959, p. 51.

hair and stroking them. A group of nursing monkeys was compared with another group that had been separated from the mothers and given a bottle propped in a wire frame at feeding time. When the two groups reached adolescence, those that had been nursed by their mothers behaved in a normal way as regards emotional development, showing normal mating instincts and interest in the opposite sex. Those fed by a propped bottle were antagonistic to the opposite sex, showed fear or anger, and retreated and fought against affectionate approaches that are normal for their age.

While people are not monkeys, it is generally accepted today that the mother who holds her baby while he takes his feeding, breast or formula, contributes to his normal capacity to give and receive love. Many mothers are not aware that the infant senses relaxation and love—or tension and anxiety. If a mother cannot hold her baby when he is formula-fed, she should select regular periods in the day to hold and caress him.

2/The baby instinctively "roots" around until he finds the nipple. Usually the mother helps him by holding the nipple between two fingers until he is started. The baby may stop at intervals or continuously nurse and swallow the milk so quickly that he practically chokes. Some mothers become anxious and tense if the baby stops nursing. They think the reason for this is that they have no milk. This is not necessarily so. Each baby is different. This shows up even in the way they nurse. As we have seen, premature babies often have difficulty nursing because of poor breathing and underdevelopment in other areas. But a premature infant desperately needs the advantages of breast-feeding. It takes courage and great patience on the part of the young mother to persist in nursing such a child. Most are inclined to give up and change to formula-feeding.

3/Babies need to be "burped," for they swallow air along with the milk and this can cause discomfort, followed by fussing. Burping should be done at the middle of the feeding and again at the end. A vigorous nurser can empty a breast in five minutes. It is important to empty the breast completely for successful breast-feeding. The baby continues to get some milk after he takes the initial supply. Thus a 15- to 20-minute feeding period is recommended for both breast-fed and formula-fed babies. It often takes more than 20 minutes to breast-feed a newborn full-term baby and still longer for a premature one. If he falls asleep after the first hunger is satisfied, he should be awakened with a gentle shake of his body and helped to start again. The mother should not be discouraged if the formula-fed baby leaves milk in the bottle. Mothers start feeding problems by overfeeding. Overweight is a condition that often starts in infancy or early childhood. Remember that infancy is a short period in a long life, but it can produce very long-lasting emotional and physical consequences.

The husband's part

The husband has an important contribution to make in promoting successful breast-feeding. He also needs preliminary preparation to help him understand the delicate relationship of the emotions to successful breast-feeding. He can help provide a good emotional climate. No discussion of controversial matters or of anything that might provoke anger, anxiety, or worry should take place at feeding time. By his expression, his tone of voice, and his actions, the husband can give his wife peace, quiet, affectionate understanding, and the confidence she needs to do this job.

The father's help in feeding and caring for the baby is a great factor in achieving a relaxed, happy atmosphere in the home.

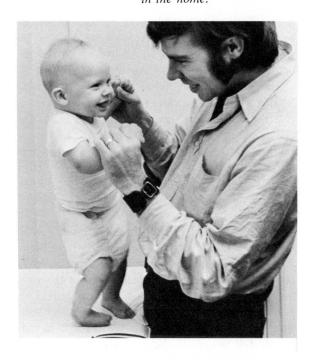

Most husbands are proud to have their wife breast-feed the baby. A few dislike or oppose it. Such an immature attitude is usually due to a lack of understanding of the advantages of breast-feeding to both mother and child.

The husband puts encouraging words into action when he takes over some of the chores the wife usually handles or provides outside help for a period. This enables the mother to rest sufficiently for her responsibility, that of feeding their child.

The aim for young parents is to establish a home free of emotional and physical stress—a generally good aim for producing healthy children and a happy marriage. This takes depth of understanding, long-range planning, patience, and mature love of the couple for each other.

Weaning the baby

Fear that the baby will be harder to wean if breast-fed is unfounded. Just the reverse is true. The mother's milk gradually diminishes and the breast-fed baby needs supplementary solid food. He usually weans himself between five and nine months and goes from breast milk directly to drinking milk from the cup along with his meals. The formula-fed baby often clings to the bottle and the mother may have difficulty getting him weaned from it, even when he has a full set of teeth and is well-prepared to take all his food from a plate and his milk from a cup.

When not to breast-feed

There are valid reasons why some women should not breast-feed their babies.

1/The mother should not nurse if she has a serious illness, such as severe anemia, tuberculosis, epilepsy, chronic fever, insanity, serious heart disease, or some types of kidney disease, such as nephritis.

2/If the baby has a harelip or a cleft palate, he cannot nurse.

3/Even primitive women in the less developed areas of the world stop nursing a baby if they become pregnant.

4/When it is desirable or necessary for the mother to return to work outside the home, she must formula-feed her baby.

Formula-feeding

Formula consists of sterilized milk, sugar, and boiled water. The sugar in human milk is lactose.

It is expensive to buy. It takes 1½ tablespoons of lactose to equal 1 tablespoon of granulated sugar. Cane sugar (white), brown sugar, or corn syrup is generally used—2 to 3 tablespoons in a 24-hour formula. Corn syrup is preferred, for it contains sugars and starch (dextrin). It takes more time for the dextrin to be converted into sugar in the intestines, and therefore it forms less gas than sugar does. Dark corn syrup, being less refined, contains more nutrients and is slightly more laxative. Powdered dextrin and maltose may be purchased, but are more expensive than corn syrup, which they resemble. It takes twice as much of either of these to equal the amount of sugar in a formula.

The newborn baby needs a great deal of fluid, but is not yet ready to digest a concentrated formula. If he weighs under 10 pounds, he is usually fed the formula recommended by his doctor, at intervals of three hours. A small baby cannot consume large quantities of food. Thus he is fed more frequently and in smaller amounts than a large baby.

When the baby weighs about 10 pounds, he receives a full-strength formula. He usually consumes a quart of formula during the 24-hour period, divided into four to six bottles, according to the individual baby's changing needs.

Different types of formulas may be purchased today ready-to-use, or to which only boiled water need be added. Some are available in sanitary disposable bottles. The cost of the formula varies according to the form of milk used and the other ingredients included.

Equipment for formula-feeding

Mothers who plan to formula-feed their babies should decide which method of sterilization to use before buying the equipment. Even those who breast-feed will need two or three bottles for water and orange juice. It is well to have the equipment before the baby arrives.

Basic materials required are 9 Pyrex nursing bottles with wide mouths (or sterilized disposable plastic bottles, which can be used only once and are therefore expensive), 12 nipples to fit the bottles, 12 caps, a large utensil with a rack and a tight-fitting lid, a 1½-quart container for mixing formula, tongs, a funnel, a nipple jar, a strainer, a set of measuring spoons, a long stirring spoon, and a bottle brush.

If the formula is sterilized in the bottle, crosscut nipples are better than those with round holes. The milk does not pour out or clog up. The crosscut nipple works like a valve, releasing the right amount of milk or liquid as the baby sucks. If nipple holes are too small or clogged, the baby must work too hard, gets too much air, and may simply fall asleep. If they are too large, he may choke or fuss later from having taken his food too quickly. If he nurses too rapidly, he also may fail to get the satisfaction he needs from sucking and might tend to suck his thumb. The nipple should be tested by turning the bottle upside down. The milk should come out in a fine spray for two to three seconds, and then fall in drops.

Choice of formula

When a mother formula-feeds her baby, she should be guided by her physician as to the kind and amount of formula to use. He will know the baby's changing needs and the needs of the mother and family as a whole.

Free bulletins on the subject can be obtained from your local, state, and federal health departments, as well as the extension division of your

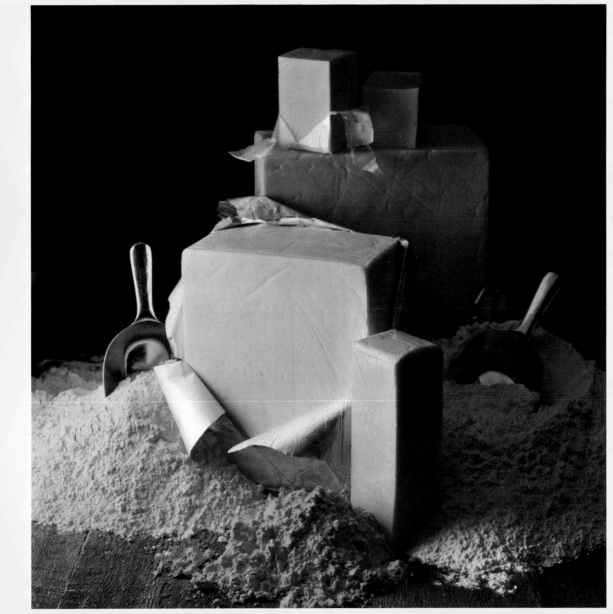

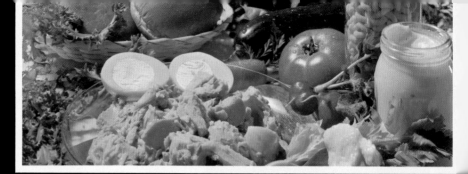

Parents and chil-ke love tuna in al-form. It is a valu-l for all ages.

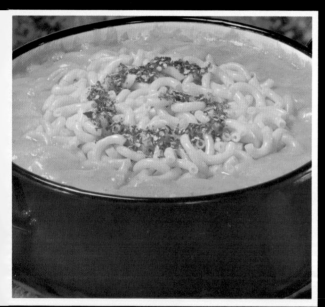

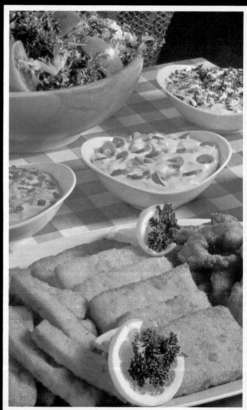

(above) *Children welcome a steaming, hearty dish of macaroni and cheese at any meal. (right) Offer a combination seafood platter with a variety of sauces and watch each person become an instant gourmet.*

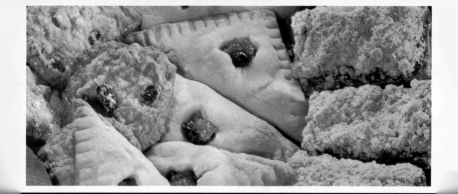

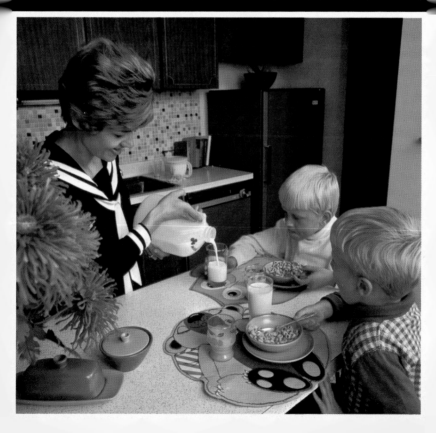

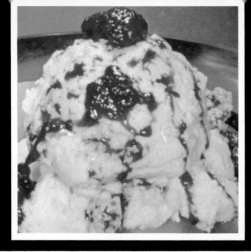

(left) *Ice cream satisfies a child's desire for sweets while providing milk nutrients to make him healthy.*
(below) *Small children like food in bite-size pieces. Turkey à la king with rice is a dish most children enjoy.*

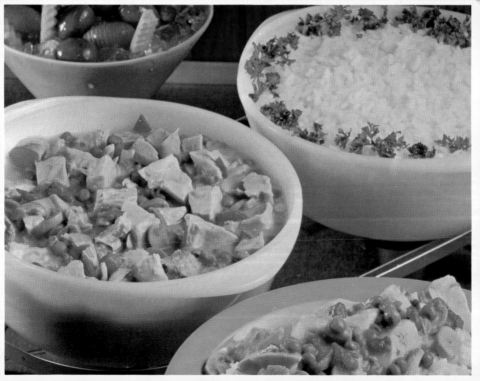

state university. These are often helpful in giving a young mother suggestions as to schedules and equipment, and also the food for infants and young children.

Since ready-to-use formulas in disposable containers are available, parents should compare the cost with that of home-prepared formula and decide whether the overall budget for family needs can cover such an expense. Ready-prepared formulas vary from three to five times the cost of home-prepared formula. Then there is the question of labeling. Parents have a right to know exactly what is in the ready-to-use formulas. They should read the label carefully and check with their physician about what is not listed. There is room for improvement in the labeling of baby foods.

Feeding schedule

A newborn baby has a small stomach and may need to nurse every two hours for a while. As he grows, his stomach gets larger and he will go longer between feedings. A baby cries for reasons other than hunger and it is not wise to feed him every time he cries. A drink of water or adjustment of some physical discomfort may be all he needs. A mother of a first baby must learn to recognize the distinctive "hungry cry," especially if she uses the self-regulating feeding schedule.

Night feedings

First the 2 A.M. feeding and then the one at 10 P.M. are eliminated, as soon as the baby can sleep through until morning. The age for omitting these feedings varies. Gradually, by the time the baby is 10 to 12 months old, however, he reaches the family meal schedule of three feedings a day.

Feeding solid foods

While milk is the most important food in the diet of the baby, he cannot live on milk alone. As soon as the baby's development warrants it, the physician begins adding new foods to the baby's diet.

Since boiling the formula destroys even the small amount of vitamin C in milk, it is necessary for the bottle-fed baby to have orange juice or another source of vitamin C by the third week. A breast-fed baby also profits by an addition of citrus juice to his diet, although a mother who eats a good source of vitamin C in each meal will provide more vitamin C in her milk than is available to a bottle-fed infant. Today, apple juice and other fruit juices are fortified with vitamin C. Apple juice is frequently recommended by doctors as an alternate for orange juice. The protopectins in apple juice also present in citrus fruits favorably affect the intestinal tract, thus aiding the digestive process.

How to introduce new foods successfully

One of the first opportunities for serious conflict between baby and mother is when the baby starts eating new foods. It is of utmost importance to his future that he learn to like a variety of foods, especially vegetables, fruits, meats, and eggs. During his first year, the child can learn to eat and like many foods in each food group. How can a parent help him establish good eating habits as he is introduced to foods other than milk?

GOOD ENVIRONMENT. Psychological factors in the child's environment often affect the establishment of good habits. The ground rules—which all members of the family should observe—are based on confidence, relaxation, and cooperation.

Solid foods are added to the baby's diet as his development warrants it— often at one month.

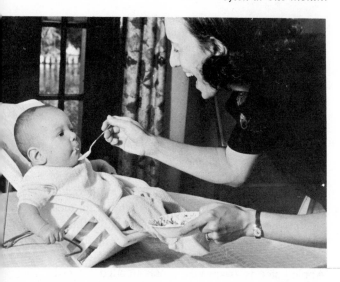

1/Recognize that the baby must get used to the different textures and flavors in foods and to eating from a spoon.

2/Praise him immediately for success in doing what they want him to. This helps him repeat desired behavior.

3/Avoid laughter or comments if he does anything that is "cute" but would be harmful for him to develop as a habit.

4/Avoid tension in following the food guides slavishly. There is great flexibility in the time of introducing different foods and in the amount individual babies eat.

5/Make all remarks positive.

6/Take quick but firm and relaxed action to stop unacceptable behavior. For instance, if the baby blows or throws food, he is either trying to get attention or is not hungry; he should be moved at once from his chair and quietly told that he may return when he is hungry and wants to eat

like a big boy. He should never be called "bad" or scolded with degrading names. It is better to take him from the room, so that he gets a clear-cut idea that his behavior is not appropriate at mealtime and is not acceptable to those he loves.

7/Never underestimate a baby. Intelligent children "catch on" quickly. They grasp the little nuances in voice and facial expression and will test their wits against those of their parents.

TECHNIQUE OF INTRODUCTION.   The technique of introducing new foods is important in developing good eating habits. The manner in which new foods are offered an infant frequently determines whether he will be flexible in his approach to food, will welcome experimentation, and will achieve variety and balance in his diet as he grows older. The suggestions that follow may serve as a guide in handling this important phase of infant development.

1/The new food should be offered at the beginning of feeding, when the baby is hungry.

2/The first food should be in liquid form. Solid food can be liquefied by adding formula—or milk, if the baby is breast-fed. For cereal, the mixture would be 1 teaspoon of cereal to 1½ teaspoons of milk. As the baby accepts the thin form, the mixture should be gradually thickened to semi-liquid and finally to normal consistency.

3/The food should be on the end of a demitasse spoon or baby spoon, placed in the approximate center of the mouth, and offered ¼ to ½ teaspoon at a time.

4/The mother should not be discouraged if the baby rejects the food at first. It is new in texture and flavor. Normally, he will spit it out. She should try again and show no anxiety or tension. If he rejects it after trying the same food for three days, the mother should wait a few days, then try again. She should control her own emotions and smile with confidence. If in three days he is taking 1 teaspoonful of the new food, that is good.

5/Only one food should be introduced at a time and the child should be allowed to enjoy it thoroughly before the next one is introduced. When the baby has learned to eat several foods, the ones he likes should be repeated while new ones are introduced.

6/Foods should be given to the baby by themselves and not mixed with others, so that he will learn to like each food for itself.

7/The temperature of his food should be kept the same as the formula, about 100°F. Many children reject food because it is too hot or too cold.

8/Home-prepared baby food should be seasoned with salt only. No fat, sugar, or spice should be used until the baby has a well-established variety of foods that he likes.

9/Chopped vegetables and other foods should be substituted for smooth strained ones when the child has teeth and can chew—at about nine months.

10/The parent must never express or allow anyone else to express by word or facial expression a dislike for a food the baby is eating. This is a vital point for success.

11/When the child refuses to eat, the food should be removed and the child excused from his table at once.

12/A child should never be forced to eat more than he wants. This is a cause of future eating problems, including overweight. If he is well, and is not allowed to snack on tidbits in-between, he will make up what he misses, to some extent, at the next meal.

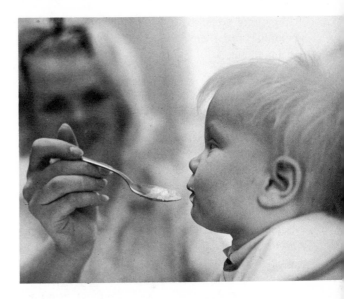

Baby foods now include the processed forms found in adult foods. They are in wide use today.

Buying and care of baby foods

The processing of baby food has become over a million-dollar business since 1928, when it was first introduced. There are on the market all of the processed forms found in adult foods. The same principles to be followed in buying, storing, and using processed foods for other members of the family apply to baby foods.

Some mothers use the processed baby foods for the young infant and change over to adult foods as the baby gets his teeth and is able to eat three meals a day. Where a family grows its own food, it is less expensive to prepare the home-grown foods for the infant. Baked or boiled potato in its skin and mashed potato or "instant dried" from the family pot may be used for the baby as an alternate for cereal at one meal.

Although glass jars are convenient and one may see what the food looks like, there is some loss of riboflavin where the light strikes the food.

If parents prefer baby food from glass jars, they should store them in a dark, cool place before using them.

What a well-nourished one-year-old is like

A well-nourished one-year-old is a healthy, attractive, active, friendly, happy child. He has tripled his birth weight, and is one and one-half times as tall as at birth. He has about six or eight teeth, can stand well, and may walk or toddle. Some can say a few words, and most are making word-sounds. He has been eating three meals a day for two to three months. His hemoglobin and protein content is now about the same as that of a well-nourished adult, and he is about to launch into a new stage of life.

Psychological characteristics of a child one to three years old

By the time the child is one year old, psychological factors are already influencing what he eats. From one to three years of age, he is becoming more independent as he learns to walk and talk and he should be encouraged in this independence.

Although he wants to feed himself and should do this as soon as possible, he tires quickly and may need some assistance without seeming to be given it. The mother needs much patience as the child goes through this period. She can make it easy for herself and for him by placing foods in bite sizes on his tray and letting him pick them up with his fingers. Our ancestors used fingers before the spoon or fork and our children go through the same primitive steps until their

muscles are coordinated. By the time he is 18 months old, the average child is quite successful in feeding himself, if he has been properly guided.

The child should not be scolded for spilling food or making a mess. When he dawdles, he may be watching something more interesting than his food. It is therefore important that the general atmosphere where he eats is calm and quiet. Highly charged emotional discussion between members of the family when the young child is eating is harmful to him.

Children learn to become good eaters with good manners through the example of sympathetic and mannerly parents who are themselves relaxed

A child should be encouraged to feed himself and should not be scolded if he makes a mess.

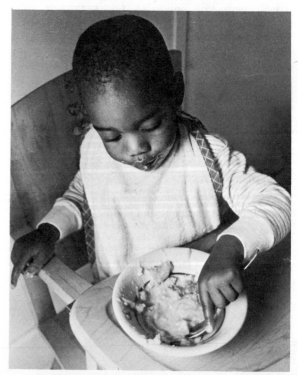

and neither overly harsh nor overly protective. The child is a great imitator. He also desires the love and approval of his parents. Parents have a great opportunity when a child is between one and three years old to guide him so that he becomes a good eater and an emotionally well-adjusted child. What are his food needs at this age?

Food needs of a child from one to three

The table of Recommended Daily Dietary Allowances on pages 446–447 gives the daily amount of nutrients recommended for the one- to three-year-old. The calorie recommendation is 1100 to 1250 daily, over half the need of a teen-ager or adult. The mother should try to keep the diet balanced and the servings small. Children do not grow evenly from month to month, but in spurts. Usually the appetite increases at the period of rapid growth, then levels off, as if the child wished to rest a bit from so much growth.

The mother who realizes that the child needs only a few more calories during this period is not so likely to be alarmed if her child does not eat much. She will direct her efforts to establishing good eating habits, rather than forcing her child to eat large amounts.

Calcium and bone mineralization

Calcium and other minerals are laid down to harden the bones. Calcium will come mainly from milk, which should be part of every meal. The mother should aim at getting the equivalent of one and one-half pints of milk into the child's diet at this age. He can surely drink a pint! If there is

difficulty in getting him to drink this much, some of his milk can be in the form of cheese cut in bite sizes for the one-year-old and also in custard, junket, and rice or bread pudding. The milk intake may also be increased by adding nonfat dry milk to the child's milk and other foods, such as cereal, mashed potatoes, and some other vegetables.

The RDA table on pages 446–447 shows that the child of one to three needs as much calcium as an adult; over half as much protein, vitamin C, riboflavin, thiamine, and niacin; more iron than an adult of 35 and over; and two-fifths the amount of vitamin A.

The mother of a preschool child helps him develop sound eating habits by offering him a variety of nutritious foods.

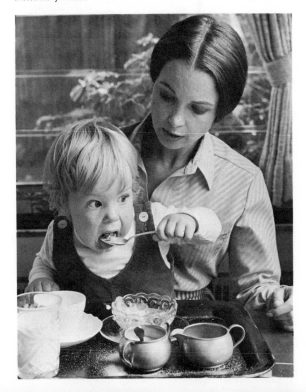

The child from one to three is a "bundle of energy." He needs a great deal of calcium and protein in his diet.

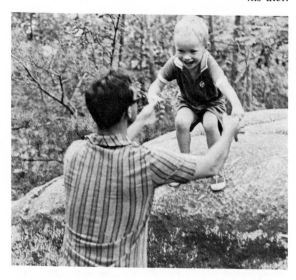

The faster a baby or child is growing, the greater the influence of nutrition, good or poor. The favorable or unfavorable effects of nutrition are more visible during periods of growth.

The mother and family of the preschool child have an obligation to help him as much as possible to learn to enjoy the variety of food he needs to eat each day, for the sake of his present and future growth and health.

The state of nutrition of the small child may affect his future development and appearance in different ways. While a well-balanced diet, whenever it is started, may not be able to undo all the harm done by a poor one in earlier years, it can help an individual achieve surprising improvement and vigor. The sooner this is started and the longer maintained, the better the results.

During periods when the child is taking only a small amount of milk, his milk may be fortified with nonfat dry milk. It may also be added to foods that he will accept, such as milk desserts, cereal, and other favorite dishes. Nonfat dry milk is low in cost. It will not take the edge off the appetite as a liquid between meals, but adds calcium, protein, and other valuable nutrients.

At one year or thereabouts, the baby starts to walk and his bones must be strong enough for the weight of his muscles, which grow rapidly. When the bones are not properly mineralized, they bend, resulting in bowed legs and misformed joints.

Protein

At this period, the child needs about 1½ grams of protein per pound of body weight. If he weighs 25 pounds, he needs about 38 grams of protein. This is over half the protein need of a girl or woman from 15 years of age upward.

At about 18 months, the baby fat begins to disappear and the child puts on much more muscle growth in the next year and a half. His muscles grow faster than bones and amount to one-half his weight. Muscle growth is particularly great in his thighs, hips, and back. This enables him to move more quickly and to become the "bundle of energy" that he is at this period.

The foods that supply high-quality protein are milk, eggs, meat, fish, poultry, and organ meats, such as liver. Three cups of milk provide 22½ grams of protein, and one egg provides 6 grams. These, with 1 to 2 tablespoons of ground meat, a serving of bread or cereal at each meal, and the small but important amount from vegetables, will easily take care of a child's protein need. When families must be on quite low-cost diets, dried beans and peas are given, along with milk and animal foods. The protein of these foods is well used when milk, egg, or meat is in the same meal.

The protein value is another reason milk should be included in every meal for the child. You recall that 1 ounce of cheddar-type or Swiss cheese or about ½ cup of cottage cheese yields 7 grams of protein. One-fourth cup of ice milk has 2½ grams of protein, and ½ cup of baked custard has 6½ grams of protein. When you add nonfat dry milk to a food, remember that ¼ cup adds 6¼ grams of protein, or about one-fifth of the daily need.

While protein and calcium are two important nutrients in the child's daily diet, observe in the RDA table on pages 446–447 that he needs 15 milligrams of iron daily from six months through three years—5 milligrams more than a grown man. This is one of the main reasons that egg is given daily and liver is added as a first meat.

Psychological traps to avoid at mealtime

Among the potentially harmful elements to be avoided at mealtime are threats, scolding, rushing, bribery, unfavorable comparison with another child, forcing, or tricks and entertainment to get him to eat. When any of these methods are used, the child turns the tables on you and controls you through various means of getting attention.

Threats

Threats set the stage for rebellion and revenge. This may have effects that go far beyond the eating of a particular food or meal.

Scolding

Scolding has different effects on different children. It may cause a feeling of shame in some, rebellion in others, and for most it does little good and much harm. That is not to say that a child should not be corrected and made to understand when he is doing something undesirable. But be sure to use a method that reaches the way he thinks and feels, so that when you correct him he feels you are fair.

Rushing

Rushing a child with statements such as "Hurry up now and eat your vegetables, we have to go out" causes a child to feel frustration and defeats your purpose. Start the meal earlier and allow more time for the slow child to eat.

Bribery

Bribing a child to eat is buying him—paying a price for something he should do and needs to do on his own, for his own sake. Such bribery as "If you eat your egg, I'll give you a dime (or buy a certain toy)" is harmful. But if the mother has a set of goals that the child understands, and is given a "star" to put on a piece of paper or is shown in some other way that he has done the desired things on this day, that is another matter. A *reward* is a just payment for an understood goal accomplished or a task done. These goals or tasks could include coming to meals promptly when called, finishing his food along with the family, and other points in learning to live comfortably as part of the family. Such daily habits are character-building, in addition to establishing good eating habits.

Comparison with another child

Comparisons with another child are cruel on the part of a parent, for they may engender jealousy toward that child and seldom accomplish your goal. Resentments are fostered that actually hurt both children.

Positive contributions to good eating habits

1/A well-balanced meal should be provided at a definite time for each meal. Then the child knows when the meal is to be served and can plan to get ready. His hunger rhythm will develop in keeping with this pattern. Mothers should not be slaves to a schedule, but should realize that temper tantrums and crying before mealtime often occur because the child is hungry. He doesn't know what is wrong. This problem is solved by serving the meal a little earlier. It is more desirable that a hungry young child eat before the family does than to have him eat with everyone and spoil the meal for all. When a child is too tired or too hungry, he may eat poorly.

When parents make comparisons between children, they foster resentment and jealousy. A warm, friendly atmosphere at meals is important.

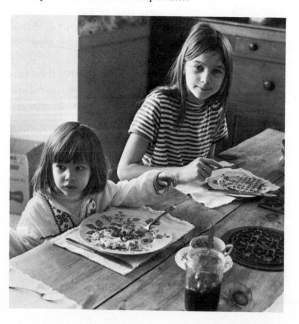

2/The food should be so prepared that it tastes and looks good to him.

3/Small portions should be served, according to the child's individual need. It is better to have him eat all of a small serving than for him to leave half of a large one. This gives him a feeling of success and of being like the grown-ups. If he wants more, he should be given a small serving. Here is the place to help him eat the balance of what he is served before he gets a second helping of a favorite food.

4/Uneaten food should be removed. The child should be excused from the table.

5/A snack between meals is needed by some children. This is more important if the child waits to eat with the family. What you learned about snacks in Part I applies also to the small child.

6/Food dislikes should not be discussed before the child. The parents' solidarity on this point can help much. By thinking ahead before the problems start, they may avert some problems altogether. They should discuss how good a food is, without pushing, and keep the conversation pleasant and their voices calm.

7/Parents should teach table manners by their own good example and by an occasional assist, instead of speeches on the subject. The child loves his parents and will want to be like them, if he knows them as lovable people.

8/When things go wrong at mealtime, the parent should first find out from the child what the problem is, from his point of view. It may be very simple. His chair may be too low. He may have tasted food that was too hot. He may be tired or worried about something. When his problem is understood, the parent can help him solve it and then go on with the meal. If this can't be done, he should be excused from the table and the room. This should be done in such a way that the child understands that it is not a punishment and that he may rejoin the family group when he is in control of himself.

9/The denial of food or a meal that a child needs as a means of punishment is unwise. Parents should help the child to feel that they are with him. He will sense their sympathy, love, and calmness, if they give them. On the other hand, he will also sense hostility, confusion, lack of understanding, and tension, if expressed.

Meal pattern for the one- to six-year-old

The pattern is the same for a young child as for any other member of the family—the variety of nutrients suggested in Chapter 2 for each meal. These are found in a variety of food that makes a tasty and emotionally satisfying meal, as well as a healthy one. Snacks for the young child should fill genuine nutritional needs for the day, such as fruit juice, fresh or dried fruit, milk, fruit-juice popsicle, or low-fat milk with a cracker or bread.

Meaningful words

adaptive food tastes
carotenoids
casein
cystine
dextrin
full-term
methionine
nephritis
weaning

Thinking and evaluating

1. What are the characteristics of a full-term baby, as compared with a premature one? Do you think most mothers- and fathers-to-be would try to eat good meals and snacks if they knew how much it would help their children and themselves? Explain.

2. What are the advantages of breast-feeding? Explain how a well-balanced diet on the part of the mother can help her breast-feed her baby well. What are some false ideas about breast-feeding? How can the father help the mother succeed in breast-feeding their child? Why is it important to hold the baby if he is bottle-fed?

3. What are the reasons for formula-feeding a baby? What are the acceptable methods of preparing a formula, and which would you prefer? Why?

4. Explain the time schedule for feeding an infant.

5. Explain the sequence of adding solid foods to the diet of the baby. Why is it so important for the mother to have good medical guidance in feeding her baby? Why is it important that she and her family be calm, patient, and persistent in a relaxed way as solid foods are introduced to the baby?

6. How can you apply what you learned about buying foods for the whole family to buying foods for the baby? How should you care for baby foods?

7. What are the physical and emotional characteristics of a well-nourished one-year-old?

8. Explain the food needs of the child from one to three years of age; three to five years of age.

9. In what ways can the mother, father, and other members of the family help the baby make a transition from baby meals to family meals?

10. What positive contributions to good eating habits can the mother and family make to the young child? What should the family avoid?

Applying and sharing

1. If you have a new baby in your family or can observe one, sit quietly and watch the way he nurses the breast or takes a bottle. If you can observe more than one infant, compare the way different babies take their milk. Discuss the differences in children in this respect with a mother who has more than one child. What did you learn?

2. Observe young children from one to three years of age as they eat. Make notes on what they eat, the time of day, and how they eat. How do they compare?

3. Talk with the mother and the father of an infant and with the parents of a child one to three years old. Ask what feeding problems they have had and how they overcame them. Make a plan to prevent feeding problems for toddlers.

4. Using the recommended diet for a lactating mother on page 264, calculate the nutrients in each meal. Is each meal balanced? Do the nutrients for the whole day measure up? How would you adjust this menu to suit your taste and individual needs for one day? For four days?

5. How would you plan to feed a baby so that he would be healthy and strong and like the food he needs? How would you try to get your husband to cooperate?

6. Visit the baby food department and note the variety. Read the labels and compare the prices. Which do you think are "best buys" in each category of food needed? Why?

7. Discuss with your teacher the possibility of having a good pediatrician in your community talk to your class on feeding infants.

part iii

the consumer
and
food protection

protecting our food from contamination

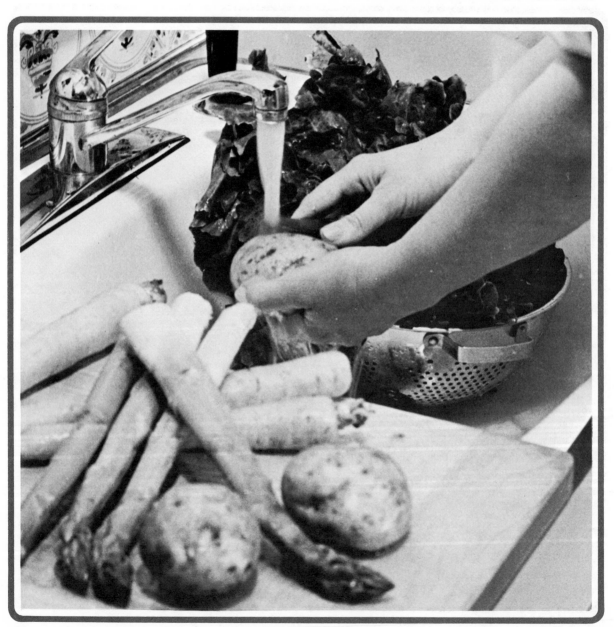

If we are to protect our own lives, we must protect our food and water supply from production source to the table. In this and the following two chapters, we shall consider (1) the different problems we face in protecting our food, (2) what is being done to solve these problems, and (3) our responsibility in their solution.

Dangers to our food supply

Dr. Carl Dauer of the U.S. Public Health Service states that the number of cases of foodborne and waterborne disease occurring annually would be somewhere in the order of 100,000 to 200,000. Other public health officials believe it may even be as high as a half million to a million cases annually.*

These diseases could, for the most part, be prevented voluntarily by food producers, processors, distributors, and all those who handle food in public eating places, as well as in the home, if we understood what to do and did it. Most persons in the food industry support the concept of a safe, wholesome food supply. Other firms and food service institutions where meals are served "barely meet minimum standards set by law. It costs no more to purchase food from firms that maintain high standards of sanitation, and it may cost less."*

As the population of our country has increased, so has the pollution of our environment. With the increased production of processed and convenience foods and of meals eaten away from home, there has been a parallel increase in the hazard of foodborne and waterborne disease and infections.

---

*Aimee N. Moore, "Meals away from Home," *Protecting our Food: The Yearbook of Agriculture 1966* (Washington, D.C.: USDA), pp. 179–190.

Hepatitis, for example, is more widespread today than in the 1930's.

Sources of contamination of our food supply

Our food supply is affected by the following major factors:

1/Contamination through the filth of the food itself or decomposition; uncleanliness in the place where it is served, in equipment, preparation, and the persons who handle the food

2/Contamination from excess pesticide residue

3/Contamination from airborne and waterborne substances, such as industrial wastes

4/Contamination from excess antibiotic or other chemical additive residue

5/Contamination from excess radioactive fallout

To allay unfounded fears and to help us see what we can do about each of these problems, let us consider them briefly.

Contamination through filth of food and uncleanliness of person

The U.S. Public Health Service lists 24 diseases producing toxin from bacteria or virus that are waterborne and foodborne. Some of these result in food poisoning, others in infections. Either may be serious to infants, older people, and those suffering from certain chronic diseases. These include salmonellosis (sal mə nel ō′ səs), staphylococcus (staf ə lō käk′ əs) infection, commonly referred to as staph, gastroenteritis (**gas trō ent ə rī′ təs**), infectious hepatitis (**hep ə tīt′ əs**), typhoid fever, undulant fever, scarlet fever, diphtheria, tuberculosis, influenza, septic sore throat, colds, and other diseases.

Table 16–1 shows that about one-third of the cases of food poisoning are caused by staph. Gastrointestinal food poisoning outbreaks accounted for more than half of the cases and 44 percent of these were of undetermined cause. Those affected didn't know their source of infection.

In the future it will be more difficult to know where we get food poisoning, Aimee N. Moore reminds us. This is because "Many convenience foods like T.V. dinners, precooked and frozen entrees, and desserts are prepared in food-processing factories and in central commissaries of large restaurant chains. Many restaurants and institutions, as well as housewives, purchase these foods." Such buyers are scattered, making the source of infection difficult to locate.

Symptoms of food poisoning

One may be slightly ill or seriously ill from food poisoning, which is characterized by acute diarrhea, nausea, vomiting, abdominal cramps, fever, and dehydration. The latter is serious for an infant. The time lag varies from a few hours after eating contaminated food to 72 hours afterward. Few persons would connect these symptoms with food eaten three days earlier. Each bacterium and virus has its own pattern of multiplication, which a

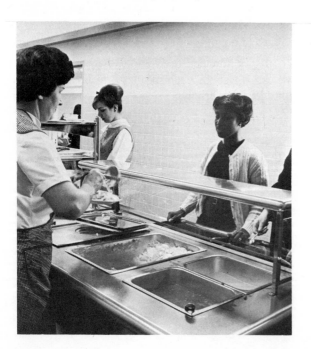

Clean food, prepared and served in clean utensils, is a safeguard against food poisoning.

table 16–1   *Summary of Foodborne and Waterborne Diseases by Types of Infections**

TYPE OF DISEASE	OUT-BREAKS	CASES	PERCENT OF CASES
Typhoid fever	65	603	0.6
Salmonellosis	209	10,699	11.7
Shigellosis	99	10,354	11.0
Botulism	56	116	0.1
Staphylococcal food poisoning	633	28,331	30.0
Gastroenteritis, undetermined cause	839	44,083	46.6
Total	1901	94,186	100.0

*Reported in 1952–60 study by Aimee N. Moore, "Meals away from Home," *Protecting Our Food: The Yearbook of Agriculture 1966* (Washington, D.C.: USDA), p. 182.

physician will understand. For this reason and because these symptoms are also symptoms of other types of illness, if you are seriously ill, see a good physician.

Ways we get
food poisoning

PEOPLE AND EQUIPMENT. People who are ill, are dirty, and have sores, boils, and infections are carriers of staph contamination. So are dishcloths, sponges, rags, and cloths that wipe up counters. Other contaminants are chopping blocks, cooking equipment, and service dishes in public eating places and at home. Food handlers contaminate food with unclean clothing and hands— even though they don't look dirty; with nose-blowing, sneezing, coughing, and the like in the presence of food or the place where it is prepared and served. In addition, feces, sewage, garbage, and failure to wash the hands after going to the toilet can contaminate food.

BACTERIA. We also get food poisoning from spore-forming bacteria, such as botulism (*Clostridia botulini*), which usually occurs in nonacid processed food. Recent outbreaks were caused by tuna in cans and smoked whitefish in plastic sealed packages. The spores are odorless, tasteless, and colorless, but deadly. They are unlike the toxins produced by staph, as they are destroyed by boiling five minutes in an open pan.

Another type of spore-forming bacterium is *Clostridia perfringens*, which has only recently been isolated. It is widespread in feces, soil, and sewage, and contaminates much food. Spores from this bacterium were found in 45 percent of the meat selected at random in the stores of one community. It shows up in much-handled meats, such as chops, ground meat, stew meat, precooked

foods—especially poultry, meats, gravies, meat dishes with vegetables and cereals—and stuffings for meats, especially when prepared and then frozen.

Leftover food should be cooled quickly and refrigerated below 40°F. When it is to be used, it should be reheated quickly to at least 140°F and served at once. Meat, especially, should be heated to a minimum temperature of 140°F, and when possible to 212°F.

Protection from food
poisoning and foodborne
and waterborne disease

LEGISLATION. The government has a responsibility to protect our food and water from contamination from sewage. But even in this we must cooperate and be our own watchdogs. We pass laws to protect us in areas of the public responsibility. We must see that these laws are obeyed.

The Model Ordinance and Code for Food Service Sanitation was improved in 1962 by recommendation of the U.S. Public Health Service. It now requires that no person be allowed to work in a public or institutional food service while "affected with any disease in a communicable form, or while a 'carrier' of such a disease, or while affected with boils, infected wounds, sores, or an acute infection."

It further states that "All employees shall wear clean outer garments, maintain a high degree of personal cleanliness, and conform to hygienic practices while on duty. They shall wash their hands thoroughly in an approved hand-washing facility before starting work, and as often as necessary to remove soil and contamination. No employee shall resume work after visiting the toilet without first washing his hands."

Our government has regulations to protect our food from filth. In this Idaho warehouse, a District Inspector checks bagged pinto beans for rodent contamination.

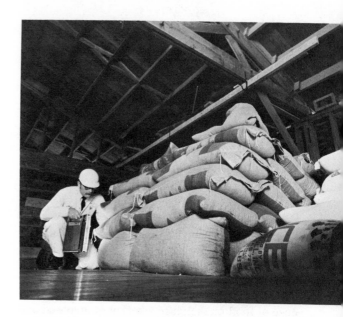

This is a fine improvement on the old law, but we must see that it is enforced by our own watchfulness, and by the standards of those who handle food. Health authorities visit food service places only every six months for inspection. There are many of these places, and indifference and laxness can slip in between visits in some eating places.

INDUSTRY SELF-REGULATION. The food industries, food-servicing places, and public eating places have a responsibility to protect the consumer from food poisoning and disease.

Most businessmen value their reputation and do not want their processed food seized by government officials and removed from the market. In self-interest, as well as concern for our welfare, the food processor aims to obey the law and protect the public. There are exceptions, and this is why we must be watchful of our own interests.

Institutions and public eating places, too, are much concerned for their own reputation and do not wish to have food poisoning traced to their place of operation. Some train their employees in the health standards and cleanliness required. Yet it is well known that many who work in the kitchens of public eating places are among the drifters in employment, and often have poor education and low health standards in their own background. Some of these do not have the habit of scrupulous cleanliness in their person or in handling food.

This was illustrated by the experience of a large American chain hotel in Istanbul. Its luxury dining rooms had to be closed because food poisoning had erupted among the guests. This hotel did give its employees special training in sanitation and health, yet the food was contaminated.

CONSUMER EDUCATION AND INDIVIDUAL VIGILANCE. Each of us has a responsibility to ourself and to others for whom we are responsible, to learn how to avoid illness from unclean food and water in the home. How can we do this? By accurately informing ourselves on food poisoning and other forms of waterborne and foodborne illness or disease; by reporting to the top authorities in a food company or business and to the proper authority in government when we observe anything that is fraudulent, false, misleading, unclean, or otherwise contrary to the letter or intent of the law.

1/When you eat out, choose a clean place where they use clean, intelligent help and an electric dishwasher. This need not necessarily be an expensive place. Reject an unclean, cracked, or broken serving dish in a public place. Reject a food that smells or tastes spoiled. Report to the manager any member of the service staff who is unclean in his person or who places his hands on food or dishes. Do this with tact.

2/Observe habitual cleanliness in your own kitchen and teach your family to acquire the same habits. For instance, if you have to prepare a meal when you have a cold, sneeze, cough, blow your nose, or spit into disposable paper with your head down toward the floor. Flush the paper through the toilet at once, and wash your hands thoroughly before you continue your work. Keep open sores bandaged and wear a rubber glove if you place a sore in water with food, as in washing lettuce or other fresh food. Keep table tops and counter tops clean by scrubbing them with a strong soap or detergent. Boil dishcloths with strong detergent and chlorine bleach. Sun kitchen towels and keep them clean. Use disposable towels.

3/ Inform yourself on things you need to know, such as

  a. Most molds in food are not harmful. Some are helpful, as in cheese. But molds have not been thoroughly researched yet, and with the exception of cheese, it is wise to discard food that is moldy.

  b. Toxins develop in some foods that stand at room temperature for as much as four hours, especially staph and salmonella. This occurs in cooked leftovers or precooked and frozen meats, poultry, fish, gravy, stuffing in frozen poultry, T.V. dinners, sliced cold cuts, smoked fish, casserole dishes, and others. The toxins can be destroyed by boiling at 212°F on top of the stove or heating to an internal temperature of 165°F in the oven.

  c. Foods containing eggs in a thick, viscous mixture should be refrigerated after preparation, unless they are eaten immediately. This includes cream puffs, éclairs, cream pies of all kinds, mayonnaise, and other foods of a similar nature. In pastry,

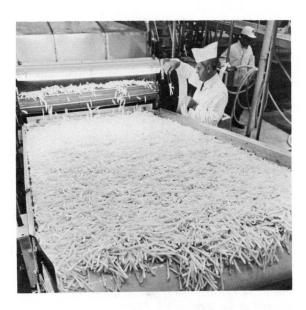

This inspector in a frozen French-fried potatoes plant is collecting an aseptic sample to check for bacterial contamination.

the texture and flavor are better if it is made fresh and eaten at once.

Studies made at Michigan State University show that the toxins and bacteria in meringue are destroyed when cooked at a temperature of 325° to 350°F for 16 minutes. Holding food at boiling temperature or just below on top of the stove achieves the same result.

Cornell University research in methods of cooking with eggs indicates that the egg and the thickening agent should be added at the same time to the hot milk when making custard, cream pies, puddings, and the like, and cooked until the mixture is smooth and thickened.

  d. When traveling away from home, especially in foreign countries, learn whether the water is safe, and if not, drink only boiled water (tea or coffee) or bottled water. Eat raw vegetable salads and cold cooked foods only in countries that have high health and cleanliness standards. Otherwise, eat fresh food that can be peeled, such as apples, pears, grapefruit, bananas, and the like. Never eat unwashed fresh fruit, such as berries and grapes, except from your own garden, if you know they are free from spray residue. The fun of eating out, whether at exotic places in our country or abroad, is spoiled if you later develop food poisoning. You can avoid this by knowing what to do and doing it.

Insecticide sprays are used on crops to destroy pests and plant diseases. The chemicals are tested for safety, as are the foods on which they are used.

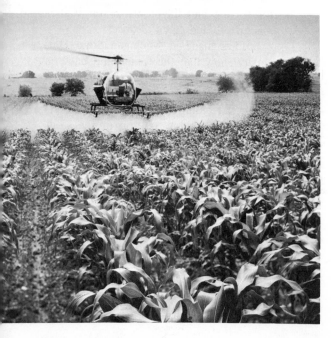

Insecticides, a chemical additive

In Part I, we discussed chemical additives to processed foods. Many people are frightened of the possible food poisoning resulting from a residue left by chemical sprays to destroy insects and plant diseases. We have a law requiring that these chemicals be tested and approved for safety before they are sold and that directions for their use be printed on the containers. Food samples are tested for safe residue levels at intervals.

Government testing

An example of how our government protects our food supply on an international level is the case of a recent shipment of cheese from Switzerland. This was rejected by the United States government, whose tests showed that it contained excessive spray toxin. Considerable research by the Swiss was required before the source of the toxicants was found. It was not the sprays used on the feed, but sprays used on the timbers of the barn to kill insects where the hay was stored. The toxicants dripped on the hay fed the cows, thus contaminating the milk and ultimately the cheese. By testing the percentage of toxin in the cheese to determine whether it exceeded the limit set by our health standards, our government agency protected not only our own health but also that of people of other nations consuming cheese from that producer.

Insecticide vs. contamination by filth

Despite the fact that many people worry about food poisoning from insecticide residue, in the year

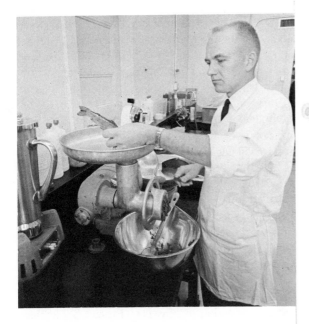

Pesticide residues have been found in wildlife, birds, fish, and other foods. A chemist grinds a fish as the first step in tests to determine the presence of residues.

immediately following the 1958 amendment to the food laws, more than four times as much food was seized by the government agents for contamination by filth, for example, than for spray residue. Only 19.6 percent of the food seized (1333 tons) was for excess spray residue, as compared with 80.4 percent (5466 tons) for contamination from filth.

Research to protect food from insect destruction

CHEMICAL CONTROL. Research is constantly going on as to the safety and application of insecticides. Without the use of insecticide sprays at present, agricultural experts tell us, we would have less animal and plant food to eat in our country, would pay more for what we do have by 50 to 75 percent, and the quality of that food

would be lower. There are, for example, some 82,500 different kinds of insects in the United States and Mexico. If you garden with flowers or vegetables, you know the problem of fighting insects and plant diseases to get a crop of food or a garden of roses. One thing that research has shown is that healthy, strong plants grown in rich, nourishing soil are more resistant to plant diseases.

Chemicals are continually being tested in the search for insecticides that will kill pests without showing up in the meat we eat or the milk we drink. Chlorinated hydrocarbons that have been used leave toxic residues that may persist in the soil and may harm wildlife and fish. Malathion and carbaryl are two chemicals being used to replace these more harmful ones. They do not show up in animal food and may be sprayed on plants up to a day or two before harvest as food for both man and animals.

In the decade 1960–70, the use of DDT (dichloro-diphenyl-trichloroethane) in our country decreased by 80 percent, or from seventy-five million pounds annually to fifteen million pounds. In August, 1970, the Agriculture Department announced further restrictions on its use on some 50 types of fruits and vegetables, forest trees, lumber, buildings, and livestock. Cotton and citrus crops will be the only remaining areas where it is used. Groups working for elimination of environmental pollution are trying to get a total ban on the use of DDT. Although it is an extremely effective and long-lasting pesticide, it does remain in soil and water for many years and has been found in birds, wildlife, fish, and other foods—even human milk. Improvements have been made on DDT, such as using a small amount in granules to help control the corn borer. No human deaths have been reported, though it is a contaminant in food and water and in tests was found to cause cancer and genetic mutations in rats.

New chemicals are being used successfully to control weeds that infest rice, corn, seed soybeans, sorghum, and alfalfa, a forage crop for cattle. Controls for rodents, which have destroyed 100 million tons of grain a year, are now being developed.

NONCHEMICAL CONTROL. A number of methods are now being tried to eliminate pests.
Sound Waves. Sound wave control of insects is potentially significant. In 1964, it was reported that the Indian meal moth could be about 75 percent controlled by exposing the adult to certain sound waves during the egg-laying period. The waves have also controlled the flour beetles—the second generation was weaker and died sooner. Research is under way to try this method on other insects.

Light Waves. Light waves have been made available, thanks to the Atomic Energy Commission, to irradiate stored grain, fresh fruits, and other foods with good effects against infestation. Light traps have also been used with success against some insects.
Biological Control. This has been successful to some extent. Biological control is accomplished by introducing a predator or parasites to destroy disease and insects, such as the Japanese beetle, weevils, corn borer, mealy-bugs, and scales.
Sterilization. Sterilization by gamma radiation has been successful on some male insects. The screwworm that infected cattle has been reduced by 99.9 percent, and pests that attack fruits, vegetables, and melons have been destroyed successfully by this method.
Hormones. Hormones are essential for the growth and reproduction of insects. Research on their

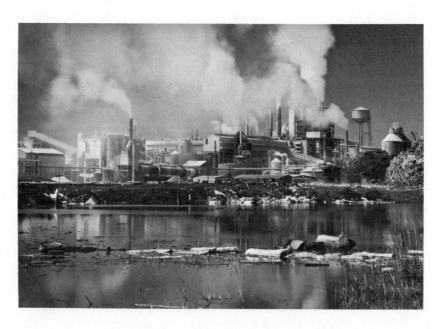

Industrial wastes pollute our air and water. Air pollution not only poisons our food, but also blocks out the ultraviolet rays of the sun that produce vitamin D.

chemical structure is now going on. Once this is learned, it will provide a key to insect control.
Plant Breeding. Research has been at work to produce seeds more resistant to pests.
Extreme Cold. This is an old-fashioned method of killing insects. Where the weather is zero and below, the farmer opens his granaries and lets in the cold air, and the weather destroys the insects. Heat kills them during cooking.

This gives us an exciting glimpse into the various scientific fields that are exploring many areas to achieve control of the pests that attack our food, while at the same time inflicting little or no harm to man or animal.

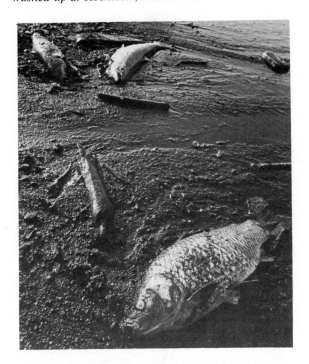

The effects of mercury pollution in the Great Lakes are visible in these fish washed up at Rochester, New York.

Environmental contamination by harmful chemical elements

The dangers to man and animals from environmental contamination have been of increasing concern to government, industry, and the public. Sewage and industrial wastes from a number of industries have caused the pollution of our air and waters. Some chemical elements, such as arsenic, lead, mercury, strontium 90, cadmium, nickel carbonyl, beryllium, and antimony, are toxic when found in excessive amounts in food or water. These may remain on plants when discharged into the air or may be washed down into streams, lakes, and oceans by rainfall. Hence, entering the "natural food chain," they are eaten by human beings.

Government vigilance

The problem of environmental pollution has been under study by the Senate Subcommittee on Energy, Natural Resources, and the Environment.

Testimony before the committee in the summer of 1970 brought out that at least 27 metals found in the air are more dangerous than organic substances, such as pesticides, weed killers, sulfur dioxide, and other similar contaminants.

LEAD POLLUTION. Lead was found in high concentrations in streams close to heavily traveled highways. Among the symptoms of chronic lead poisoning are colic, nausea, anemia, sometimes a grey-blue skin coloration, and coma.

MERCURY POLLUTION. Mercury pollution emerged as a new hazard to food and water during 1970. In the past, mercury had been considered an inert metallic element. However, in the spring of 1970, government chemical analysis of foods revealed it in potentially poisonous quantities in the Great Lakes, some of which were then closed to resort fishing. It is known that, like other pesticides, it moves along the food chain from water to fish, birds, plants, animals, and human beings. As early as 1960, it was learned that 111 persons had been poisoned between 1953 and 1960 from eating fish caught in Minimata Bay, Japan, where compounds from a plastic factory were discharged into the water. Of these, 43 persons died. But the fish and shellfish eaten contained 10 to 80 times the level considered "safe" by the U.S. Food and Drug Administration.

Mercury is a substance that attacks the brain and can cause blindness, paralysis, and even insanity. It also attacks vital internal organs, particularly the liver. It easily passes the placental barrier to become concentrated in the fetus. It has also been known to cause chromosome damage.

In our country, mercury pollution comes mainly from the manufacture of chlorine-caustic soda (chloralkali), paper, and paint, and from agriculture and lumbering. There are many secondary sources, including sewage, newsprint, moonshine liquor, and mercury fallout from industry, automobile fumes, and incinerators. About 5000 tons of mercury move through our environment annually by the natural process of erosion from the cinnabar ore from which it originates.

Federal scientists reported toxic levels of mercury in the livers of Alaskan fur seals (*The New York Times*, October 30, 1970) "up to 116 times the amount of mercury considered safe for human consumption." Here is an example of follow-through by the Food and Drug Administration. It examined products made from seal livers and found "contamination at up to 60 times the safe level in iron supplement pills . . . that are sold in health and specialty food shops." The quantity of mercury considered safe by the F.D.A. is one part per two million of any substance for human consumption. However, the amount cited as safe by the World Health Organization is only one-tenth as great.

Steps are being taken to halt this pollution. The Department of Agriculture has suspended the use of mercury on seeds and various state legislatures and governors have taken measures to stop the flow of industrial wastes carrying mercury into streams. New York State, for example, effected a decrease in the mercury discharge into its streams from 71 pounds a day in May, 1970 to 3 pounds in August, and a further drop to 12 ounces per day was expected by the summer of 1971. The FDA had more than 1000 inspectors and chemical analysts working on the problem. During December, over two million cans of tuna were ordered withdrawn from the market because levels of mercury in certain lots were found to exceed the minimum levels set by the government. Dr. Charles C. Edwards, Jr., Commissioner of Food and Drugs, explained that this was merely a precautionary measure and should not be considered an absolute level of tolerance for the substance. He added that the tuna was actually "absolutely safe to eat."

Continued research and investigation are proceeding, under the supervision of the Food and Drug Administration, the National Oceanic and Atmospheric Agency, and the fish canning industry, both on fish already canned and on new catches before processing, as well as on imported fish. Another "precautionary" measure was the removal in December, 1970 of frozen swordfish from the market because tests disclosed excessively high mercury levels. Since 98 percent of the swordfish consumed in this country is imported, provisions were made for testing of fish at the source.

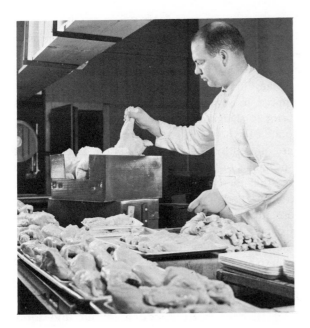

The USDA stamp on poultry means that it has been inspected for cleanliness, wholesomeness, and safety for human consumption, and also that it is accurately labeled.

Individual vigilance

For our own protection, we should keep well-informed about the pollution situation through reliable sources and follow the instructions of our local, state, and federal authorities. In this way, we can safeguard our own health and that of our family and community. We should, however, avoid panic. As Dr. Jesse Steinfeld, the U.S. Surgeon General, said in the Congressional inquiry, "The problem of health defects of toxic materials is a legitimate area of concern, but not a legitimate cause for hysteria."

Antibiotics and food

Research has been under way since 1943, testing how antibiotics may be used to improve our food supply in cost, quality, and quantity without injury to those who eat it. Some interesting things have already been learned and more will be learned as the research proceeds.

The law aims to give both the producer and the consumer the benefit of "food additives under conditions of marketing and use that will assure safety." Most commercial feeds now contain some type of medication, including hormones. An antibiotic is a chemical substance used in the practice of medicine with human beings and animals. They are produced by yeast molds and bacteria. Drugs fed to animals have (a) helped control disease in these animals—an advantage for us; (b) sped up growth and shortened the feeding period—saving money for both the producer and the consumer; (c) produced more meat per pound, with improved texture and tenderness.

Because poultry grows so rapidly and we can see the results, many people think it is the only meat which has been fed antibiotics and hormones. Some have a prejudice against these additives, an attitude which is not sound. A consumer who buys poultry inspected by the USDA for wholesomeness can be sure that it does not contain hormones or any other substances that would make it unsafe.

Antibiotics are also added to the slush ice when poultry or fish are eviscerated. When poultry is held in this ice one to two hours, it acquires a longer market life without spoiling. Whole fresh fish and fillets are dipped into brine containing an antibiotic during the holding, transporting, processing, and marketing of fresh fish when it is partially processed at sea.

Red meats, milk, and baked foods with cream and custard fillings have an enhanced market life through the use of these drugs, but not fresh or canned fruits or vegetables.

Laws on drug additives

What protection does the consumer have under the law on drug additives? We have stringent laws to protect us. The Federal Government, via the Food and Drug Administration, must approve every chemical added to the food of livestock. To gain approval for use of a chemical additive,

1/It must be shown that the proposed use will not leave any residue in milk, meat, or eggs, if the directions for use are followed.

2/If any residue is left, it will be safe for human beings to eat the product.

3/The feed must be accurately and honestly labeled as to contents and amount to feed each animal.

4/The manufacturer must conduct tests in feeding his product to at least two species of animals, and one species for the entire life span.

5/A wide margin of safety is required between animal and man to allow for low tolerance of some individuals for the drug additive.

6/The manufacturer of such foods must show that he has the equipment and controls to measure and mix the feed and drugs properly.

7/The farmer must follow the directions for feeding with drug and hormone additives and take the animal off the feed long enough before slaughter to be sure that any residue in his body is cleared out. The government finds that farmers usually accept their full responsibility.

Our laws regarding food additives are very strict and do much to protect us. One example of this careful scrutiny is the Food and Drug Administration's ban on the use of synthetic diethylstilbestrol (dī eth əl stil bes′ trōl), a hormone additive, in the feed of poultry and swine and the restric-

tions on its use for cattle. Farmers add this hormone to the feed of animals to fatten them faster for the market. As of September, 1970, the farmers may add up to 20 milligrams per pound (the former limit was 10 milligrams). But they are required to stop feeding it to the cattle two days prior to slaughtering, to ensure complete elimination of the hormone from their systems before they are offered for human consumption. Scientists test specimens of food by spot-checking the markets to see that these foods are safe. If they are not, the food is withdrawn and the persons responsible are prosecuted under the law. You recall from Chapter 8 that studies have been under way on the addition of antibiotics such as nisin and subtilin to canned food.

Radioactive fallout and food

Our government has been quietly looking ahead, working to learn ways to detect radioactive fallout and protect its citizens and our food supply from the hazards to health in the atomic age. In our discussion of milk in Chapter 5, some results of this research were reported. The person who is armed with the facts has the best chance of taking care of himself and his family in any age.

Nuclear research

The probability is that many nations in the future will continue nuclear research. When nations test nuclear-type explosions, the air above all citizens of the world is polluted with radioactive isotopes of different kinds, commonly referred to as radioactive fallout. This condition is with us now, and has been for years. Thus let us face up to what is real, unpleasant as the facts may be.

Research has provided some good suggestions as to what we can do to protect ourselves so that we may face the future with some understanding, instead of blind fear. You recall that the soil, open water, and all plants above the soil are immediately affected by nuclear explosions, and hence contaminated. This is because radioactive fallout settles to the earth like fine dust. Tests show that people can be protected in an attack by seeking adequate shelter before the fallout arrives in large doses, and that some food and water can be similarly protected for emergency or immediate use. The problem, then, becomes one of "scientific housecleaning," as it were, and long-term management to protect water, food, and ourselves.

How to protect the family from radioactive fallout

Research shows that radioactive isotopes enter our bodies through the food we eat and the water or other contaminated beverages we drink. The food that is growing on the land is the first to be affected. Fruits and vegetables above the earth catch and hold some of the fallout. Rough or sticky leaves hold more than smooth surfaces, especially of strontium 90 and 89 and ruthenium, but cesium 137 and iodine 131 move at once. All are moved by wind and rain and are eventually taken throughout the plant, because the soil retains some. More is found in soil with a heavy rainfall than in arid districts.

Table 16–2 gives the fallout isotopes that are most serious to human beings and to the animals and plants that provide our food, because the earth is contaminated with them. Food and water are most contaminated in the heaviest fallout zones.

Research indicates that about 1 percent of the strontium 90 is removed by one crop of food grown on most soils. Sandy soils remove as much as 5 percent a crop. Thus on sandy soil it would require about 40 years to remove 90 percent of the contamination.

table 16–2 *Important Fallout Isotopes in Food and Water**

NAME OF ELEMENT	HALF-LIFE SPAN**	CHARACTERISTICS
IODINE 133	22 hours	Chemically similar to iodine, which is an essential nutrient.
IODINE 131	8 days	Accumulates in the thyroid gland.
CESIUM 137	29.7 years	Chemically similar to potassium, which is an essential nutrient. Locates in muscles and can cause cell damage, including genetic. Not contained in the body long, as it enters and leaves the body continually, like potassium.
STRONTIUM 89	50.5 days	Both behave chemically like calcium in plants and animals.
STRONTIUM 90	27.7 years	Laid down in the bones, as explained in Chapter 5. Can cause serious illness, such as bone cancer. Children more affected than adults, because of influence on growth.

*From A. B. Park, "Fallout and Food," *Protecting Our Food: The Yearbook of Agriculture 1966* (Washington, D.C.: USDA), pp. 340–41.
**When the reading of radioactive fallout is measured, the term "half-life" is used to measure the rate of radioactive decay. It is the time lapse during which a radioactive mass loses one-half its radioactivity.

You recall from our study of milk that the more calcium available in the diet, the more it "beats out" strontium in the race for being laid down in the bones. This is an incentive for all age groups to include some milk in meals and snacks.

The principle of protecting human food and water is to prevent the fallout from becoming mixed with them. If the fallout is removed, the food and water are safe. An example of this is a haystack simply covered with a tarpaulin. The fallout is on the tarpaulin, and if it is carefully removed, the hay is safe for animals. The same is true of animal food in a silo. This may be used at once. Well water is safest at first. But if open water is covered, the covering is contaminated, not the water. Studies show that dilution of the radioactive fallout in water is less serious as time passes, because some of it is absorbed in the earth around and below the water. It is important to remember that fallout can be removed in much the same way as dust—by washing, vacuum cleaning, and brushing. While fallout is being removed, every precaution should be taken to avoid inhaling or swallowing particles of the material.

Thus we see that part of the hazard is removed for the family that has facts and thinks and plans ahead. Food that is canned in tin or other types of sealed packages, preferably metal—which does not break or become contaminated by water in case of fire-fighting—are best choices. The problem is to decontaminate fresh food and the cans and covers of tinned foods without self-contamination or spreading it to the clean, safe food.

Studies show that peel-covered food in the field (such as orchard fruit and melons) may be washed and peeled and the inside eaten, even right after contamination. Even head lettuce and cabbage may be made safe by such a procedure. But strontium 89 and 90 and ruthenium 106, when de-

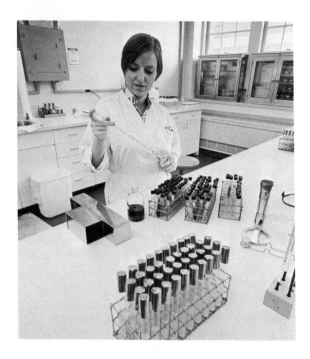

A technician tests a prepared potato product for fallout and microbiological contamination.

posited on leaves, are absorbed. Animals or man should not eat the exposed leaf soon after a nearby nuclear explosion.

Some of the crops above the ground are unsafe. Root and tuber vegetables, such as potatoes, carrots, beets, and others that grow under the ground, and seeds are immediately safe after contamination by most fallout, if properly peeled and/or washed. Eventually, through rainfall or irrigation, the long-lived isotopes shown in Table 16–2 find their way into the soil.

Steps in decontaminating food from fallout

1/Vacuum the outside of cardboard boxes and other materials containing food or water.

2/Wash utensils, paring knives, or other equipment that comes in contact with radioactive fallout. This means frequent washing of some equipment to prevent contamination of safe food.

3/Wash all food that can be peeled, husked, shelled, or pared, such as cabbage, before peeling it. Wash your hands after the food is washed, and before peeling it. Use well water, if possible.

4/Peel and remove all outside shells of foods such as root and tuber vegetables, beans and peas in the pod, corn in husks, uncrushed fruit, or vegetables in skins.

5/Washing is not effective in removing fallout from contaminated meat that is exposed on the surface. Meat in cans and unbroken sealed packages is safe for immediate use.

6/Decontaminate cans by washing and rewashing. Simple plastic film, such as polyethylene, is effective in covering food, but the covering should be vacuumed before the container is opened.

7/Cooking does not destroy radioactive isotopes. However, studies show that the radioactive materials will leach from food into the water in which it is boiled. This occurs with all types, and in this case it is safe to use the food, but not the liquid. Drain the liquid carefully from the food, even meat.

8/Radioactive food loses contamination if held in storage before it is eaten. You would need to use a measuring instrument to detect radioactive isotopes before eating such food from storage, because the time element will relate to the degree of contamination and the kind.

9/Discard any tinned foods in swelling cans, for this indicates bacterial spoilage.

10/Food covered with porous paper or unlined cloth is not safe from contamination.

Reserve food supply

A good manager of family meals has on hand a reserve supply of foods that enables her to prepare a balanced meal for her family three times a day for as long as a week. She can use it right along, replacing it as it is used and keeping the oldest food rotating to the front or top of her shelf for use first.

The most important thing to remember is that you have a responsibility to assure yourself and your family that it is ridiculous to be afraid of the food in our markets, and to refrain from eating any specific food lest it "poison" you in some way. Malnutrition and starvation are not the answers to the problem of exposure of foods to fallout or other forms of contamination. Your government

Meat in unbroken sealed packages is safe from contamination.

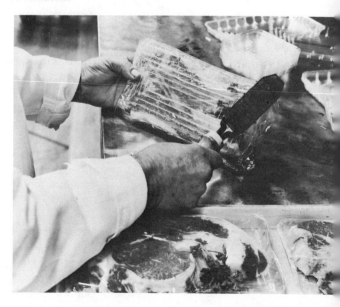

is on guard for you in testing and inspecting all types of foods to see if they are safe for human consumption.

In every section of our country, the diets of selected teen-agers are being tested all the time, to learn if the amount of pesticide residue and isotopes from radioactive fallout exceed the safe level. To date on each score we have a wide margin of safety, authorities tell us.

When we take our personal responsibility to do our best to protect our food in the home from contamination by filth and disease, and to wash carefully all fresh fruits and vegetables to remove further spray residue or radioactive fallout from it, we should then use our food with confidence in its safety. As consumers, we have the responsibility to be the watchdogs of irregularities in protecting our food supply from contamination, and to make our voices heard with the facts to the government and the food industry, from the highest level right down to our local places of business and government.

Meaningful words

botulism
carbaryl
cesium 137
chemical additives
chlorinated hydro-
    carbons
chlortetracycline
decontamination
dehydration
diethylstilbestrol
gastroenteritis
infectious hepatitis
leaching
Malathion
oxytetracycline
radioactive fallout
ruthenium 106
salmonellosis
staphylococcus

Thinking and evaluating

1. In what ways does this chapter have meaning for your life now? How can it help you and your family when you have your own home?

2. How does understanding the problems of food contamination help eliminate fear of food poisoning? Help you prevent it?

3. In what different ways can one get food poisoning? Which ways are most dangerous? How do they differ? Why is staph-type food poisoning so serious? Salmonella?

4. On the basis of your own experience, would you connect the characteristics of food poisoning with a specific food you ate three days earlier? How does food poisoning affect a person? To which members of a family might it be quite serious?

5. With your family and friends, discuss what each person can do to protect himself from food poisoning.

6. What do you consider safer as a whole, the meals and snacks prepared at home or those you eat out? Explain your answer. How do convenience foods fit into this picture? Which are the safest convenience foods? The least safe? Why?

7. What basic facts that research has revealed can help guide you in protecting yourself and others from food poisoning? Why is cleanliness at every step so important?

8. What are the advantages and disadvantages of using sprays and insecticides in growing food? What can you do to protect yourself from remaining residue from their use? What do you consider the outlook in the research in this area? Explain.

9. How would you sum up the problem of contamination of our food and water supply, and what we can do about it as individuals? As families? As a community? As a nation?

Applying and sharing

1. In your public library, conduct some independent research on the most recent material available to help you get a broader understanding of food contamination and its control. Be prepared to share your information with the class.

2. The teacher may divide the class into groups and have each write to one of the following: your local, state, and federal health departments, and your county extension office of the state agricultural university, for related information.

3. If a specialist in this area of public health lives in your community, discuss with your teacher the possibility of arranging for an illustrated lecture on this subject.

4. Share with your family what you have learned and make plans for improvements in preventing food contamination in your own home.

5. Investigate, insofar as you can, the food markets and eating places in your vicinity. Decide which you consider safest with respect to food protection from contamination. Be prepared to state your reasons for this choice. Would you prefer to eat in a restaurant that has an electric dishwasher? Why? What steps would you take to try to improve cleanliness in public eating places, including school cafeterias?

6. Plan balanced meals for your family for one week, using processed foods which may be stored and used in emergency. How would you store these? Decontaminate them?

fads, fallacies, and consumer protection

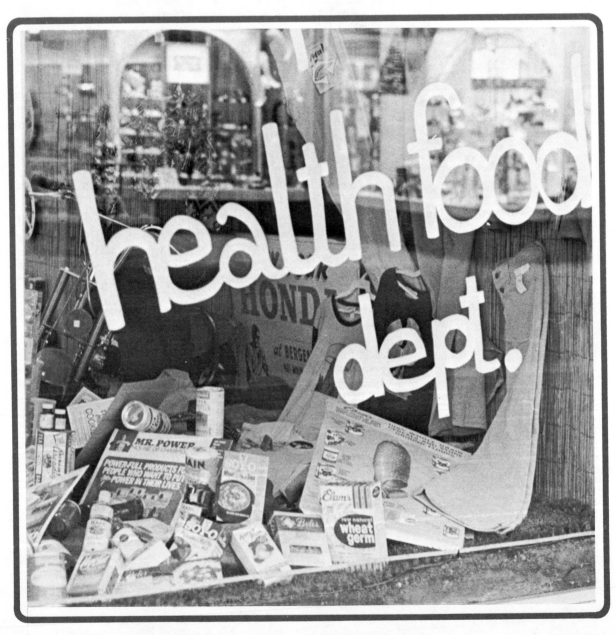

Food quackery

A half-billion dollars is an enormous price to pay for nutritional quackery annually. Yet 10 million Americans are doing just that, according to the American Medical Association. It would be less serious if it were only a matter of wasted money. The personal dangers are even greater.

You, as a consumer, have the right to expect that your food will not only be safe and wholesome when you buy it, but that you will get a fair return on your money. That the food is honestly represented in advertising, packaging, labeling, and weights and measures. That you are not exploited in any way by twisted, evasive, or misleading information on food or in its advertising in any form. Before we spell out the more personal dangers, let us define a few terms.

A **fad food** is one thought to have "magical" powers and used with fanatic zeal. It may be used for a short period or a long one. Among such foods are yeast, yogurt, wheat germ, and blackstrap molasses—all good foods when used in their proper place in cooking and meal planning.

A **fad diet** is one that is followed with unjustifiable zeal and that lacks a sound nutritional base. It may accomplish a temporary goal, but lacks the quality for long-term success, if followed indefinitely.

A **food fallacy** is a belief about food based on misinformation, with no scientific facts to support it. Fad diets are usually based on fad foods and food fallacies.

Why food fads and fad diets are dangerous

As the above definitions indicate, the food faddist is headed for trouble. In what ways?

Hazard to health

MALNUTRITION. Food fads and fad diets undermine health. Each year, millions of people, from teen-agers to senior citizens, aggravate health disorders or afflict themselves with new ones by getting involved in fad diets. This fact is not well understood by those who most need to know it. But it is vividly illustrated by the case of the 36-year-old woman who followed the Zen Diet for eight months in 1967. She ended up in the hospital with a full-blown case of scurvy, severe protein deficiency, folic acid deficiency, and general malnutrition. On this diet, she ate no meat, milk, or fruit, but only ground oatmeal, cornmeal, buckwheat, bread made from rice, and 12 ounces of soup or tea daily. For eight months she refused medical treatment, fanatically believing that the Zen Diet would overcome her "temporary" disability, though she was bedridden. Once hospitalized, her life was saved by nothing more dramatic than adequate diet therapy.

THE SHORTCUT FALLACY. The concept is all wrong. The food fad and the fad diet rest on the idea that you can take a quick shortcut in dieting and get better results than those who eat the recommended balanced daily diet. The central message of this book is, first, that there is no substitute for the knowledge of food and nutrition necessary to be well-fed; and, second, that there is no substitute for managing the daily diet so as to benefit from this knowledge. Shortcuts are harmful, because they deprive the dieter of necessary foods and result in undernourishment. But they are also not effective, since a return to a normal diet will bring back all the pounds lost.

FALSE SECURITY. Fad diets and foods give a false sense of security. They give us the illusion of knowing more about food and nutrition than we actually do. They afford a temporary escape from facing our real diet problem. They excite our imagination with their promise of a quick magical solution to a serious problem that can be solved only by a balanced diet, over a long stretch of time. Food is an area in which scientific knowledge operates, not magic.

When we allow our natural desire for quick results to overrule our better judgment, we are behaving like our six-year-old friend, Jack, who wanted to plant some corn in his garden. His father explained what was needed and how to accomplish his goal, so that by August he would have corn to eat. Jack planted the seed after school, covered it with a rich mulch of soil and fertilizer, watered it, and went to bed. The next day, the sun shone and after school Jack rushed

Fad diets don't work. For sensible, permanent weight control add eight ounces of skim milk to this lunch of green lettuce, shrimp, grapefruit salad, and toast.

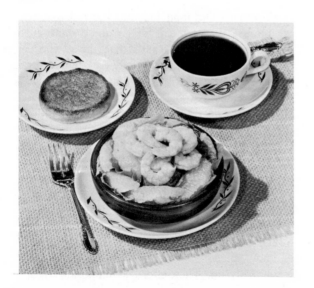

to see if his corn had come up. It hadn't. He dug it up to see why. It looked just the way it had when he had planted it. He complained to his father, who explained that he must let the corn grow in its own way and be patient. This he could not do, such was his eagerness. So each day after school he dug up the seed to see why the corn had not come up. In defying the slow, gentle way that nature works, he never was able to enjoy any corn from his garden.

Exploitation

Fad diets exploit the consumer. Some are promoted and followed by honest, sincere people, but, for the most part, the promoter is a deliberate and shrewd swindler. The sale of special foods as "health foods" is misbranding, and is so regarded by the Food and Drug Administration. In Part I we learned that there is no one food that is all-sufficient, or that could be called a health food. It is the combination of a variety of foods that produces sound nutrition—the basis of good health. The exploiter, or quack, has "special" foods, vitamin combinations, formulas, gadgets, gimmicks, diet schemes, cooking utensils, printed matter, and lectures to sell. This is big business that attracts the quack.

George P. Larrick*, who was long with the Food and Drug Administration, reports the case of the health lecturer who invited the public to an introductory free lecture, during which he sold tickets to a paid series. Though his audience paid a tuition fee, they spent 90 percent more on foods that he sold—"his own brand" of whole wheat

*George P. Larrick, "The Pure Food Law," *Food: The Yearbook of Agriculture, 1959* (Washington, D.C.: USDA), pp. 444–451.

Nutrition is front-page news and big business today. The consumer must learn to distinguish between sound principles and fads in the products and literature offered him.

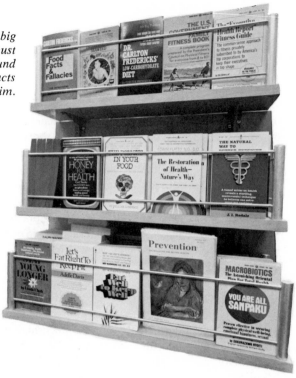

flour, peppermint tea, wheat germ, and honey. He urged them to buy only his brand. He claimed these foods would prevent and cure arthritis, cancer, liver trouble, heart disease, and most other ills, and would "put off death to the very last minute."

After a nine-month trial, the jury found him guilty of fraud. While out on bail, he conducted another lecture tour and solicited funds to "continue his struggle against persecution" by "the medical trust, the Better Business Bureau, and the Food and Drug Administration." Do you think people believed his claims? They did. He was against the Establishment. He was clever in methods of deceit. A jury sentenced him to a year and a day in the penitentiary. He appealed and sued the judge. The appeal court upheld the verdict.

Larrick points out that fanatic food faddists of this type build up a fanatic zeal in their followers. Such nutritional quackery not only wastes millions of dollars, but it also endangers the lives of people who are in need of competent medical diagnosis and treatment. What is the answer? It is to teach all age groups the facts about sound nutrition and competent medical care.

Quacks thrive on those who are suffering and those who desire to lose weight. The woman cited on the Zen Diet lost 35 pounds and nearly lost her life. The problem of overweight is so important that special attention is given to it in the next part of this book.

Scare psychology and fallacies

"Soil depletion"

Soil depletion is a favorite topic of the food faddists. They would have us believe that our farmland is so eroded and deprived of nutrients that it cannot provide foods with sufficient vitamins, minerals, and protein.

In the light of scientific facts, this nonsense simply doesn't stand up. You recall that the green leaf utilizes the radiant energy of the sunshine and oxygen from air and water to bring about photosynthesis in which vitamins, sugars, and starches are made, and later fat; and that proteins are made by the plants in this fashion, with the added help of the nitrogen from the soil. We depend on the soil for minerals. The only mineral that is thoroughly depleted in our soil is iodine, which is added to table salt to compensate for the deficiency.

The fact is that a cow on a poor diet will not give as much milk as one on a good diet, but she maintains the level of calcium in her milk, even if it is not in the food. She takes it from her bones. A hen on a poor diet will not lay as many eggs as one on a good diet, but she keeps the nutrient standard the same in minerals, protein, and other nutrients. Both the cow and the hen are dependent on some green leaves or yellow foods for the vitamin A content in the diet, which they convert to pure vitamin A, and, like us, they depend on sunshine or another source for vitamin D. The chief value of adding fertilizer to the soil is to increase crop production, not the nutrients in the plants. When more nitrogen or other minerals are in the soil, the plant will take up only what it needs.

PLANT BREEDING. Plant breeding is doing far more to increase the nutrients in foods than elements added to the soil. You recall from preceding chapters that corn, wheat, and rice have been bred to produce cereal grains of much higher protein content, and that fruits and vegetables have increased in vitamin C content through breeding.

Food processing

According to the faddist, processing food deprives it of its more important nutrients. While it is true that highly refined foods lose some vitamins, minerals, and protein, as in milling flour, these are restored to a great extent (though not completely) by enrichment.

You remember from our study of fruits and vegetables that frozen and canned foods are processed in the field at the peak of maturity, when the nutrients are highest in the plant; that the heat in canning destroys no more nutrients than the heat of cooking fresh foods in your kitchen; and that often these foods are higher in vitamin and mineral content than so-called fresh ones. Highly sophisticated processed foods will be discussed in

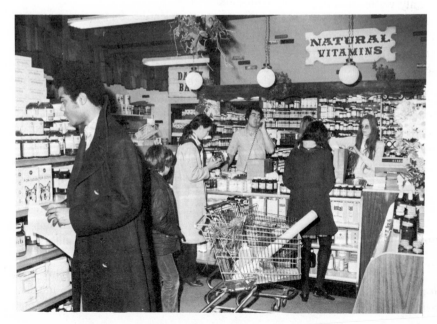

Properly chosen food will supply all the nutrients you need. Food supplements are not necessary for the normal person on a well-balanced diet. Note the display of bottled vitamins (called "natural") in this food shop. This sign is misleading.

the next chapter. But let us say here that these are not the basic foods, but fringe ones. Hence this argument of the faddist is false.

Liquefied foods

The faddist has made a cult out of liquefied vegetables and fruits. All of us enjoy tomato juice and various fruit juices. But the idea that carrots and other vegetables are better for you if you liquefy them is ridiculous for those who have teeth and a normal digestion. Indeed, too much carotene from liquefied carrots causes discoloration of the skin. Usually, the faddists sell the gadget that does the liquefying. Again, their real interest is in your money, not your health. Some faddists go so far as to decry pasteurized milk. These truly belong to the dark ages.

Nutritional deficiencies

Subclinical nutritional deficiencies and the fetish that all disease is caused by a poor diet are two myths that faddists and quacks present to ensure sales of "health foods." Here we see them presenting half-truths and twisting the minds of their audience to suit their purpose—to scare the unknowing into parting with their money for the product at hand. They take advantage of studies made to show how so many people are suffering from poor nutrition. They take a truth, then twist and exaggerate it to make the prospective buyer feel that his life depends on his purchase of the product. If a person is really suffering from malnutrition, or even a poor diet, he needs competent nutritional guidance to help him understand his problem and learn how to correct it on a successful long-term basis of eating a balanced diet at moderate cost.

The charlatan's bank account grows by playing on our fears and ignorance, and these are often found among people with advanced academic degrees, but with inadequate and inaccurate knowledge of nutrition.

How to detect a food faddist

One way is to ask yourself the following questions:

1/Does he have something to sell?

2/Is the price high? He appeals to snobbery and enriches himself by setting a high price. The case of the "Vermont maple syrup" which sold for $10 a gallon, but cost about 50 cents a gallon (as made from sugar, water, flavoring, and coloring), illustrates this point.

3/Does he exaggerate, quote out of context, and sprinkle in a few high-flown scientific terms to impress you?

4/Does he claim superiority for his product and downgrade the competition?

5/Does he advocate "natural" hand-ground grains, honey, raw milk, and liquefied vegetables and fruits?

6/Is his psychological approach one of creating fear if you don't do what he says?

7/Does he condemn the Food and Drug Administration? The USDA? The American Medical Association?

8/Does the title of a book, periodical, or magazine article he has written have a misleading or dishonest title or substance?

A "Yes" answer to these questions indicates that it is wise to take his message with caution. These are characteristics of the faddist or of the unscrupulous quack. If he belongs to a recognized professional group, such as the American Medical Association, and if competent people in in his field have evaluated what he is selling, in reliable professional literature, he is probably not a food faddist.

Dr. Herman Taller's book on weight reduction, *Calories Don't Count*, published in 1961, became a best seller, partly because of the misleading title. The physician's books and the safflower oil capsules sold in conjunction with them were seized by the Food and Drug Administration. He was brought to trial and given a jail sentence. In a book review, Dr. P. L. White of the Council on Foods and Nutrition of the American Medical Association stated, "This book is a grave injustice to the intelligent public and can only result in considerable damage to the prestige of the medical profession, of which Dr. Taller is a member."

Sources of protection for our food supply

More than any other consumer goods, our food is protected by law. In the preceding chapters, we noted how many steps are taken to protect us from contamination of our food supply. What are some of these agencies and how do they help us?

Federal

The Department of Health, Education, and Welfare is a division of the Federal Government. It is a cabinet post concerned with protecting our food. A division of this department is The United States Food and Drug Administration, and it is this division that has the closest supervision of

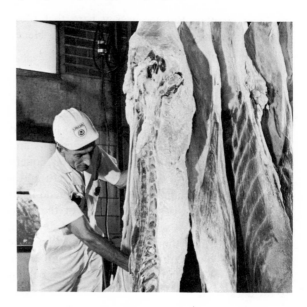

USDA's Consumer and Marketing Service meat inspectors check sides of beef at a packing company.

our food by law. Cooperating with this division and supplementing it are The United States Department of Agriculture and the United States Public Health Department. In the Department of Agriculture we have the Meat Inspection Agency and the Marketing Program. Then we have the United States Interstate Commerce Commission, the Federal Trade Commission, and the United States Fish and Wildlife Services.

Others

Many states have set up their own divisions of protections similar to the national ones, and some cities have these, too. Then there are nongovernmental agencies. It is quite an impressive lineup on the side of safe, wholesome, honest food by all phases of government, semiofficial organizations, world health organizations, professional groups, and food industry-supported studies.

How these agencies help us

Tests and laws

Let us take a few examples of how these agencies help us. One is the 1958 amendment to the Food, Drug, and Cosmetic Law of 1938 for better control and protection of our food. In the congressional investigation that brought forth this new law, we learned that of 704 additives to processed foods in use at that time "only 428 were definitely known to be safe." Many additives being used in food at that time got by without being tested; now the law requires that before the food industry can make a chemical addition to a food, it must first be tested on two sets of animals, one through a complete life span. These tests are submitted to scientists in the Food and Drug Administration, which decides on the basis of the evidence whether the additive is safe for human consumption. If not, it is rejected. Such tests led to the ban on cyclamates, discussed in Chapter 12, as well as re-evaluation of the safety of saccharin and monosodium glutamate for human consumption.

Bread, which once molded quickly in hot, humid weather, now does not mold, because of the additive propionates that inhibit the growth of mold. These are legally used in most commercial baked goods today. Another example is the antioxidants used to prevent rancidity in fats, bleaching agents to whiten flour, emulsifiers to prevent the separation of oil from liquid in salad dressing, artificial coloring and flavoring, and other chemicals to prevent lumping and caking in mixes.

Sample testing of food products in our stores goes on constantly to learn whether the food producer is living up to the law. In the fall of 1959, cranberries were withdrawn from the market by the authority of the 1958 law, because of excess spray residue. The Food and Drug Administration seized 824 shipments of food and filed 91 criminal cases of prosecution the first year the law was amended.

Federal trade commission

The Federal Trade Commission performs the following services for the public:

1/It sees that prices do not discriminate against the consumer in the long chain of distribution.

2/It keeps an eye on advertising to see that false claims are not made for the advertised items. It is hard to police this job, for there is much evasive, fraudulent advertising that we, as consumers, must recognize and reject. A not uncommon example of deceptive advertising was a large supermarket that advertised in the spring of 1969 "Veal, Lamb chops, USDA choice grade, 69¢ per pound." When the homemaker went for these, along with her $35 food order, she couldn't find them and was told, "They are just out. Come back tomorrow." She did, and was told the same thing and offered an inferior alternate. She wrote the manager and sent a copy of her letter to the Federal Trade Commission. She stated that this was fraudulent and deceptive advertising, and that this was not the first time it had occurred. The store manager answered her letter with apologies, and the federal agency with appreciation. The latter said the matter would be investigated. The only way to correct such practices is to inform the proper authorities.

3/It prohibits cooking equipment promoters from making false or unfair claims about their competitors, such as "Aluminum is porous and foods cooked in it are poisonous."

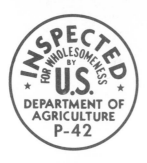

fig. 17–1 *Inspection stamp for poultry and egg products.*

4/It prevents price trickery in sales, such as advertising "3 8-oz. packages of a cold meat product for a dollar." Ordinarily, it sold for 33 cents each.

5/It regulates trade to provide fair competition in foods for buyers of raw products. The aim of this regulation is to prevent the large companies from pushing the smaller ones out of business by unfair methods of buying. One type of business practice the FTC seeks to prevent is the one illustrated by the spiraling cost of coffee some years ago, because of "a restrictive contract used by a New York Coffee and Sugar Exchange." This was corrected, and the price of coffee went down.

Inspection of meat and poultry

In federally inspected meats and poultry, the animals are inspected live, before slaughtering, and sick animals are eliminated. After the animal is slaughtered, the whole carcass is inspected, including the internal organs, to insure the good health and cleanliness of the meat. The surroundings at each step of preparing the meat or poultry for the retail trade are also inspected. Anything added to the meat must be clean and wholesome. Thus inspection marks are placed on meats and poultry to indicate cleanliness and wholesomeness.

The inspectors are veterinarians with special training for this work. To illustrate how this law, with well-trained inspectors, protects us, consider the year 1964. There were 5,493 animals condemned before slaughter and 113,637,893 passed inspection. After slaughter, another 274,156 were condemned. The rejected animals are destroyed.

Learn to recognize the inspection stamp in Figure 17–1. Look for it and buy meat that has it, for it is your symbol of meat that was clean and healthy at the time the stamp was placed there. Investigate your state and local laws on this aspect of consumer protection and learn how they compare with the federal regulations. Patronize only clean meat markets with adequate refrigeration. Meat of all kinds deteriorates rapidly when not frozen or adequately refrigerated. This can also happen at home.

Wholesome meat act and consumer protection

The Wholesome Meat Act of 1967 is an example of how the government is alert to changing needs and moves to protect all the consumers if the states fail to act. This act enables every homemaker to feel assured that what she serves her family "is pure, that it has been packed and it has been processed in a sanitary plant," as President Lyndon B. Johnson stated when he signed the bill.

This bill means that by law the total meat supply in the United States will be equally well-inspected, either by the federal or the state government. The Meat Act of 1906 required inspection of only that meat that entered interstate or foreign commerce. It left the inspection of meat sold within the state to the individual states to inspect. As it worked out, the standards used by the states were not as high, in some instances, as those for the federally inspected meat—or were nonexistent. Since 1967, the states either comply by passing their own laws and setting up a state meat inspection program with equally high standards or the federal government is authorized to take over.

This law was sorely needed. Only 29 states had mandatory inspection laws governing intrastate meat (that is, sold within the state); 12 states had

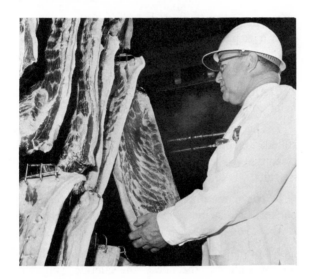

A USDA meat inspector examines bacon in a smokehouse during processing. All meat and meat products are checked to make sure the approved formulas and procedures are followed.

voluntary inspection laws; 2 required licensing of meat packers; and 7 had no inspection laws at all. Of course, this does not mean that all the uninspected meat was unfit for human consumption. It does mean that there were no controls to assure the healthiest, cleanest, purest meat possible. The 1967 law was designed to give uniform protection by meat inspection throughout the nation—a landmark for consumer protection.

Food standards

MEANING OF FOOD STANDARDS. Standards are both a goal for achievement and a yardstick to measure progress. In the preceding discussion, we have seen how our standards have improved since the first law to protect the consumer's food was enacted in 1906. And in Part I, we noted standards set for enriched bread-cereal products of all kinds, for addition of vitamin A to margarine, and of vitamins A and D to fortify skim milk.

Nathan Koenig, the United States delegate to the first three sessions of the International Commission (1962–65) which set the first worldwide standards for many staple foods, points out that "Standards for food that are properly drafted are a yardstick for the buyer, the seller, and the enforcement official alike." They promote confidence in the food trade.

WHAT OUR STANDARDS INCLUDE. Some aspects of food standards are the following:

1/They define the product, giving the name, additives, description, and some aspects of quality, such as minimum figures for important ingredients, and sometimes the maximum figures.

2/They set forth hygiene requirements—the product must be sanitary, safe from excessive pesticides and other contaminants, wholesome in all respects for eating, and in marketable form.

3/They specify weight and measure requirements—these must be accurate as stated, and the fill of the container or the count of units must not be deceptive.

4/They establish labeling requirements—the label (including pictures) must present specifically and accurately what is in the product. Imported products must be labeled in English.

5/They provide for sampling, testing, and analysis of products. This is a government safeguard to ensure that the food meets the standards set to protect the consumer.

HOW WE GET OUR FOOD STANDARDS. Standards for many staple foods are agreed upon in our country by government technicians working with consumers and members of a food industry. Thus we are given an opportunity and a responsibility to help set standards. When standards are set, they become legal regulations. This was illustrated in the 1967 Wholesome Meat Act, which was passed to protect consumers in the 31 states that had no mandatory laws to assure cleanliness, safety, and wholesomeness of meats. Another example of improving standards by testing and analysis is the banning of the chemical additive sodium cyclamate and the restrictions on the use of the pesticide spray DDT. Analysis of water, fish, and wildlife for mercury content has led to restrictions on industry and agriculture, limiting the amount released into air and water.

Food labels

LABELS NEED CONTINUOUS IMPROVEMENT. The law on food labeling illustrates how standards are applied in concrete action to help the consumer. The labeling law is under the supervision of the Federal Food and Drug Administration and covers foods in interstate commerce. When products do not measure up to the law, the entire shipments are seized from the market and the processors prosecuted. The law requires that:

1/The label must accurately represent the contents of the package or can.

2/It must not make false or misleading statements and must be easily read in English. This also applies to imported foods.

3/The ingredients must be listed with the largest amount first and the balance in descending order. For instance, if there is more liquid safflower oil than hydrogenated oil in a margarine, the safflower oil is listed first. Or if there is more gravy than chicken in a chicken product, the gravy must be listed first.

4/The net contents must be stated in units of measure that we use.

5/The product must fill the container at the time it is packaged. Packaging must not be misleading, as representing more in amount than there is.

6/All chemical additives, preservatives, artificial coloring, and flavoring must be listed.

7/The variety and style of the food must be stated, together with the name of the product, in clear type—such as thick, thin, or medium syrup in fruits; whole or kernel corn; and so on.

8/The name and address of the manufacturer, packer, or distributor must be on the label. This is where you can write if the product is substandard.

9/Special dietary foods for diabetics, heart disease sufferers, the obese, the allergic, and others, such as low-sodium products, must specify on the label the amount of ingredients for a given measure.

10/When nutrients such as vitamins or minerals are added to a food, the label must state the amount in a recommended serving, in relation to the daily recommended amount.

Although the label law is a fine thing for the consumer, it is useful to you only when you take the time to read the labels and understand what they mean. For instance, when you see chemical additives listed on the label, you may not know what that listing means. For practical purposes, it means that the additive has been tested according to law for safe human consumption over a lifetime. This is quite an important piece of information for you. If the food does not live up to the label, the processor is prosecuted to protect you.

Good as this is, many consumers think that the labels should be further improved. For instance, the consumer wants to know—and has the right to know, for the sake of intelligent meal

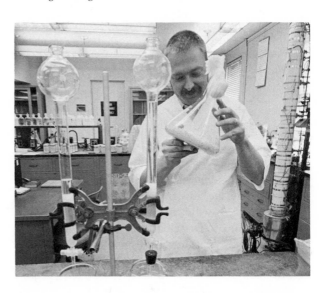

A chemist in the Food and Drug Administration checks a corn extraction to make sure the quality and labeling meet government standards.

planning—what kind and percentage of fat is contained in "low-fat" cottage cheese, other cheese, milk, yogurt, imitation ice cream, or ice milk. She should know that "nondairy creamer" for coffee contains as much saturated fat as dairy coffee cream, and sometimes more. Only with such knowledge can she evaluate products, and (where necessary) work to change the labeling or improve the product.

Brand names

A brand name is owned by a company and no one else can use that name. The standards for their product are agreed upon between the food industry and the government, and the industry must follow these standards like a recipe. When this is not done, the product is removed from the market and those responsible are penalized. Occasionally this happens. But those who own brand names value them in the same way that a family values its crest or coat of arms. The reputation of their brand is what they expect the consumer to respect and want, because of its consistently high standards of quality.

A product with a well-known brand name may cost a few cents more for a given weight than one with a lesser-known brand. It may also give you more solid food and less water for the money. Only you, the consumer, can determine which to buy and what to pay, by comparing the amount of solid food and the number of servings for a given price. Check the cost per serving of solid food. Keep a record of what you learn. Refer to this information to save money.

Dr. J. A. Bayton, president of Universal Marketing Research, Inc., made this comment: "The low-income housewife seems to have an abiding faith in the product she has heard the most about. Upper-income purchasers, however, are leaning more and more to less expensive and less well-known products." A wise homemaker judges a product by its merit, not its name.

What the consumer can do to improve food standards

The consumer has much more power to improve our food standards than many of us realize. The lone battle of one young lawyer, Ralph Nader, for safety standards in cars and other products, in the consumer's interests, is just one example of what an individual can accomplish, and how public support can be summoned to improve the safety, honesty, and quality of our products. This includes the nutrients in our food supply. As individuals, consumers should

1/Learn the laws that protect our food. You have had a brief glimpse of federal regulations

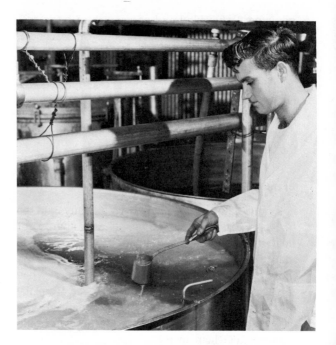

A laboratory technician samples the mixture in a blending tank at a Florida orange juice plant. The food industry watches carefully to protect the quality and purity of products.

designed for consumer protection. Study your state and local laws, and see to it that they meet or surpass the federal standards.

2/Watch carefully for violations of the laws and report them at once, whether they are in a public eating place, on a food label, in fraudulent and misleading advertising, or in some other area.

3/Report the violations you have found, and the reasons for your objections, to the FDA (Food and Drug Administration). Send copies to the manager of the store or restaurant, requesting him to forward it to the proper authority in his company; to the USDA Consumer Marketing Service, to your state consumer adviser (if you have one), and to the National Consumer Adviser to the President.

4/Make specific suggestions on how to improve the laws on labeling. If you think some of the standards agreed upon between the government and a food company should be stated on the label to guide the consumer when he buys, work to have this accomplished. If you feel that the label or the advertising of a product is misleading (such as "low-fat" or "polyunsaturated," when the food does not actually live up to these claims), protest in writing and work to have the situation corrected.

5/Use your influence to set standards for all types of processed foods, especially highly refined convenience foods. Labels on these foods should contain full information on the nutrient content of these foods and meals.

6/Seek accurate information. Don't get upset over every newspaper or magazine report on a food danger. Depending on the particular publication, these may present only half-truths or twisted information. Some reliable sources of information are the following:

a. Biochemists or nutritionists in colleges; health officers; hospital consultants, state and county extension nutritionists; national, state, and local Health and Welfare nutritionists

b. Your family physician and the American Medical Association's Council on Food and Nutrition, especially the latter

c. Books and articles written by recognized authorities in good standing in their profession and published by reliable publishers.

d. Teachers and research workers in the field of nutrition and food

e. The Federal Trade Commission (regarding fraudulent advertising and misleading and doubtful statements about food in advertising media and elsewhere)

f. The Federal Food and Drug Administration (for advice and help on labels and contamination of food in any form, from filth to pesticide residue)

g. The United States Department of Agriculture, Consumer and Food Economics Research Division

h. The National Consumer Representative and the state one, if you have such an official

If in doubt, write to the FDA, which will forward your letter to the proper source if it is not in their category. Weigh all the facts.

7/Take all the precautions discussed in Chapter 16 to remove contamination of food in your home. Wash food carefully and take the greatest care of it at every step. Remember that you are the guardian (as is every other member of the family) of all food when it enters your home. Remember, too, that the food you need to provide a well-balanced diet is sold right in your everyday food stores, not in the so-called health stores. Dishonest "promoters," quacks, and faddists thrive on the public's fears and ignorance about the safety and nutrients of our food supply. They will not flourish at your expense, for you will be accurately informed. You understand why Dr. P. L. White, secretary of the Food and Nutrition Council of the American Medical Association, points out that "Nutrition authorities are in agreement that needed vitamins and minerals can best be obtained from vegetables, fruits, milk, eggs, meat, and whole-grain and enriched cereals." These can be combined in a balanced diet.

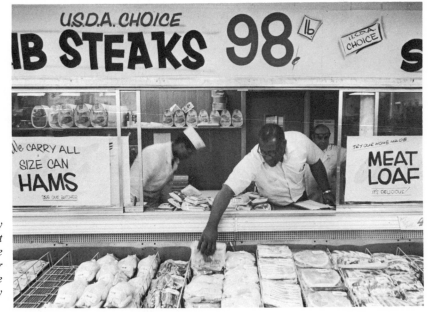

The consumer is protected by regulations ensuring honest weights and measures in the foods he buys. This inspector is weighing meat to determine whether weight is properly marked.

Meaningful words

brand labels
brand names
fad diet
food fad
food fallacy
"health foods"
nutritional advertising
nutritional quackery
standardized foods

Thinking and evaluating

1. Explain why food fads and fad diets are dangerous.

2. What is the technique of the food faddist? How can you detect a food faddist?

3. What is an additive? Are all additives harmful? Give examples of useful ones.

4. In the Congressional investigation which led to the 1958 law to provide better control of our food, it was learned that only one-half of these additives to food were known to be safe. How has the 1958 law helped in this respect?

5. What are the advantages, aside from saving money on the food budget, for the homemaker who can cook her own meals?

6. In what ways does the Department of Health, Education, and Welfare function to help you and your family have a healthier diet?

7. Explain how the 1967 Meat Inspection Law helps all consumers.

8. In what ways does the Federal Trade Commission help the consumer with family food?

9. In what different ways do the food faddist and the nutritional quack mislead the person who does not have depth of knowledge concerning foods and nutrition?

10. Why was the book *Calories Don't Count*, by Dr. Herman Taller, condemned by the American Medical Association? In what ways does the title appeal to and mislead many in nutritional matters? Why was Dr. Taller prosecuted by the courts and convicted?

11. New processed foods are constantly coming into our markets. How can you evaluate them accurately?

12. Why is the accurate labeling of food so important? What role do you have to play in improving labeling and making it work? Give examples.

Applying and sharing

1. Analyze the information about foods and nutrition that comes into your home on TV, radio, newspaper columns, news reports, magazines, and other media, to learn if the information is accurate. How many use half-truths and/or slanted or twisted information to

sell a product? How would you decide on an accurate basis? Do such techniques influence small children for better or worse? Teen-agers? Adults? You?

2. What do you think of food fads and fad diets as a means of controlling one's weight over a lifetime? Explain how fad "reducing" diets can undermine your health, make you less attractive, and hurt you on a long-term basis.

3. Do you or any member of your family or any of your friends follow food fads or fad diets? If so, examine them and see if they measure up in helping you achieve your long-term goals, such as controlling your weight. Learn what fad foods or diets cost you or your friends in terms of money and other things you value. Share with your mother and family or with a friend what you have learned in this chapter.

4. Some nutritional supplements cost as much as $20 per month for adults and $10 per child. Show how this money might be used more wisely for a balanced diet.

5. Write to your federal government and your local health department to learn what laws in your county, state, nation, and community protect the consumer. Share this with your family.

6. What suggestions do you have for the improvement of food labeling? Do you read labels before you buy and compare prices on the basis of the contents listed? What have you learned that can help you now? Later?

convenience
foods and meals

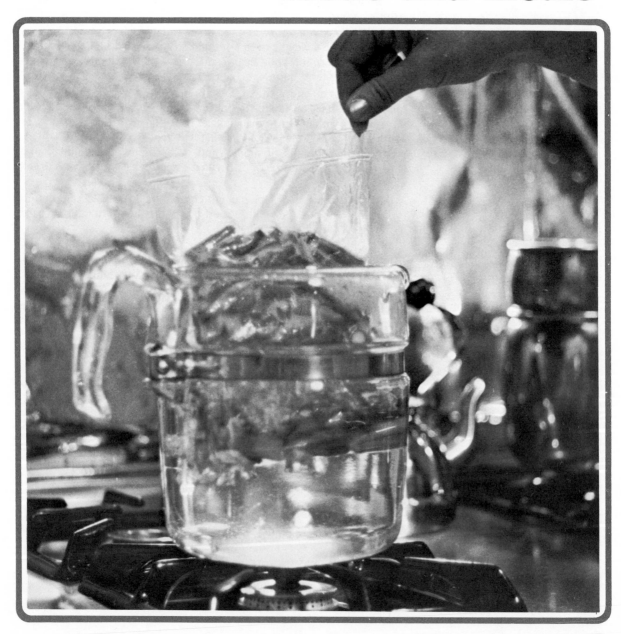

Consumers are expressing grave concern over the trend toward increased use of more sophisticated convenience foods and lack of nutritional information about them. This topic was discussed at the International Congress of Home Economics by delegates from 62 nations, meeting at the University of Bristol, England, in 1968. It is discussed in national meetings, in our homes, and elsewhere.

George P. Larrick, Commissioner of the Food and Drug Administration, strikes at the heart of the matter in his statement, "It is becoming easier to conceal substitution or inferiority from ordinary observation in today's processed, compounded, packaged foods."*

Nature of the problem

The inventive genius of the people in this country and elsewhere has made food our largest business —and a highly competitive one. In 1967, for instance, 74 billion dollars went from our pockets over the food market counters. People are in this business to make money—a legitimate aim. You, the consumer, will determine which convenience foods will succeed by demanding value for your dollar. The food industry is highly sensitive to your desires and criticisms.

Bewildering variety

In 1968, 7500 new food items were launched in our markets, according to a report made that year. High on the list were convenience foods. Low-calorie foods and those with an international appeal were also numerous. We have not yet

---

*George P. Larrick in *Food: The Yearbook of Agriculture, 1959* (Washington, D.C.: USDA), p. 445.

reached the peak in the number of food companies that will compete for our dollar, or the number of convenience foods available, the report stated. Two billion dollars were spent on snack foods alone in 1967.

To some homemakers, this increasing number of foods from which to choose is a nightmare. They are frightened, lest they become dependent on trivial new items which appropriate money that should be used for foods to maintain basic health. This was reported at the 1968 meeting of the American Home Economics Association. Some of the people in the group work with food companies. They are in a position to exercise influence on the production of convenience foods.

A survey was made of all age groups, from teen-agers to older persons. In each of these groups, consumers were frightened. They felt that the food companies were forcing on them a multitude of new products, very few of which were necessary or important to them.

Only half of the new foods introduced in 1968 were successful and remained on the market. In contrast to the frightened food shopper, there are also discriminating shoppers among us.

The informed food shopper knows what she is about in the world of food. She makes out her menu for the week, writes down the foods she needs, sticks to the list, and moves through the store with speed and confidence, knowing what to buy and why she buys it. She does not slip into her food basket alluring new items that take the food money and leave basic needs unmet.

Inadequate consumer information

The problem, then, arises from the flood of new food items in a sophisticated form on the one hand, and, on the other hand, the millions of homemakers who lack adequate information to make wise choices about these foods. Naturally, it is a frightening experience to be constantly exposed to more foods from which to choose and not to know how to evaluate these foods.

Standards for convenience foods

Convenience in a new food item is a fine thing, but as the homemakers made clear to the food companies in 1968 by rejecting over 3000 of the items introduced, convenience alone is not enough.

What do you need to know to be able to evaluate convenience foods and meals? You need an understanding of the strengths and weaknesses of

Frozen convenience foods appear in overwhelming variety in our markets. We must learn to evaluate them and use only those that are practical and valuable.

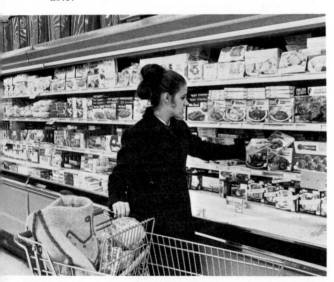

the different foods we need daily for sound health and an attractive person, and how to combine these foods in meals so that the strengths of one balance the weaknesses of the other. When taken together, the foods you choose should provide a balanced meal that pleases your taste and fits into your food budget. You have acquired this basic knowledge in the preceding chapters.

Thus it is quite important that, as new foods come on the market, adequate information be given about them. What will one serving, for instance, contribute to the day's nutritional need?

Advantages of convenience foods

Each of us, whether a full-time homemaker, a working wife, a single girl, or a bachelor, often needs to prepare a quick and easy meal. A convenience food makes a meal easy to prepare and saves time and energy. These are the two big selling points for the busy homemaker. But if we continue to buy the product, it must taste good and the flavor and texture must please us. These are subjective or personal evaluations and will not be the same for each person.

BASIC FOODS. Basic convenience foods have met these tests. Many have been on the market so long that we take them for granted. Some of these foods are:

1/All forms of cereal foods ready to eat, such as fresh-baked bread, brown-and-serve baked products, whole wheat flour, refined enriched cereals, flour, and flour and cereal products

2/Pasteurized milk in many forms and at different prices

3/High-quality fresh or cured meats, poultry, and fish ready to cook or to use from a can or to thaw and heat

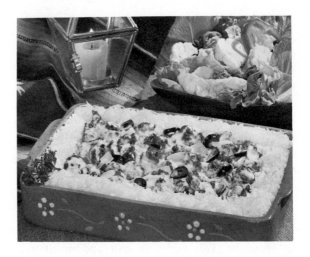

Convenience meals may be made at home for future use. When making a beef and rice casserole, prepare twice the quantity needed for one meal and freeze half.

4/Vegetables and fruits that are canned and ready to eat, frozen, dried, freeze-dried, pickled, or preserved

5/Canned, frozen, and dried soups to begin a meal or use as a convenience in making a casserole

6/Butter, margarine, oil, shortening, lard, and sugar

These are all convenience foods that are ready to use and save us hours of hard work. They have proved their worth by the test of time. They are worth the price we pay for them. From these foods and fresh vegetables and fruits we make dull or delightful meals and become poorly-fed or well-fed.

COST. In an indirect way, convenience foods lower the total money spent for food. This sounds like a paradox, but it isn't.

In developing nations, some of the fresh fruit and vegetables in season may rot while people starve in the same nation, because of lack of processing equipment and knowledge of processing methods that would enable them to preserve surplus food, or the transportation and storage facilities to make it available to all the people. Because of our advanced food technology, from the field and factory to the kitchen, our surplus foods are made available for use the year round in convenience forms. We are not dependent on a good growing season to eat well. This large volume of food helps reduce total costs, and at the same time provides the choices for a better diet.

SPACE SAVING. The fact that convenience foods are often reduced in weight and bulk means that it costs less to transport and store them. This is another factor in reducing the total cost of food. Flour, for instance, weighs two-thirds as much as wheat; canned corn, one-third as much as corn on the cob; frozen orange juice, one-fourth as

much as fresh; dehydrated or frozen vegetables, fruits, and other foods, about half as much; and dried fruit crystals a very small percentage of the weight of fresh fruit.

CONVENIENCE MEALS. Ready-to-eat meals are the ultimate in convenience foods. Nevertheless, they should be evaluated in comparison with home-cooked meals. There are many types that fall into two general classes: the ready-to-eat meal that is served at home and the one prepared and eaten away from home. The convenience of both types is well worth paying for in an emergency situation, even on a low budget.

Such an emergency might occur when a young mother comes home from the hospital with a baby, if her husband can't prepare the meal and there is no outside help; or when guests come for meals and the mother is unable to prepare a meal but wishes to have one at home. Older people are often provided for in this way, too, when they have no facilities to cook properly or are unable to do so.

There are choices between the frozen-type TV dinner that may be heated and served, eliminating some dishwashing, and other types of prepared food. "Meals on Wheels" are being provided in increasing numbers, particularly for older people and shut-ins. The meals are prepared in a central kitchen, according to the individual's order from a choice of menus, then delivered to his home at an appointed time, being kept hot in an electronic oven. This type must be kept in a low oven until it is served.

MEALS EATEN OUT. Most couples enjoy eating out, and families like to take their children out to eat occasionally. It is often a convenient way to entertain. This varies in cost and nutritional adequacy according to how well you know what to select—including the place. Snack bars are popular among young people. Vending machines that sell beverages and foods are doing between 2 and 3 billion dollars business, studies show. There are automats, cafeterias, drive-ins, and good and poor restaurants. Every home should have a variety of convenience foods from which a quick meal may be prepared.

Disadvantages

FLAVOR AND TEXTURE. Let us consider first the disadvantage of the ready-to-eat meal that you serve at home. The chief criticism is that the flavor is like that of warmed-over food. The texture may be too soft. Often there is too much bone and fat in the meat and too little lean, or more gravy than meat.

NUTRIENTS LACKING. An important question to ask yourself is: Is this a balanced meal? Usually it isn't. You need to provide milk or cheese and a raw salad or fruit. Often these meals do not provide a third of the day's vitamin C requirement; they may or may not provide any vitamin A; little iron or calcium; and too little protein. Too often they are high in starch, fat, and sweets. The flavor and appearance may be excellent and still it may be a poor meal nutritionally.

A disadvantage of convenience foods is that some food companies are more concerned with the appearance, flavor, color, texture, and their profit than they are with the nutrients in the food, especially in the sophisticated or fringe foods. Not all are, by any means. When the company will place on the label or wrapping the amount of nutrients a serving will provide toward meeting the day's recommended need, you will have an accurate basis for comparison that is more valid than an emotional reaction to flavor, texture, and appearance.

As consumers, we may be able to help eliminate these weaknesses in the future. If you demand it and there is a great enough need for this type of food, meals can be calibrated (kal' ə brāt əd) for the nutrients they provide toward the day's need. We can know the total calories from fat, protein, and carbohydrate in the meal, and the approximate quantities of vitamins and minerals.

COST. In figuring out the cost of this type of service, be sure that you add to the cost of the meal the price of the beverage and fruit or salad it may require to be balanced nutritionally. You are paying for service, as well as food, and this makes the meal cost more.

At a restaurant, the cost of the meat often determines the cost of the meal. The meal can be expensive and still be poor nutritionally, serving no more than a salad or soup, the meat, a potato —often French-fried—and rolls. You may have to pay extra for a cooked vegetable, a beverage, and dessert. There are some moderate-price eating places that serve balanced meals. These are popular in any country or state. There is no doubt that a good cook and manager can prepare the menu of an expensive restaurant at home for much less, and in addition provide a better meal. Still, we do enjoy eating out if we can get a good meal at a fair price.

Another factor in cost is what you add to complete the recipe for a convenience food. Take mixes, for example. In popovers, there is nothing but salt and flour, but you add milk and eggs—the expensive items. Fresh eggs are usually required as an addition to most mixes. Milk, nuts, dried fruits, and other ingredients may be called for. In a fair comparison, every item that you add must be added to the total cost of that convenience food. It is wise to make a record of these costs. Then you know the facts and can make your comparison accurately. This technique is used by the best food managers.

ADDITIVES. Chemical additives are used in most convenience foods. This does not necessarily mean they are undesirable. It does mean that you have to pay for them, and that a homemaker who uses many processed foods, especially the more sophisticated ones, gets more additives than she would by preparing meals from basic foods. The food and drug laws are now more stringent, for your protection, as you noted in Chapter 17.

Let us take a convenience form of potatoes to illustrate how additives are used to sell you what you want and make money for the processor. In making the flakes for mashed potatoes, the potatoes are washed, peeled, trimmed, cut into slabs a half-inch thick, and immersed in hot water to gelatinize the starch. Then they are plunged into

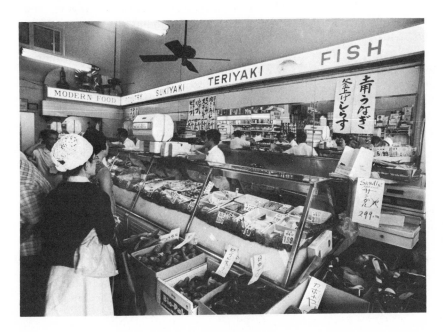

This Little Tokyo food store offers both raw and precooked foods. The buyer must determine which prepared foods are wise purchases on the basis of nutrition and price.

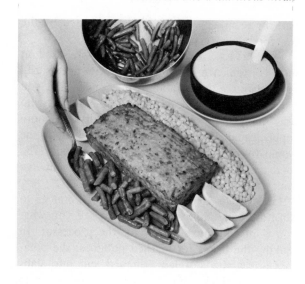

Canned salmon or tuna is a convenience food that is easily and quickly converted into a nutritious meal.

cold water to make them less pasty. Next, they are cooked in steam until tender, and riced to a mash.

The consumer likes fluffy mashed potatoes. Therefore, the producer, trying to give the public what it likes, adds the chemical glycerolmonostearate (**glis′ ə rol män ə stē ə rāt**) in small amounts, and the convenience potato is fluffy—just the way we like it—when it is completed by the addition of hot water or hot milk in our kitchen. But first an antioxidant is added to prevent the small amount of fat in the potatoes from spoiling the flavor. Again, this is done to please our sense of taste and to help sell the product. Then the mixture is dried in a drum, coming off in continuous sheets that are broken into flakes. Tests show that good flakes can be made from 12 different varieties of potatoes tested from the West Coast to Maine.

This product was so successful that in about a year after the first commercial tests were made, 6 million bushels of potatoes were made into 50 million pounds of flakes annually. They are now sold all over the world.

Chemical additives are not new in the diet. In most nations in the world, people have long added salt, vinegar, pepper, spices, sugar, and other chemicals to foods to improve their flavor and increase the supply, by preserving them. Salt was added to meat to cure it, and to cabbage, cucumbers, tomatoes, and other foods to pickle them, before we had modern technology. The principle is simple. Salt produces fermentation in which a healthy acetic acid develops that destroys the growth of microorganisms in curing meats and pickling vegetables and fruits, and makes these foods usable for a long time. Similarly, when sweet milk sours, the sugar is changed to lactic acid, which preserves buttermilk, yogurt, sour cream, and cheese. It inhibits the growth of bacteria that spoil milk. Hence the popularity of yogurt, buttermilk, and cheese in hot countries.

Women all over the world have added sugar to fruit and by cooking it to a syrupy concentration could preserve it, but they did not know why the process succeeded in preserving the fruit. We know the reason now. It is the sugar concentration. When the syrup reaches 62.5 percent sugar, sugar draws water from bacteria by osmotic pressure and prevents their growth, thus preventing spoilage.

An innovation in the process of fruit preserving, achieved by pioneer research in the USDA studies at Wyndmoor, Pennsylvania, is a method to catch and hold the volatile flavors that boil off in the making of jellies and jams. These can now be added back to produce a more flavorsome product than our grandmothers could make.

Our new knowledge of nutrition and biochemistry enables us to add nutrients back to processed foods, compensating to some extent for the losses suffered when they are being highly processed.

Another development in food processing is the use of chemical additives to produce the desired texture and flavor in some foods, as well as to preserve them—features that the consumer wants.

What does processing do to the nutrients in convenience foods?

This question is often asked. It has been discussed in connection with each food group as we studied it in Part I. You may wish to browse through this again. You recall that the vitamin C content in fresh-cooked new potatoes is three to five times as high as in convenience forms; that the B and C vitamins are soluble in water, as are all minerals. There is also a loss of these vitamins and minerals when they are placed in water, hot or cold.

B vitamins, vitamin E, some protein, and probably other nutrients still unidentified are removed in refining whole grains and other foods. Though three B vitamins and iron (in some instances) are added back to cereal grains, not all nutrients removed are restored. Vitamin B_6, B_{12}, vitamin E, and some amino acids are examples of this. However, the "enriched" white bread is so much better than the unenriched refined type that pellagra, a niacin-deficiency disease, has been eliminated in our country.

The processing of dried eggs does not harm the nutrients. Research has unsnarled the problem of flavor and keeping quality in this food by preventing the small trace of sugar in eggs from combining with protein. Now, when you eat dried eggs in commercially prepared scrambled eggs and baked products, you are not aware of any difference between the dried egg product and that made with fresh, whole eggs. Processing milk into dried forms makes no significant change in its food value beyond that of pasteurized fluid milk. Think what this convenience food has meant to humanity all over the world!

Importance of labels

Read labels on convenience foods. Learn what is added back before you buy and the price you pay for the additions, as compared with the plain form of whole-grain cereals, for example. Usually, the additions make the food more expensive in highly processed or sophisticated forms. In some

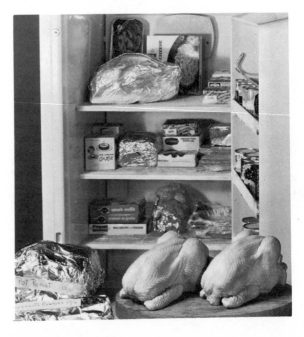

Foods prepared and frozen during winter provide easy meals and party fare in hot weather. Which foods are best for freezing?

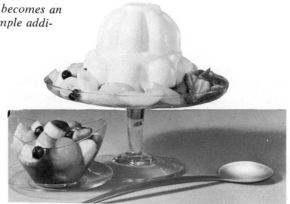

Prepared instant pudding becomes an elegant dessert with the simple addition of fruit.

cases, as the addition of vitamin D to milk, vitamin A to margarine, and the B vitamins to breads, flours, and basic cereals, this extra cost is negligible.

In general, the more highly processed a convenience food is, the greater the loss of nutrients and the greater the cost per serving. But foods must be judged individually.

Processed foods vs. homemade foods

Flavor

Despite the fact that desirable flavor and appearance are important things that food companies try

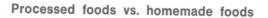

Canned applesauce is the surprise ingredient in the sauce that makes Shrimp Temptation a special treat. This easy dish uses canned shrimp and quick-cooking rice.

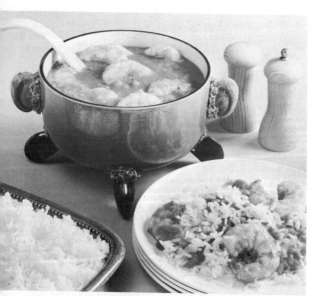

to achieve in convenience foods, most people prefer the flavor of home-cooked food and meals, when they are well prepared. Listen to the sounds of approval when your family or friends at the table learn that you baked the cake or made the bread!

Appearance

While another big selling point in convenience foods is appearance, homemade dishes and meals can surpass the ordinary and equal the best when you give thought to their appearance. What is more pleasing to smell and see than a home-baked loaf of bread or a glazed ham with pineapple; a pork roast surrounded by crabapples; a golden-brown turkey or chicken garnished with orange slices? The salads you make at home can far surpass in appearance those bought from a special food store or eaten in the most expensive restaurant.

Evaluating new products

As new food items that appeal to you come on the market, evaluate them on the basis of factual information. Some will be excellent, others poor. Consider the cost, the nutrients, and the calories each brings to a meal or a snack. Remember that many of the snack tidbits are quite high in fat or in sugar, or both—and in calories. What are you paying for the flavor of the jam-filled pastry that you toast, as compared with a slice of whole wheat or enriched toast with margarine and jam? What are you getting for your money? Ask fair questions and answer them, before you create a desire in yourself and your family for new foods you may not need and cannot afford.

If you think that more information is required on a product's label, state your point, in writing, to the store manager and the food company. Genuine intelligent interest in food brings results, if we go to the proper place with our complaint or idea. By such informed buying on your part, you will keep on the market foods that are convenient and at the same time important in nourishment, as well as flavor.

Many desirable foods will come to us in the future. Recently, a fat-free milk containing more protein than regular milk was introduced. Another product was an imitation sour cream made with vegetable oil—so desirable for those who need to limit intake of animal fats, if the oil is high in linoleic acid.

In evaluating a convenience meal that you prepare or buy, it may help if you ask these questions: Is there three to four ounces of lean meat per serving? Is there a green or yellow vegetable or fruit? How large are the servings of vegetables— ½ to ¾ cup? Is there a good source of vitamin C in the meal? A third of the day's calcium requirement, in the form of milk or milk products? How does it rate when compared with the plan for a balanced meal given in Chapter 2? It shows important growth if you answer these and other questions of your own. It is important to know how the cost of homemade convenience foods and meals compares with that of ready-to-eat ones, taking all costs and considerations into account.

By using the information you have gained, you will be able to make the wise decisions in buying convenience food, and purchase only what is well worth its cost to you. Thus you separate the worthwhile foods from the frills. You will know that the convenience form of potato, for instance, can be supplemented for any lack in vitamin C by a serving of cabbage, a green salad, a citrus fruit for dessert, or another seasonal food high in this vitamin. You can prepare nutritionally balanced meals at little cost and with little expenditure of energy, if you keep yourself informed on sound nutrition, and if you plan and shop carefully.

Compare a homemade beef stew with a frozen TV dinner for taste, nutrients, and price. How much is the convenience worth to you?

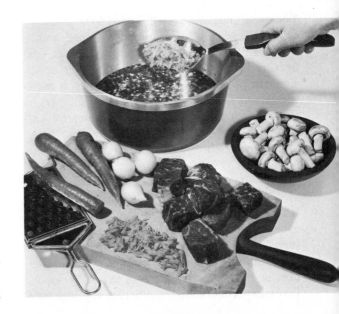

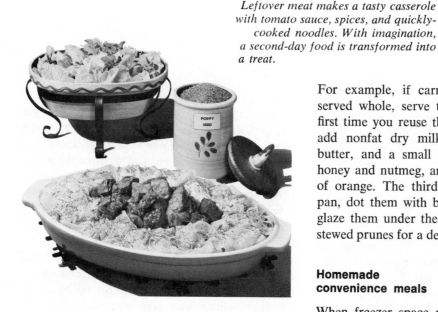

Leftover meat makes a tasty casserole with tomato sauce, spices, and quickly-cooked noodles. With imagination, a second-day food is transformed into a treat.

For example, if carrots have been cooked and served whole, serve them in buttered circles the first time you reuse them. Next time, mash them, add nonfat dry milk, some margarine, oil, or butter, and a small amount of brown sugar or honey and nutmeg, and garnish them with a slice of orange. The third time, place them in a flat pan, dot them with butter and brown sugar, and glaze them under the broiler, or serve them with stewed prunes for a delightful flavor.

Homemade convenience meals

When freezer space permits, it is good management to freeze a home-prepared meal that a child or man could serve quickly in an emergency. A vegetable-meat soup can be used in this way; so can a meat-vegetable-cereal casserole or a stew. Add to this carrot sticks, celery, or raw sliced onions, bread, milk, and a canned fruit for dessert, and you achieve a tasty and well-balanced meal with little effort and at low cost.

Studies made by the USDA show that "Most processed foods . . . are not equal to strictly farm-fresh foods or freshly caught fish or home-baked cake. But when we cannot get the farm-fresh foods and do not have the time to bake the cake, we are glad to have the processed foods."

You may find, along with many others, that the family is better fed for less money when we do a good share of the cooking ourselves. And besides, we derive great satisfaction from going into our kitchen, taking a group of low-cost foods and some basic convenience foods, and creating a meal that we know provides what our family needs in good nutritional balance. We like to see our family eat it with enjoyment, and to hear them say, "Everything in this meal tastes good."

Make your own convenience foods and meals

Quantity cooking for future use

You recall that as we studied each food group we considered how to save time, energy, and money by cooking some foods in large amounts and freezing them in family portions for later meals. You can precook a large roast, a turkey, a meat-vegetable soup that makes a main dish, various meats (such as pot roast), vegetable-cereal casseroles, boiled and baked beans, carrots, beets, tomato-meat sauce, white sauce, and other foods for later use.

Varying leftover foods

It takes no more fuel and little more time to cook enough tomato-meat sauce, rhubarb, or applesauce for three meals at one time than it does for one meal. Use your cookbooks and your imagination, and cater to your family's tastes, by serving the extra portions of food a different way each time.

Meaningful words

acetic acid
antioxidant
calibrate
gelatinize
glycerolmonostearate
meals on wheels
quick-cooking food
sophisticated foods
volatile flavors

Thinking and evaluating

1. What is a convenience food? In what different forms do they appear? Which convenience foods do almost all of us use? Which convenience foods do you use most? Your family?

2. What do you need to know to evaluate convenience foods intelligently?

3. What are the advantages of convenience foods? The disadvantages?

4. How would you compare the food or meal made from basic materials at home with a similar one that is "convenient" in (a) cost per serving; (b) nutritive values that you need in your daily diet; (c) flavor; (d) appearance?

5. Which convenience foods do not lose nutrients in processing? Which do?

6. Why do additives in convenience foods need to be tested?

7. Does the type of package of a convenience food influence your choice? Explain which type of packaging you prefer and why. How much may packaging increase the cost of a food product?

8. What are the advantages of preparing your own convenience foods at home? Which foods are well suited to this type of preparation? Which foods may be precooked and ready for a quick convenience meal at home? Do you consider it a matter of food management if a homemaker can prepare her own convenience foods and meals? Explain your answer.

Applying and sharing

1. Visit a large supermarket to learn the different convenience foods on the market in each food group by listing them and noting the following information: (a) cost per package; (b) weight per package; (c) size of package (measure with a flexible tape); (d) label listing ingredients—note additives that are necessary for processing only; (e) what you consider essential and nonessential in the packaging of convenience foods.

2. Do the same for convenience meals.

3. Be prepared to discuss in class what you have learned from the above comparison. On the basis of what you learned, make a plan showing how your family now could save money and have a better diet by changing the foods you buy.

4. If you had your own home, which convenience foods would you try to keep in reserve for emergencies? In what emergencies would you use convenience foods? Under what circumstances would you make your own convenience foods? Convenience meals?

5. Suppose you were a young married woman. In this imaginary role, go to different types of eating places. Make notes on what you get to eat in a meal and the price charged. Compare this with your nutrition requirement for that meal or snack. Compare it with what you would pay per serving to prepare the same meal at home. Note the time it takes for each. Which is a wiser use of money? Time? Energy? When would you use each? Why?

part iv

the science
and art of
meal management

19

managing family meals

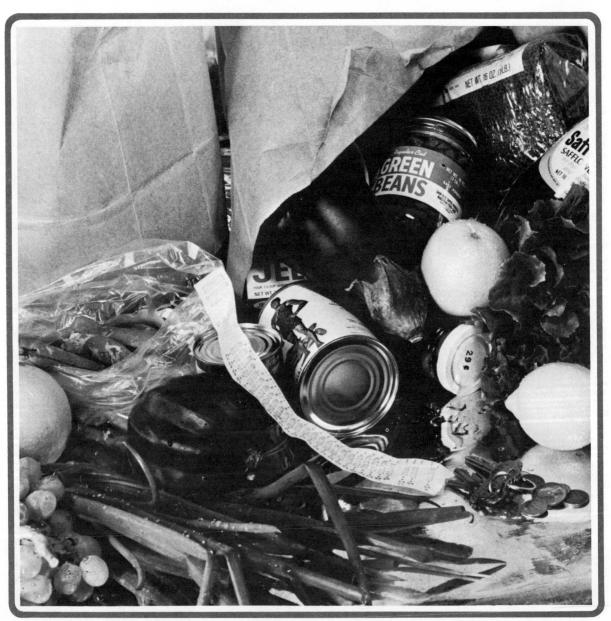

Most men agree with Samuel Johnson, the noted English writer and lexicographer, who said, "A man in general is better pleased when he has a good dinner on the table than when his wife talks Greek." One of the skills men admire most highly in a wife is the ability to prepare and serve a good dinner. Most women and girls aspire to please their husbands in this respect. It is a feminine desire as old as the ages and as strong as the family that is sustained by both food and affection.

To accomplish this feat in modern life is both a science and an art. The manner in which we accomplish it is changing, for today more and more wives are working full or part time outside the home, with less time to do the traditional jobs that must be done for the family inside the home. In the past, these duties have been her primary responsibility. They still are. But when a woman works, most men wish to help her with her traditional work, for she is sharing in the responsibility of his traditional role of providing the income. As children grow, they, too, can assume much of the responsibility that contributes to family life, and at the same time add to their development in family management.

The spirit of this chapter is expressed in the dedication of *Practical Housekeeping*, a nineteenth century cookbook, "To those lucky Housewives who master their work, instead of allowing it to master them."

How to succeed in managing your meals

When you succeed in managing family meals, you have the technique for managing all meals—for guests, for special occasions, or for a modified diet that may be needed by an ailing member of the family. We can learn a great deal from the way executives in business succeed. We are the executives in managing the meals in the family. What principles do these most highly paid business men follow that can help us? There are several.

1/The first principle is to acquire accurate, up-to-date information about all aspects of the job. You have been doing this in the preceding chapters.

2/Organize this information so that it applies to you and your family. And organize the different jobs that must be done in order to apply it. Assign these jobs to different members of the family and hold them responsible for when the job is to be done and how it is done. Do this by family conference. Help them see and feel with you that they are involved in the most important business in society—making a successful family life, the basis of our civilization. And that the payment each member receives for success cannot be measured in money—it is far more precious.

3/Give clear, simple, and accurate directions to those who help you with shopping, food storage, meal preparation, and meal service. Let each member of the family feel that you are not there to criticize, but to help solve problems that arise. Share what you know, in solving these problems.

4/Set an example of high standards in each phase of meal preparation, from making menus, reading recipes and deciding which to use, to the actual wise shopping and scientific cooking of food that will taste good.

5/Set an example of enthusiasm about the worthwhile adventure of feeding a family adequately on the amount of money you have to spend. A successful executive projects his belief in, and his enthusiasm for, the business that he directs to those who work with him. It is teamwork that spells success, not solo flights. In time, family members will see a job to be done and do it without having to be asked. Such an attitude gives the wife and mother a deeper desire to do a good job in feeding her family.

The food budget and total income

Every young couple should talk over both the fixed and the flexible expenses they will have in relation to their income from all sources before they marry. Many fail to do this. Money matters often cause the breakup of a marriage. It is important that both partners be mentally flexible, adjust to facts, and change as conditions change.

Every young couple should work together to plan a budget and keep expenses within the total income.

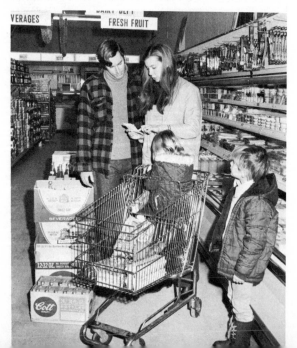

Preparing a budget

Begin with total available income. Then make a column for fixed expenses. These include such items as food, housing and cost of operation, furnishings, and clothing. The flexible items include cost of transportation, dues such as insurance and clubs that are necessary for professional or social reasons, medical care, recreation, and education. There is a certain flexibility even in fixed items. The mentally flexible couple tries different methods with open minds to find the best division of their total income for them and their family.

Priorities in the use of income will vary with family tastes, background, sense of values, and total income. However, no matter how a family places its priorities, it cannot afford to sacrifice a balanced diet in favor of higher-priced living quarters, furnishings, clothing, and other items important to them.

How the food dollar is spent

As you have learned in the preceding parts of this book, there is great flexibility in the choice of foods which can provide a well-balanced day's diet at low, moderate, or liberal cost.

Americans are not spending their food dollar as wisely as they might. This is shown in the 1965 survey of the national diet. If you apply the standards of good nutrition, you will find that the diet can be well-balanced at an economical price by including more milk (especially nonfat) and milk products, more green vegetables, yellow vegetables and fruits, and more citrus fruits.

CALORIES. It is not wise to derive the largest share of calories from fats and oils, but rather

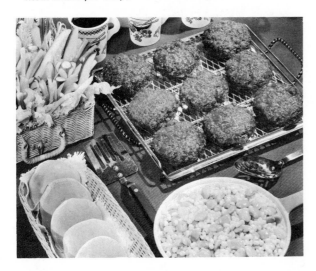

Dovetailing the preparation chores and assembling the various parts of a meal make for easy, relaxed serving.

from bread-cereal, vegetables, fruits, and milk and milk products, for reasons explained in Part I of this book, indicating again that we need to know more than the cost of a food to understand its value to us.

VITAMIN C. Citrus fruits in any form are the most economical source of vitamin C and we also depend on tomatoes, potatoes, raw cabbage, and dark green and other vegetables and fruits to help balance each meal in this nutrient.

VITAMIN A. We depend on the dark green vegetables and deep yellow vegetables and fruits to provide the most economical source of vitamin A as carotenes.

PROTEIN. Meat, poultry, and fish yield less protein for the dollar spent than five other foods or food groups studied, but they yield complete protein, as do milk and milk products and eggs—the latter for lower cost per dollar. We see afresh why those on a low income can be well-nourished in protein. They can lean heavily on dry beans, peas, bread-cereal, and potatoes, and add some milk, eggs, meat, fish, and poultry to balance the lower quantity of complete protein in the more economical foods.

CALCIUM. No other food compares with milk and milk products as an economical source of calcium. The vegetables and fruits recommended in Part I as an important part of each meal help supplement milk.

IRON. Dry beans, peas, and nuts rate another first place as the most economical food sources of iron, with potatoes second, bread-cereals third, and the deep green and yellow vegetables fourth.

RIBOFLAVIN. Milk, cheese, and ice cream as a group provide more riboflavin than any other food for the dollar spent. Other foods, such as bread-cereals, eggs, and vegetables play a supporting role.

THIAMINE. Potatoes rank first in the thiamine provided for the dollar spent, with bread-cereal a close second and dried beans, peas, and nuts third. This further illustrates that, when we know the nutritive values in foods, we can be well-fed on a low income as well as on a high one.

NIACIN. Dry beans, peas, and nuts rate a third first place, this time as the foods that provide the most niacin for the money spent, with potatoes second, and bread-cereal third.

While the prices of food change as the economy changes, the tables in this book illustrate that the cost of food does not relate to its contribution to a good diet.

Food in the budget

Food is the Number One fixed expense. The lower the income, the larger the percentage of it that goes for food—up to 50 percent and more for those below $3,000 annually. In 1966, it was 30 to 40 percent and more for those with an income of between $3100 and $5500. As the income gets higher, a smaller percentage is spent on food. The food budget should include all money spent on meals and snacks paid for away from home, and also that spent on entertaining.

Studies show that 37 percent of our citizens had good diets in 1966 (survey as illustrated in Figure 1–1) who had an income under $3000. By comparison, only 63 percent whose incomes were $10,000 and over had good diets—an illustration of the fact that good eating habits are more important than a fat purse and an indifferent attitude toward the values in foods.

ADJUSTING TO A LOWER FOOD BUDGET. What a young couple faces on a low income in the first years of marriage is what many retired people are facing: they must become accustomed to eating lower-priced and often lower-quality food than that which they have formerly enjoyed. Those who know the nutritional values of foods and have become imaginative cooks—or are trying to reach that goal—can be very well nourished with careful menu planning, shopping, and cooking on a low income.

An example of the success of inexpensive foods is the fame gained by a well-known chain of self-service restaurants and food stores, which built its reputation on two excellent low-cost meat substitutes—baked beans, made according to its own recipe, and macaroni and cheese.

Family sharing in menu planning

The more a husband and wife have in common to talk about, the more fun they have in their marriage. As children come, they can be important members in the family group. It is wise and enjoyable for the family to sit down together and think through the menus they would like to have for the week. Where do you begin?

1/Begin with the nutritional needs of each member of the family to provide a balanced diet. Use your background study of Parts I and II to guide you.

2/Set down the total amount of money you can spend in one week on all meals and lunches that are prepared and eaten at home or carried to work. Set aside money to be spent on meals and snacks to be paid for away from home.

3/Consider the favorite foods of each member of the family and use some in the menus each week. When high cost or poor nutritive value for-

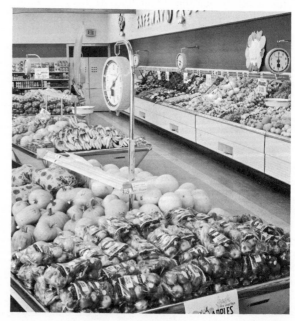

The modern supermarket offers a convenient, quick method of obtaining all types of food under one roof. Food is the Number One fixed expense.

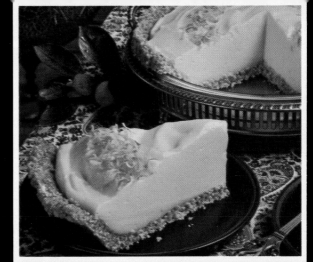

(right) *Lemon cream pie has the right combination of tart and sweet to follow a hearty meal. A graham cracker crust adds lightness to this dessert.*
(below) *You can display a buffet supper attractively and keep it warm at the same time.*

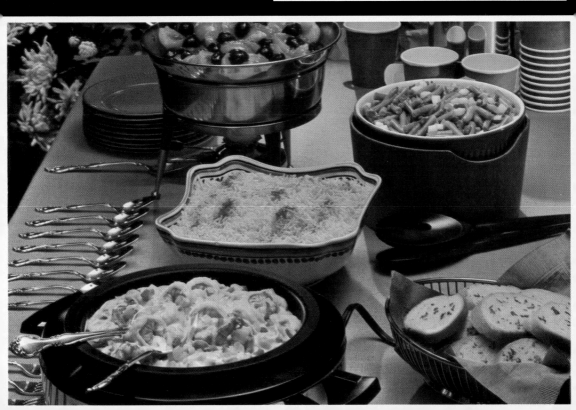

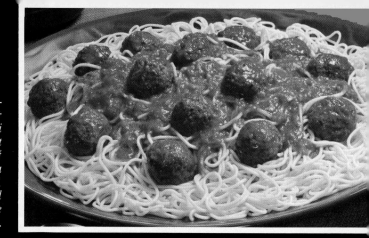

(right) *To satisfy the appetite developed during a day of hard work or play, serve your family spaghetti and meatballs.* (below, left) *What family would fail to enjoy a roast of beef with rich brown gravy? It is a universal favorite.* (below, right) *A Chinese dinner is a delightful and relatively inexpensive change of pace in meal planning.*

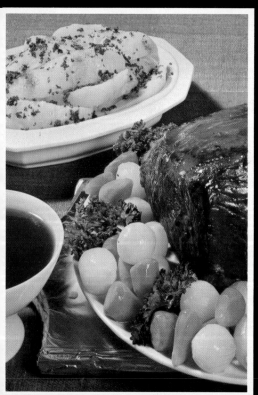

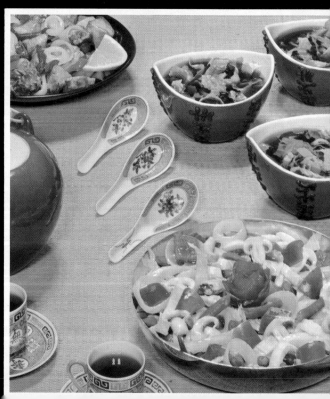

Spices, used properly, can make an artist out of a cook. They make meals exciting.

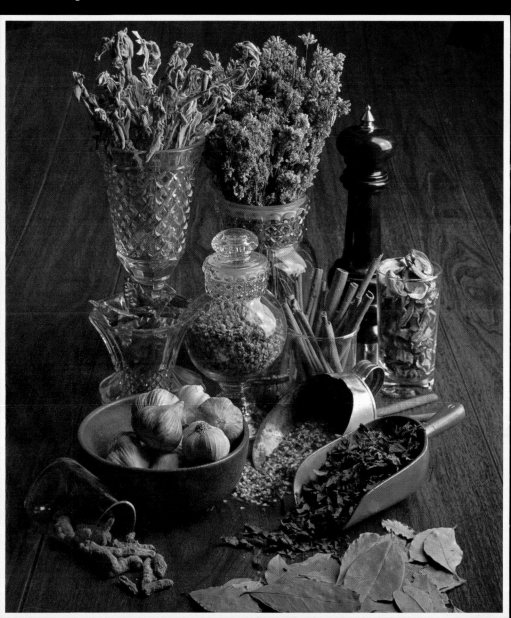

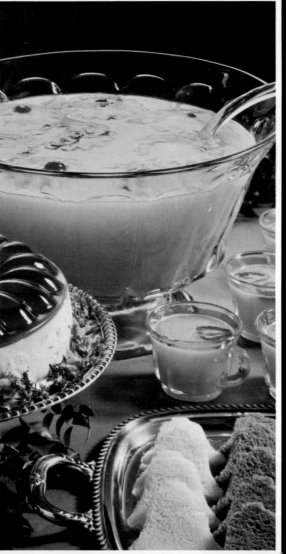

(left) *Eye-catching refreshments enhance the pleasure of any party.*
(below) *Mexican food is popular in many parts of our country. This is another example of the variety available to the menu planner.*

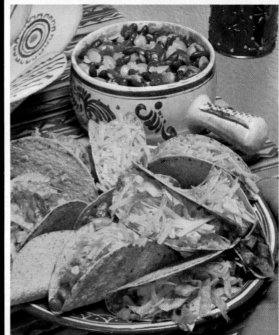

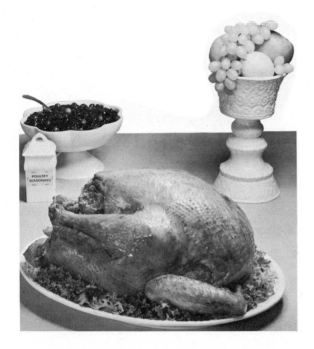

bids the expenditure, explain this to the person making the request. It helps each member of the family to learn to adjust to the reality of controlling our desires to fit our purse. When the family is willing to share a child's favorite food, the child is more willing to try new foods that you wish to introduce and that he needs.

4/Use foods in season. These cost the least per serving. For instance, fresh corn at the peak of the season (August) in San Diego during the summer of 1970 was 5¢ an ear, but in December, 15¢ an ear. Fresh strawberries in May were 25¢ per pint, but in March they were 69¢ per pint. At the peak of the season, cantaloupes were 8 for $1, but out of season they were 49¢ each—and not so tasty.

Families learn by discussing the advertised price of food together and are more critical when in the store. Those on a low budget can enjoy a wide variety of delicious foods, if they take advantage of the peak low prices in season. It is wise to buy out-of-season foods in cheaper forms, such as canned, dried, or frozen. Fresh citrus fruits, for instance, are usually cheapest from January to

What are the advantages of buying a large turkey, even for a small family? How would you use it for future meals?

April and canned and frozen ones are cheaper during the rest of the year.

5/Watch the specials each week and adjust your menus to take advantage of them. This may mean giving up sirloin steak for roast loin of pork. For instance, in one city in the summer of 1969, pork loin roasts were 79¢ to 89¢ per pound. Then in late August there was a special on these at 69¢ per pound. It is wise food buying and good menu planning to buy a large roast on special and have it cut in two parts, or buy two or three smaller ones, according to your freezer space. The same is true for turkeys, which are year-round meats. During the year the price on turkeys varies. Buy the specials, if you can use them, and save money.

Remember that perishable foods are usually placed on specials when they are most plentiful,

Beef Stroganoff is a delectable dish. It is equally delicious the second time around.

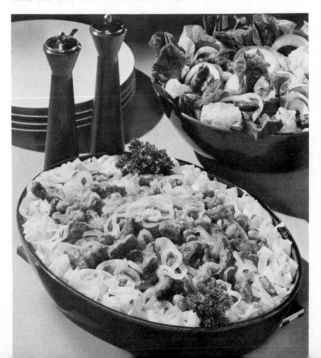

and that the price in general is lower at this time, too. Not all specials are worth buying. Some stores run a special to attract a crowd, hoping they will buy all their food order at the same time and thus make up on other items any loss there might be on the special. In marketing, this is called a loss leader. Too often, they may have a short supply of a desirable special, and will tell the customer that they "had it this morning," when food is advertised for a particular day, but "it is all gone now." This is fraudulent advertising and should not be accepted by the consumer, particularly if the clerk shows you another food that is 10 to 30 cents more per pound than the one advertised. This is the time to be firm and express disapproval of fraudulent advertising, to the store manager and the state appointee in charge of consumer affairs, in writing.

6/Write down your menus for each meal in the week and allow space for comments on each item as to how the dish or meal was accepted and how you think it might be improved. Such a record can become highly prized by all members of the family for future use. You will see growth in your record, if you keep it faithfully.

7/Make your shopping list on the basis of the menus planned. Allow for flexibility, so that you may change your mind and buy a higher-quality alternate for less money when you see one. This often occurs in fresh green vegetables, fresh fruits, and meats. It may occur in unadvertised specials.

Before you market

Keep a shopping list pad in the kitchen and write on it each food that is low, before you run out of it. This is good management in time, money, and energy and saves frustration in running to the store for one or two items.

Before you market, clean the refrigerator with warm water and soda. Place unused food to the front, so that it will be used first. Wash all dishes, put them away, clean the counter tops and the sink, and sweep the floor before you shop. This saves annoyances in putting the food away, saves time, and enables young children or other members of the family to help with this job.

Select a time to shop for food when the store is least crowded, if possible, and when the food is freshest.

The refrigerator should be thoroughly cleaned before you market.

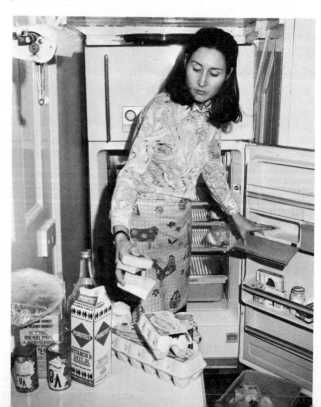

Effective food marketing

Do you ever wonder whether you are getting your dollar's worth on the food you buy? Most of us do. How can we tell whether we are getting full value for our money?

You have made good use of your food dollar when you buy foods that provide the best flavor, best quality, and most nutrients for the lowest cost, to meet the nutritional needs of each member of your family. In studying each food group in Part I, you learned how to reach this goal. Now apply this knowledge at the food market. How will you divide the food dollar among the different foods you need?

Milk

A good way to begin is with the foods required from each group as a minimum. This is given in Table 2–2. You can calculate the amount of milk, for instance, that each member of your family needs each day, by taking the recommendations for each age. Add the amounts for the whole family and multiply the total by 7. This gives the amount of milk the family needs for one week. But this does not tell you what kind to buy. Let us take some examples.

You can save approximately 63¢ per week for a family of four that uses 21 quarts a week, by buying milk by the half-gallon at the store, instead of having it delivered—and you save more if you buy by the gallon. A saving can be made by buying skim milk instead of whole—adding up to about $1.30 a week. You can save another $1.65 by mixing a half-gallon of whole milk (bought at the store) with a half-gallon of reconstituted nonfat dry milk. By using reconstituted nonfat dry milk, you can save about one-half or more, meas-

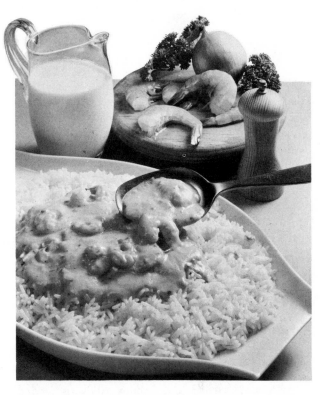

Seafood with a spiced white sauce and fluffy rice gives rich nourishment with little effort.

ure by measure, as compared with the cost of whole milk. Evaporated milk when reconstituted is about one-third less per quart.

Since all the nutrients we need from milk are present in nonfat forms, except the vitamin A (and this may be added), nonfat milk is a good buy, especially since it contains no saturated fat.

Meat group

In cost per serving, the best buys are fish, liver, chicken, and turkey for lean meat, low-saturated fat, and nutrients, as well as price. While the price range per serving is from 12 to 69 cents, the lower-priced meats are just as valuable for good health as the more costly ones. They are more valuable when the saturated fat is low, as in all of those mentioned above, and liver is exceptionally high in many nutrients. Remember that, while prices per pound change in meats, the nutrients remain the same. We allow two servings of meat, fish, and poultry daily (about 3 ounces each, when cooked), and liver once per week.

Vegetables and fruits

List these in separate categories for efficient shopping.

Citrus fruits and other foods rich in vitamin C: Buy at least one serving per person per day.

Green leafy and yellow vegetables and fruits: Remember that we depend on these for three-fifths of our daily need for vitamin A; therefore, allow a serving at least every other day—more often, if possible.

Potatoes, white and yellow: Allow a serving per day (or an alternate) for everyone, from the baby to older people.

Other vegetables and fruits: Use these in season to save money and spark up the flavor of meals.

Be sure that at least one serving is raw daily, and if possible use fresh fruits in season for desserts, to help control weight and promote sound health. Price per serving does not indicate the true value of food. We can learn to think in terms of food value for each food, asking the question: What does it yield in total nutrients? You recall that we depend on fruits and vegetables especially for vitamins C and A.

Bread-cereal

Normal, vigorous people should have four servings of these foods daily in whole-grain or enriched form as bread, cereals, or macaroni products.

Eggs

For normal persons, use six to seven per week. The nutritive value of eggs is outstanding and there are many ways to use them, as suggested in Chapter 4.

Fats

Use about two parts of polyunsaturated fats in your meals to one part of saturated. Remember that for the normal person it is desirable to hold the fat level in the diet to between 30 and 35 percent of the total calories, and that much saturated fat is hidden in some types of convenience foods, the fat of meat, whole milk, and whole milk products. Vegetable oils, with the exception of coconut and peanut, provide the richest source of the linoleic acid desired. Among table spreads, margarine with liquid safflower oil listed as its first ingredient is the most desirable for linoleic acid content.

Sweets

Some sweet is needed to round out the emotional satisfaction of a meal—one teaspoon of jam on toast at breakfast, the natural sweets in fruits, and small servings of your favorite sweets when your weight control program permits it. Sugar made into foods is costly. For instance, 100 calories of sugar costs about 2 cents, but 100 calories of sugar made into candy costs about 10 cents.

Value of records

Keep a record of the amount of money you spend in each food group for one month during each season, for the first year of marriage. Keep this in a permanent notebook and refer to it for future use. This can serve two valuable purposes:

List foods by category to save time in shopping, and stick to your list. Resist impulse purchases.

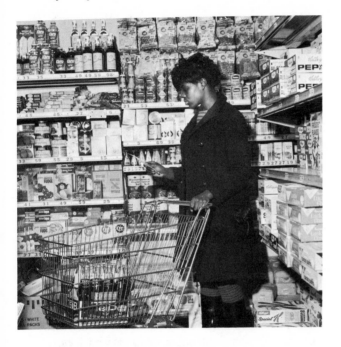

1/You can quickly see whether you are spending too much of the food budget on one food group and neglecting others that should be included to meet family needs.

2/You can see whether too much of the money is going for fringe beverages, convenience foods, fresh foods out of season, or expensive foods, so that you may learn where you need to change your buying practices. This can help you become a shopper who gets the most flavor, quality, and nutrients for your food dollar spent.

Other factors affecting enjoyment of meals

No matter how good a food is for you, or what a great "bargain" it is, it can't help you or your family if you don't eat it. Thus the final test for good meal management is to cook all kinds of food so that they taste good and you enjoy eating them. **Balanced meals that you enjoy eating are made up of separate dishes.** All taste good. Each provides about one-third of the nutrients to meet the body's need for the day.

A meal you enjoy eating (1) blends in **flavor** as a whole; (2) has contrast in **texture** with some crisp, firm foods, and some soft ones; (3) has **color contrast** to whet the appetite and please your artistic senses; (4) has food **temperature** that is pleasing for flavor, with hot foods hot, and cold foods cold; (5) tantalizes your taste buds with the **individual taste** of each dish.

The flavor of food is a personal matter. What one man thinks is delicious—be it caviar, liver pâté, chitlings, raw fish, blood pudding, or gooseberry pie—another abhors. Anthropologists have found that appreciation for the taste of a food is learned by exposure to eating it.

To illustrate the above points, consider the following menu: Cream of celery soup, chicken à la king on mashed potatoes, creamed cauliflower, a wedge of iceberg lettuce with mayonnaise dressing, milk, bread, margarine, and vanilla pudding. Nutritionally, it is a good meal, but one that is poorly planned. What is wrong?

The *color is too white* for all dishes; and the texture is too soft. The meal does not blend as a whole. How can we improve it? Add some red bits of pimento to the chicken in white sauce, and serve it on crisp whole wheat toast. To the mashed potatoes, add 1 cup of finely minced parsley or onion tops when you are mashing them. This not only adds color, but also vitamins A and C, and gives an Irish fillip to the meal. Omit the celery soup and use tomato juice, improving the nutrients and adding color, snappy flavor, and contrast in

Would this meal have appetizing contrast in flavor? color? texture? Would it supply all the nutrients you need?

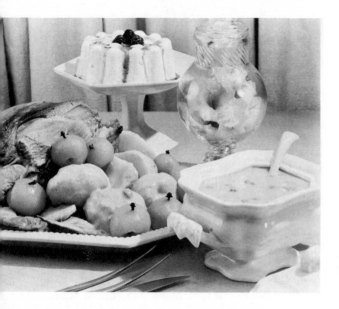

texture, with fewer calories. Use mixed green lettuce salad with radish and pickled beets grated on top and a French dressing. These give contrasts in flavor, texture, and color—and higher nutrients. Cook the cauliflower simply with soft margarine, then garnish it with strips of green pepper. Change the dessert to fresh cold watermelon in season or other fresh fruit.

Taste depends on our taste buds, which are located in the papillae (**pa pil′ ē**—little bumps) on the tongue. Their life span is about seven days. They are constantly being rebuilt. As some people get older, their taste buds become less acute. Then, if the nerve fibers are destroyed, they completely degenerate. Alcohol, when taken in excess, diminishes the ability to distinguish subtle flavors. Hot peppers and heavy spices overpower subtle flavors in food, instead of enhancing them. When you hear a person say that "Food doesn't taste as

good as it used to," the fault probably lies in his own taste buds.

We distinguish four basic flavors: sweet, sour, salty, and bitter. Yet we can distinguish hundreds of subtle flavors. This is due to the delicate mixing of the basic flavors. A. C. Guyton has compared taste to the color spectrum: a few primary colors shade into hundreds of new ones, related and unrelated. This comparison helps us realize our broad potential in preparing meals with innumerable delicate flavors. An example of combining the four basic flavors and more is in the salad dressing and a green salad when endive, a slightly bitter lettuce, is used. A well-prepared salad and dressing can add just the right exciting taste fillip to the whole meal. Lemon juice on a cooked green vegetable, on melon, or on fish adds to the flavor.

Combine foods in each meal to blend as a whole. You can become a great success in managing meals and a hostess from whom others wish to learn, by proper blending of foods and flavors. Here are some examples of how you can plan balanced meals nutritionally with foods that go together in flavor, color contrast, texture, and temperature. Since you share the dinner meal more often with guests, let us begin with it.

Balanced dinners that blend

In any meal bread, soft margarine, and coffee or tea are served, if desired.

These suggested dinner menus at moderate cost can be scaled down or up for a lower- or higher-cost meal, if you wish. They will delight your family or guests. Remember to include liver and fish in the week's menus. You can then feel assured that you are off to a good start on your dinner menus.

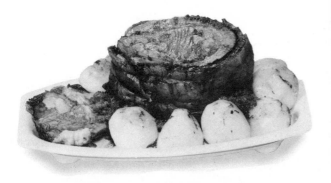
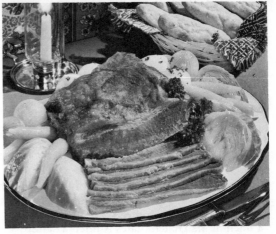

ROLLED ROAST BEEF
FRANCONIA POTATOES
WHOLE BABY CARROTS
MIXED GREEN SALAD
ANGEL FOOD CAKE   MILK

ROAST FRESH PORK
BAKED SWEET POTATOES   SAUERKRAUT
FINGER SALAD
BAKED APPLE   MILK

POT ROAST OF BEEF
SMALL WHITE POTATOES   SMALL ONIONS
CARROTS   TOSSED GREEN SALAD
BUTTERSCOTCH PUDDING   MILK

ROAST TURKEY OR CHICKEN
BROWN RICE   SWEET-SOUR CABBAGE
CRANBERRY SAUCE
FRESH FRUIT SALAD   COOKIE   MILK

BAKED BONELESS FISH FILLET
BROWN RICE PILAF   STEWED TOMATOES
GREEN PEPPER   ORANGE-SLICED ONION SALAD
YOGURT TOPPED WITH FRESH STRAWBERRIES
MILK

BROILED LIVER WITH BACON
HARVARD BEETS   BRUSSELS SPROUTS
TOSSED SALAD
PECAN OR WALNUT PIE   MILK

CORNED BEEF OR BOILED TONGUE
CABBAGE SECTIONS   WHOLE POTATOES
PEARL ONIONS   CARROT STICKS
FRESH FRUIT IN SEASON   MILK

BAKED BEANS
CORN MUFFINS OR STICKS
BROCCOLI   SLICED RED ONIONS ON LETTUCE
CHERRY CHEESECAKE   MILK

BROILED HAM STEAK
COLLARDS   WINTER SQUASH   PEARL ONIONS
PINEAPPLE UPSIDE-DOWN CAKE
MILK

BROILED TENDERIZED ROUND STEAK
MASHED POTATOES   GREEN PEAS
LETTUCE AND TOMATO SALAD
PEACH MELBA   MILK

LAMB STEW
TOMATOES   RICE   RED BEANS
ONIONS
CHILI PEPPERS   COLESLAW
BANANA   MILK

MEAT LOAF
SCALLOPED POTATOES   SPINACH
CUCUMBER, TOMATO, AND LETTUCE SALAD
GINGERBREAD   MILK

OVEN-FRIED CHICKEN
BAKED POTATOES   GREEN BEANS AND ONIONS
WALDORF SALAD
CRANBERRY SAUCE MIXED WITH APPLESAUCE
CUPCAKES   MILK

Casseroles make tasty fare at a party brunch and can be prepared the day before.

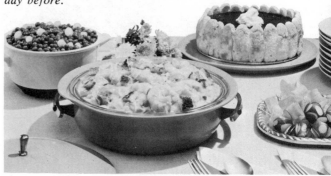

Balanced lunches
or brunches that blend

Lunch in the United States is often a skimpy meal. In most European countries and other parts of the world, lunch is the main meal in the day and is eaten in a leisurely manner. It is often followed by a nap, even for the business man, who usually comes home. The pubs in Britain serve a full-course, hot, well-balanced meal at noon for the business person. In the evening, many people serve a cold buffet. In some countries, lunch and dinner are both hearty meals. For American families that have the main meal at noon, the evening meal is usually a light supper or leftovers.

Lunch in our country can be well-balanced. It need not be rich foods that down cut efficiency for afternoon work. This can be so whether you eat at home or away from home.

Many homemakers lean quite heavily on cold cuts as the main protein dish at noon, not realizing that many are far heavier in saturated fat calories than in protein, as shown in the table of Nutritive Value of Foods in the Appendix. Lunch is a good time to use up nourishing leftovers in soups, casseroles, sandwiches, or salads. Suggestions for a good lunch at home, or that you can carry or buy away from home, are as follows:

SOUP: Bean; pea; lentil; potato; vegetable; vegetable-meat; chicken or turkey with vegetable, noodles, or rice; fish or shellfish with vegetables and milk. Add a salad or finger salad, crackers or bread, milk, and fresh fruit or another dessert.

SALADS: Chef's salad with fruit and cheese, shellfish, meat, or hard-cooked eggs and mixed raw and cooked vegetables. Serve with hot bread or fruit-nut bread, milk, and caramel custard.

SANDWICHES: Fat-trimmed roast lean beef, veal, lamb, ham, fresh pork, chicken, turkey, tuna, sardine, egg, tongue, corned beef, hamburger, frankfurter, cheese, baked bean, or peanut butter. Serve on whole wheat, rye, pumpernickel, or enriched white bread, according to preference; add milk and fresh fruit.

CASSEROLES: Meat, fish, or poultry with vegetables and white sauce or cheese sauce plus noodles, rice, bulgur, or macaroni products, if desired; macaroni and cheese; spaghetti and meat balls; pizza; or baked beans. Add milk, bread and spread (if desired), and fresh fruit for dessert.

SAUCES: Welsh rarebit; chicken à la king; creamed meat, poultry, or fish with vegetables. Serve on toast, toasted English muffins, hot biscuits, or toasted corn bread. Add milk, a tossed or fruit salad, and fresh or canned fruit or deep-dish fruit pie.

Any of these combinations could be used for family or guests for brunch. In addition, a soufflé —cheese, chicken, or fish—or a spoon bread as the main dish adds a more elegant touch for a brunch. A brunch may be a stand-up meal or a sit-down one. Usually people prefer sitting, but a young group enjoys the informality of finger foods eaten standing.

Need for better breakfasts

Many surveys indicate that one reason the American is not as well-nourished as he can be is that he skips breakfast or eats a poor one. This author, with two of her senior nutrition classes at Fort Lee High School, New Jersey, made a one-day survey of 686 high school students and their teachers during the homeroom period. The study was prompted by teachers' reports of a lag in attention from about 10:30 A.M. to lunch time and also by the fact that some girls had fainted in gym classes.

The 168 who reported that they had eaten no breakfast that morning and usually ate none gave the following reasons:

Not hungry.
Too sleepy to get up in time.
Too tired to get breakfast.
Mother slept in and did not prepare breakfast for the family.
No one to eat with.
Not enough time.
On a diet and skipped breakfast to lose weight.

Of those who ate breakfast, only 168 had an adequate breakfast. The teachers ate poorer breakfasts than the students. Of the students, 580 had breakfasts that were too low in either total calories or one or more nutrients. About one-third had no milk, no egg, no citrus fruit or juice; about one-sixth had no bread or cereal.

This one-day sampling confirmed a study of 1200 school children in Iowa from first grade through twelfth. The most intensive study of breakfast to date is the 10-year study of both sexes in all age groups in Iowa. Here are some highlights:

1/What you eat at breakfast is not as important as that the foods provide the combination of nutrients in the amounts you need. This can be baked beans, corn bread, two tomatoes and a glass of milk, if that is what you have and like!

2/Skipping breakfast does not help a person lose weight or control it. "In fact, it is a disadvantage in that those who skip breakfast not only accentuate their hunger, but suffer a significant loss of efficiency in the late morning hours," the study report stated.

3/It was found that we need 20 to 25 grams of protein at breakfast to help maintain adequate energy for the late morning hours, and that 15 grams was borderline, while 10 grams produced symptoms of fasting in late morning (which can account for fainting and weakness).

4/The aged, as well as others, will eat the same nutritionally sound breakfast, if it is available and if they are properly motivated.

5/When breakfast was skipped, the ability to work physically and mentally, the attention span, the attitude toward work, and the scholastic level were lowered and fatigue set in more quickly.

6/An adequate breakfast is a better economy for producing a normal morning work load than either a coffee break or a midmorning breakfast.

A good breakfast is one that provides one-fourth to one-third of the day's calories and total nutrients to meet individual needs. Many countries do not have the foods to provide good nutritional balance. Breakfast is the most neglected meal in many areas. It should concern us all.

Here are some suggestions to help you prepare breakfast within different time limits. These can also be adjusted according to your income.

Balanced breakfasts that blend

Use tea or instant coffee with any of these, if desired.

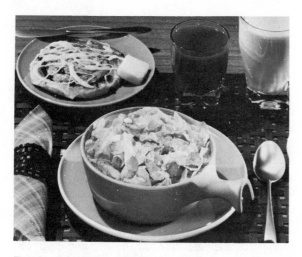

Ready-to-eat breakfasts

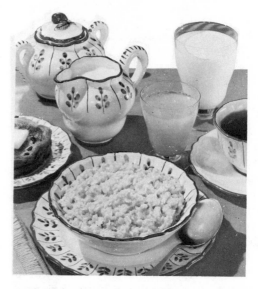

Quickly prepared breakfasts

CITRUS JUICE READY-TO-EAT WHOLE-GRAIN OR ENRICHED CEREAL BANANA GLASS OF MILK WITH ½ CUP NONFAT DRY MILK	HALF-GRAPEFRUIT SOFT-BOILED EGG WHOLE-GRAIN OR ENRICHED WHITE TOAST SOFT MARGARINE MILK
CITRUS JUICE OR WHOLE ORANGE "INSTANT" HOT CEREAL BANANA MILK FORTIFIED WITH NONFAT DRY MILK	WHOLE ORANGE, SLICED SCRAMBLED EGG WITH ¼ CUP COTTAGE CHEESE TOAST SOFT MARGARINE MILK
CITRUS FRUIT OR JUICE CHEESE SANDWICH MILK	HALF CANTALOUPE POACHED EGG 2 SLICES CRISP BACON TOAST SOFT MARGARINE MILK
WHOLE PEELED ORANGE OR ½ GRAPEFRUIT READY-TO-EAT WHOLE-GRAIN OR ENRICHED CEREAL BANANA GLASS OF MILK WITH ½ CUP NONFAT DRY MILK	CITRUS JUICE QUICK-COOKING OATMEAL RAISINS CINNAMON 1 TEASPOON VEGETABLE OIL TOAST SOFT MARGARINE MILK
CITRUS FRUIT OR JUICE PEANUT BUTTER AND JELLY SANDWICH MILK	FRESH BERRIES IN SEASON WITH ½ CUP MILK PANCAKES (made from mix) SOFT MARGARINE SYRUP MILK

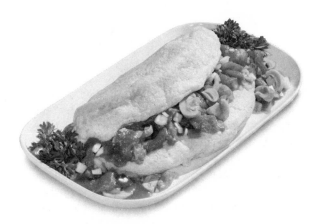

**Leisurely breakfast or brunch
for family or guests**

FRESH STRAWBERRIES IN SEASON
WAFFLES   SOFT MARGARINE
SYRUP OR MARMALADE   MILK

MELON IN SEASON
CHICKEN LIVER OMELET
BLUEBERRY MUFFINS   MILK

FRESH SLICED PEACHES IN SEASON
SPOON BREAD   CANADIAN BACON
CREAMED HONEY   MILK

MIXED FRESH FRUIT COMPOTE
HAM KABOB WITH CHERRY TOMATOES
BROWN RICE   MILK

WHOLE ORANGE, SLICED IN CIRCLES
HAM   HOT POPOVERS
HONEY OR PRESERVES   MILK

ORANGE-GRAPEFRUIT COMPOTE
LEAN BROILED HAMBURGER ON TOASTED
ENGLISH MUFFIN
MILK

MIXED DRIED FRUIT SOUP
PANCAKES   HOT SYRUP
MILK

Timing in the preparation and service of a meal

Timing in meal preparation is a point that confuses, frustrates, and discourages many young brides. Good timing can be learned so that every dish served in a meal is at its peak of perfection. This is accomplished by learning to do each separate part well, a step at a time. When you put the parts together through repeated experience, your timing will smooth out. Once this technique is well learned, you can make an art of serving a well-prepared meal. What are these steps? Most of them you have already learned in Parts I and IV. Here are some additional steps that may help you.

1/Begin simply. Select a menu within your budget, using recipes that incorporate the nutrients you need and that you can prepare in the amount of time you have. These should require a minimum of stress at the last few minutes.

2/Select menus that blend in flavor, contrast in color and texture, and provide a third of each day's nutrients. Be sure you have ready each item you plan to use.

3/Start the preparation of a meal with the dish that requires the longest time: putting a roast in the oven, making a gelatin salad the day before, making a dessert the day before or the morning before the dinner—or the preliminary steps for it. Suppose you plan to have franconia potatoes with a roast and carrots. Cook the potatoes whole in their skins ahead of time, until they are just tender. Cool and peel them. Roll them in brown drippings from the roast, season and lay them on a cookie sheet ready to brown in the broiler on each side, 20 to 30 minutes before the meal is to be served. Then place them around the roast after the fat has been drained from it and allow them to keep hot and further soak in the delicious dripping flavor.

Since carrots are not high in vitamin C or the B vitamins, little is lost here by preparation. They are high in vitamin A, which is more stable to heat. Hence scrape the carrots and place them in a plastic bag well ahead of time. Cook, season, and mash them before the last few minutes, or serve them in round slices seasoned after they are cooked with soft margarine, salt, a pinch of brown sugar, and mint leaves. The fat encases each piece and retains the vitamins.

With planning and practice, you will learn to prepare all the ingredients in a meal so that everything is ready and perfect when you serve.

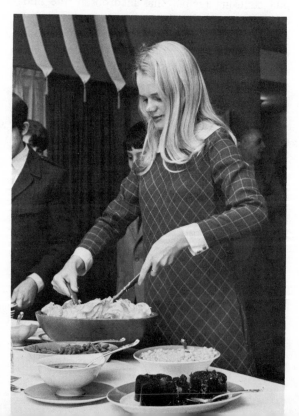

For a tossed green salad, grate or slice a whole fresh onion fine and cut radishes in circles and celery in cubes or semicircles. Break the lettuce in bite-sized pieces. Place all these vegetables loosely in a plastic bag in the coldest part of the refrigerator. When you are ready to serve, put the mixture in a salad bowl, top it with tomato sections, and toss it with dressing at the table. Have the salad dressing ready in a dish to place on the table. The same can be done for coleslaw, an all-lettuce salad, or a fruit salad.

If cake, pie, or a rich dessert is to be served, you might omit bread, if this is desired for weight control. If the dessert is low in calories, have the bread ready to heat or cook in the last few minutes. This is thinking, planning, and working ahead to establish good techniques in meal preparation and service. Soon it becomes automatic.

4/As a bride or beginner in managing meals for the family or guests, learn to prepare at least seven different menus for each meal, in which you can succeed on every point, including that the food is enjoyed by your family. Then widen your menu list by trying different meats and different vegetable combinations. Fit together the separate jobs so that the total work is smooth.

5/Dovetail your work. If you are in the kitchen waiting for the pressure to rise in your pressure cooker and be adjusted for cooking dry beans, for instance, get ready the seasoning that will be added after the "soak and hold" period. If apples are to be baked with a pork roast, prepare them while the roast is in the first period of cooking and cook them ahead of time. If potatoes are to be baked, get them ready. Keep your counter tops clean and dishes washed up or in the dishwasher. Set your table for guests well ahead of time; for the family breakfast, the night before.

Arrange the table centerpiece well ahead of time. Dovetailing your work reduces time, expenditure of energy, and fatigue. This helps make a smoother-running home.

6/Meal service can be simple, yet attractive, even elegant, when you plan it. The basis for good meal service is the setting of the table and the appointments.*

A good plan to save energy and time and give a feeling of relaxation to all is to have much of the meal on the table or near it when the meal is served. Most young people are not fortunate enough to have a heated cart for side-table service, but a hot tray makes a good wedding gift. It enables the hostess to bring most of the meal to or near the table. The dessert may serve as an attractive centerpiece for the meal.

7/The style of table service can save time and energy, yet be artistic. Families that feel rushed often serve the food on the plate from the kitchen, cutting down on the total time spent at the table. Other families like the father to serve the food with assistance, and enjoy good conversation, especially at dinner. Some families put all the food on the table and pass it, letting each serve himself. Children need help from adults in this type of service when they are small.

8/The serving time for each meal should be agreed upon by the family. Then every member should consider it an obligation to be at that meal on time. It is not only discouraging, but also a discourtesy to the homemaker, when the meal is ready to be served at the appointed time and family or guests are not ready to be seated for it.

A meal's peak of flavor and appearance can be lost by waiting for thoughtless people.

9/Good table manners are learned as part of life by cultivated people. In Part II, we noted that children adopt the eating habits and table manners of their parents. It is good manners to eat cereal or stew and other foods with the fingers on the west coast of Africa, with chopsticks in China and Japan, and with a knife, fork, and spoon in western countries and elsewhere. However, the approved way of using the fork and knife varies in the latter countries. Good table manners, like other good manners, are basically the same everywhere. They are expressed by kindness and consideration toward the other people at the table.

Kitchen: work and play center of the home

The modern kitchen is one of the most beautiful and delightful rooms in the home. True, meals are still prepared there, but in addition, young people study at the breakfast table, dance to the record player or radio, or sew up a costume for the school play when the kitchen is also a combined family room in size. The excellent lighting, color and texture on walls and floors, labor-saving equipment conveniently placed, and the abundance of food within reach leave no room for self-pity for the time spent in meal preparation.

The U-shaped kitchen

Photographic illustrations of well-planned kitchens indicate how versatile this room can be. For food preparation and meal service, the U-shaped kitchen has long been a favorite for its use of space to save time and energy.

---

*See *You and Your Food*, by Ruth Bennett White (Englewood Cliffs, N.J.: Prentice-Hall, Inc., 1971), Ch. 25.

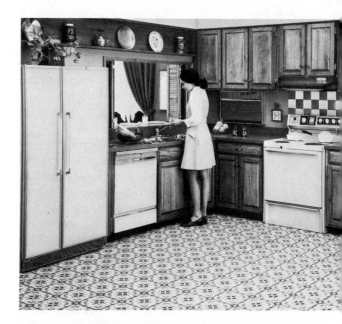

This modern L-shaped kitchen has an energy- and timesaving arrangement of appliances.

The square kitchen

The square kitchen has its advantage, too, in that the center can provide a wall refrigerator on one side and a bookcase-desk on the other for the use of the homemaker and small children. This divider can separate a wall of storage space and laundry equipment.

Other kitchen arrangements

The galley-type kitchen with two parallel lines of equipment close together saves steps and is favored by some, but not by big families. The L-shaped kitchen is very popular because it is comfortable and useful.

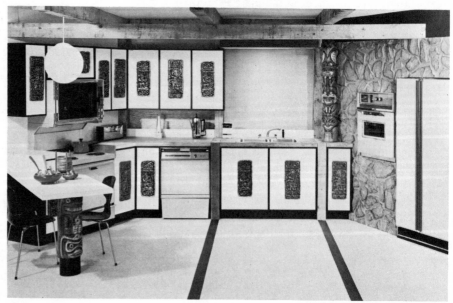

A modified U-shaped kitchen is efficient, compact, and economical.

(above) *Poor posture when working causes fatigue.* (below) *To save energy, learn to work with your body erect.*

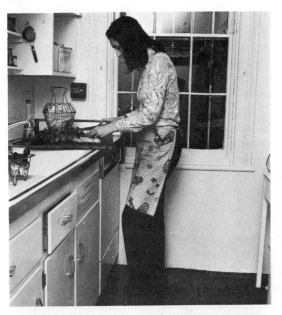

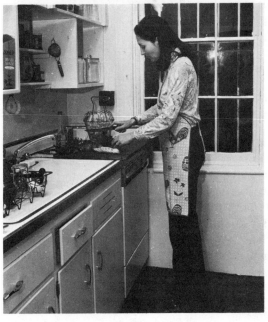

Work centers

Whatever the shape of your kitchen, it is important to have good work centers. The highest reach for cabinets should be fingertip height at the base of the top shelf. Newer-type base cabinets have drawers with fingertip control that slide out easily so that the homemaker can select any pot or pan with a minimum of stooping. This saves time and energy. The counter tops should be at a comfortable height for her to work without stooping or raising her elbows.

Posture and fatigue

The height of working surfaces affects posture and hence fatigue, as well as appearance. Test the correct height for you by standing with your arms forward; when your hands rest comfortably on the surface and your back is straight, you have the correct placement of work surfaces. A few inches of toe space beneath cabinets improve standing posture. There should be one place where you can sit comfortably with your lower back straight against a chair and work with your feet and legs under the counter or table.

Remember, when standing, that if you can drop an imaginary line from your ear to pass through your shoulder, hip, and ankle in a straight line, that is good posture. To save energy, stoop by bending the knees instead of the back.

Work centers are needed around the sink, range, and refrigerator. A good arrangement requires no more than 22 feet in the triangle formed by these three. All equipment and food supplies should be arranged within convenient reach of the mixing center, where a 36-inch counter space is needed for food preparation; 24 inches of this should be near the stove burners.

Basic kitchen equipment

A stove, a refrigerator-freezer, a sink, and cabinets are usually standard equipment in modern apartments, houses for rent, and often houses for purchase. A garbage disposal unit and a dishwasher may also be included. Such rapid changes are being made that by the time you are ready to buy your own, an electronic oven may be within financial reach of the average homeowner. One of the best ways to learn and keep up on kitchen equipment is to visit large department stores or specialty stores that sell different makes. Look at them. Then get the literature on each make and model and compare and study the pamphlets to see which is the "best buy" for you. See what you are getting in each case for the price, and how much of the price goes into nonessentials. Also learn how much extra electrical expense is for automatic defrosting and the automatic icemaker, as compared with the conventional type of refrigerator, and see if it is worth the extra cost.

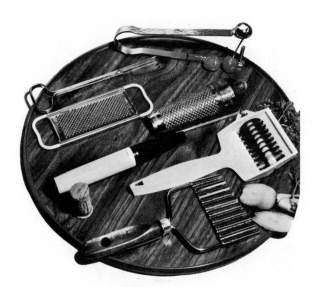

Buying small kitchen utensils and equipment

Too many homemakers spend too much on large equipment and tend to slight the small equipment that is the key to successful and comfortable meal preparation. A stove will cook, whether it costs $150 or $1500, but it is hard to get along without a set of sharp knives and basic cooking utensils.

The following are questions to ask when buying small equipment. They will help guide you in making wise choices.

1/Can you use this piece of equipment in more than one way?

2/Is the size right for your family needs now? Can you continue to use it as your needs change?

3/Is the construction good? Does it have a long life? What is the warranty?

4/Is it easy to clean? Is it safe and easy to use when directions are followed?

5/Do you have adequate storage space for it? Will it fit in with what you have?

6/Can you remove ovenware easily from your oven without strain or danger?

7/Does the cost justify the expenditure in relation to your total needs for meal preparation and service equipment?

8/Will you be happy to use it for many years?

9/What pieces of electrical equipment do you consider basic? Which can you put on a list for addition as you can afford to purchase them or for special gifts? A person can spend a small fortune in this category and seldom use much of what she buys. On the other hand, an electric mixer is a first requirement for most homemakers and many brides get one as a wedding present. The small whisk or eggbeater is a handy low-cost beater to have, even if you have an electric mixer.

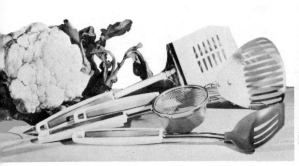
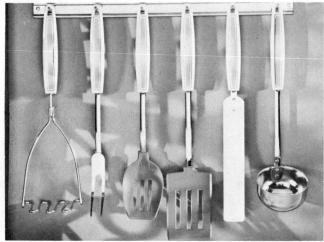

table 19–1   *Small Kitchen Utensils and Appliances*

BASIC MEAL PREPARATION EQUIPMENT		TO BE ADDED LATER
1 set graduated mixing bowls	1 set: long-handled fork, slotted spoon, solid spoon	1 double boiler
1 set graduated sauce-pans, with handles and tight-fitting lids	1 pancake turner with raised handle	1 6-qt. pot, with lid
1 10-in. frying pan	2 spatulas (1 metal, 1 rubber)	1 12-in. iron skillet
1 7-in. frying pan	1 eggbeater	1 chicken fryer— Dutch oven
1 4-qt. pressure saucepan	1 colander	6 custard cups
1 1-qt. casserole, with lid	1 sifter	Casseroles (additional)
1 2-qt. casserole, with lid	1 rolling pin	1 angel food cake pan
2 layer cake pans, 8″ × 1½″	1 can opener— bottle opener	Molds
2 9-in. pie pans	1 knife sharpener	2 muffin tins, 6 sections each
1 muffin pan (Teflon), 12 sections	1 grater—shredder	1 cookie sheet (additional)
1 cookie sheet	1 wide wooden spoon	1 loaf pan (additional)
1 loaf pan (Teflon), 9″ × 5″ × 3″	1 wooden mixing spoon	1 pancake griddle
1 shallow roasting pan with rack	1 potato masher	1 2-qt. pressure saucepan
1 teakettle	1 vegetable brush	1 pr. kitchen shears
1 coffeepot	1 fruit juicer	1 kitchen stool, with steps
1 chopping block (small and light)	1 set of sharp knives (a 5-in. blade French type, an 8-in. blade for slicing bread and meat, and a paring knife)	1 food grinder
1 pastry blender		1 garlic press
1 set graduated measuring spoons	1 peeler	Electrical equipment as needed and allowed for in budget
1 set graduated measuring cups for dry ingredients	4 graduated refrigerator storage containers	
1 1-cup (Pyrex cup)	1 toaster	
1 1-pt. (Pyrex cup) for liquid ingredients	1 timer	
1 1-qt. (Pyrex cup)	Pot holders	
	Tea towels	
	Dishcloths	

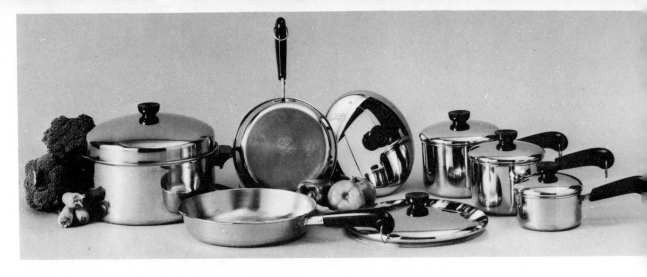

table 19–2   *Evaluation of Types of Cooking Equipment*

MATERIAL	ADVANTAGES	DISADVANTAGES
ALUMINUM	Attractive, strong, light in weight. Next to copper in spreading heat evenly. Cast aluminum better than light-weight product. Nontoxic and can be used for any kind of food. Moderate in cost. Stain does no harm. Anodizing provides better wear and heat-spread surface than polished equipment. Long life.	Thin, cheap grades dent easily and warp. Discolors and pits when alkaline foods are cooked in it or it is cleaned with alkaline compounds.
STAINLESS STEEL	Resists stains. Easy to clean. More useful if copper or other material is used in base to help spread heat. Holds heat well when hot.	Expensive. Conducts heat slowly. Spot-burns, making cleaning hard. Shows water spots.
GLASS	Holds heat well. Attractive. Permits watching food cook. Cost inexpensive to moderate. Absorbs heat quickly.	Conducts heat slowly. Sensitive to sudden change of temperature. Breaks easily and must be replaced. More loss of riboflavin because of exposure of food to light.
EARTHENWARE	Conducts heat evenly and holds it well. May double to serve food on table. Does not discolor foods and is not discolored by them. Moderate cost.	Absorbs heat slowly. Needs to be glazed. Quick change in temperature may cause breakage. Lead in glaze may be hazardous to health, if not properly fired.
IRON	Cast iron heats evenly, is thick and durable. Holds heat and shape well. Inexpensive. Sheet iron is thin, light-weight, and used as frying pans.	Cast iron heats slowly. Rusts easily when iron oxide coating wears off. Discolors acid foods. Heavy to handle. Sheet iron pans heat unevenly, warp, rust.

MATERIAL	ADVANTAGES	DISADVANTAGES
TIN	Conducts heat well. Light. Easy to clean. Inexpensive.	Not durable when tin coating is cut. Affected by acid foods. Turns dark, unattractive. Cuts easily. Bends.
NICKEL ALLOY	Strong, attractive. Doesn't scratch or dent easily. Doesn't rust. Affects color, flavor, and keeping properties of food very little, if at all. Extremely easy to keep clean and shining.	Doesn't conduct heat as well as copper. Costs more than aluminum. Will spot unless thoroughly dried.
TEFLON-FINISHED COOKWARE	Teflon is a finish that is coated on aluminum cookware usually, but might be applied to others. Its chief virtues are that foods don't stick in cooking and it requires no scouring. Some companies will replace the Teflon finish, if the guarantee covers it. Gives excellent browning.	Requires special care with hot temperatures or a quick change in temperature, such as pouring cold water in a hot pan. The finish is destructible.
ENAMELWARE	Made by fusing a glasslike material on iron. Best ones are acid-resistant, have several coats of baked-on enamel. Absorbs and holds heat well. Colorful and decorative. Good grade expensive, others moderate in cost. Does not discolor food or affect its taste or keeping properties. Easy to clean.	Conducts heat slowly. Chips when dropped or exposed to sudden temperature change. Hard to clean if food burns. Marked by metal spoons and beaters. Food scorches easily. Some heavy, hard to handle.
COPPER	Quick, even heat. Sturdy. Attractive when kept highly polished.	Expensive. Must be lined with another metal. Tarnishes and discolors readily. Extremely difficult to keep clean.

Meaningful words

budget
fixed expenses
flexible expenses
food specials
loss leader
papillae
work centers

Thinking and evaluating

1. What did you learn in this chapter that meant most to you?

2. Do you think it is as important for a girl to prepare herself so that she can succeed in managing family meals as it is for her to prepare herself so that she can succeed in a career outside the home? Explain your answer.

3. Do you think young people should discuss their total budget before they are married and consider the amount of money they can afford to spend on food? What difference will this make? Do you have a food budget in the home of your parents? If so, how does it work? Do you know now how much money you spend for meals and snacks eaten away from home? How would you decide the amount of money to allow for these?

4. What points would guide you in planning the food budget for your own home? The day's meals? The week's menus? Snacks? What advantages are there in planning meals in terms of a week?

5. Is income the most important factor in determining whether you and your family are well-fed? Explain your answer and show how on a low budget you may have adequate meals and tasty ones.

6. What principles can we learn from successful business executives to help us make an art of managing family meals?

7. What principles will you follow in planning meals when you have your own home? Explain.

8. On the basis of what you have learned in this and preceding chapters, how may advertising help you shop effectively for food? How may it cause some homemakers to waste food money? Time?

9. What do you consider the key points to remember in effective shopping for family food? What preliminary preparation do you need to do at home before you shop? What would influence you in selecting the place where you shop? The time? How would you organize your shopping list to be sure you buy at one time all the foods you need for a week?

10. Explain how you would correlate your work with the time available, in preparing a meal.

Applying and sharing

1. Analyze the work habits of someone you know and consider a good manager of family meals. One who is a poor manager. What did you learn that can help you?

2. Discuss with your parents and with another married couple you know how they manage their food budget. Do they have a plan? If so, do you consider it as good as it might be? Could you find a tactful way to share with them what you have learned to help them succeed in managing family meals? Think it through and try.

3. List menus that you would like to serve your husband the first week of marriage on a low food budget. On a moderate budget. Learn to prepare each dish in these menus until you and your family enjoy them.

4. Make a shopping order for the menus you planned and buy the food, if possible. Did you stick to your plan? If not, why not? Were the changes made to save money? Time? Energy? How would you improve on your second try?

5. In a notebook, keep an account of your successes in cooking, trying different seasonings with the same food. Write notes indicating how you can improve, after you have performed a task in meal management. It is by critical evaluation of your work by yourself and members of your family that you can improve. Make a plan to do this.

preventing and controlling overweight

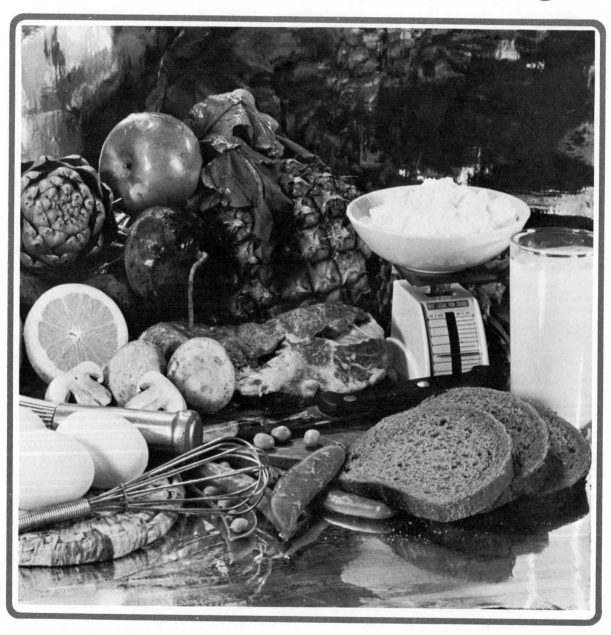

The problem

Managing food to prevent and control overweight was a problem considered with the study of each food group in Part I. Dr. Jean Mayer of Harvard, who has spent almost a quarter of a century studying this subject, points out that we in the United States in our generation are the pampered of our planet and that "nowhere else in the world have such huge numbers of human beings eaten so much, exerted themselves so little, and become and remained so fat."

One can scarcely pick up a newspaper or a magazine or turn on the television or radio without being exposed to shrewd advertising of some "secret" formula or special food, pill, or beverage that promises to help the purchaser achieve the desired weight. When one listens to the dieters' conversation and looks at the unsuccessful ones who repeatedly try the latest diet food or plan, one begins to see the truth of the findings that obesity is America's Number One nutritional problem. At least one person in five is affected, and many of these are poorly nourished. This is due to the way they become fat and the way they try to lose the excess weight.

Studies show that self-selected reducing regimes don't work. Most people regain most of the pounds lost. Let us see if we can achieve an interpretation of the research which can help us attain and maintain desirable weight.

What is desirable weight?

Desirable weight is one at which you look, feel, and can be your best self. Dr. Herbert Pollack, a physician who has worked on the problem of over-weight for more than twenty-five years, defines overweight as 10 percent above the recommended figure for your height and weight. Obesity ($\bar{o}$ bē′ sət ē) he defines as being 15 to 20 percent above your height-weight figure.

Dr. Mayer defines obesity as the excessive accumulation of body fat. Overweight is weight in excess of normal range. But this does not necessarily mean fat. It can mean excess lean tissue, as is the case of athletes in training, and it can mean excess fluid in certain types of disease.

Guidelines for weight control

Height-weight tables

No one should slavishly follow the height-weight tables, as they are simply guidelines and nothing more. The tables in use today are more meaningful than those of the past. They consider the body frame, or bone structure, which is classified as small, medium, or large, on the basis of chest breadth and hip breadth. Weights and heights are usually given for fully clothed persons. The nude weights for women are four to six pounds less than those given in most tables and those for men seven to nine pounds less, the authors of the study estimated. Thus, if you use the guide and take off a light dress jacket, it is cheating.

On the height-weight table in the Appendix (page 456), you will note that for a woman 5 feet 6 inches tall, the weight range for a small frame is 114 to 123 pounds; for a medium frame, 120 to 135 pounds; and for a large frame, 129 to 146 pounds. This allows for individual differences.

Note that age beyond 25 is not given. The modern concept is that the healthy weight for a woman at 22 years of age is the one that should be maintained for the rest of her life. For a man, the desirable weight is the one reached at age 25. Understanding this when we are young helps us gradually reduce the total calories we eat after we reach our full growth. Reduced activity with increasing age requires a reduction of caloric intake.

Other guides

There are other tests for desirable weight, besides the height-weight tables. For example, Dr. Mayer suggests as practical but "unscientific" tests the following.*

THE MIRROR TEST. "Looking at yourself naked in a mirror is often a more reliable guide for estimating obesity than body weight. If you *look* fat, you probably *are* fat."

THE PINCH TEST. "In persons under 50, at least half of the body fat is found directly under the skin," at locations such as the arms, back, calf of legs, abdomen, and below the shoulder blade. If the layer of fold between your fingers when you pinch the skin and tissue beneath it together on the back of the arm is more than one inch, this indicates excessive body fatness. For desirable weight, it should be between one-half to one inch thick. Thickness markedly below one-half inch indicates abnormal thinness.

THE BELTLINE TEST. "In men the circumference of the chest at the level of the nipples should exceed that of the abdomen at the level of the navel. If the latter is greater, it usually means that abdominal fat is excessive."

---

*Dr. Jean Mayer, *Overweight: Causes, Cost, and Control* (Englewood Cliffs, N.J.: Prentice-Hall, Inc., 1968), pp. 29–30.

Why overweight and obesity are undesirable

"Medical frauds are today more lucrative than any other criminal activity. . . . Reducing schemes are perhaps the most lucrative of such schemes," a Post Office release states. According to the American Medical Association, one single company grossed eight million dollars in ten months on one "worthless" reducing drug. It spent two million dollars on TV advertising alone, and this on some of the best shows.

All the so-called health foods that are said to be "slimming" are planned to catch the uninformed. You don't need "low-calorie" or other high-priced breads, beers, or yogurts to "slim." You need to know your foods and read the labels, and to understand what they mean. Special "slimming" foods are costly. They are not the answer to the overweight problem. Many women spend on these foods money needed for basic foods for their families. You will not make that mistake.

Excessive overweight is associated with a greater risk of heart disease and other diseases. Table 20–1 shows the effect of overweight on the life span: the greater the overweight, the greater the mortality. Table 20–2 shows that obese persons have a high incidence of mortality from heart disease, cerebral hemorrhage, diabetes, digestive diseases, and cancer. Excess weight also contributes to circulatory disease, high blood pressure, gout, some types of kidney disease, liver disease, and degenerative arthritis and lowers resistance to other diseases. There is a greater risk from anesthesia in surgery, and also in pregnancy and childbirth.

The obese are likely to feel less at ease in social situations, discriminated against in getting a job and holding it, unhappy with the way they look,

table 20–1   The Greater the Overweight,
            the Shorter the Life Span*

PERSONS	OVERWEIGHT Percent	EXCESS IN MORTALITY OVER STANDARD RISKS Percent
MEN	10	13
WOMEN	10	9
MEN	20	25
WOMEN	20	21
MEN	30	42
WOMEN	30	30

*Metropolitan Life Insurance Company, "Overweight—Its Significance and Prevention" (from *The Build and Blood Pressure Study,* Society of Actuaries, 1959).

unhappy with the difficulty and the cost in buying clothes, unhappy with being the victim of rude jokes, and often held in low regard by associates, as if they were gluttonous. In George Orwell's *Coming Up for Air*, the fat man says, "They all think a fat man doesn't have any feelings."

Understanding the causes of overweight and obesity

To understand the cause of a disease is the first step towards curing it. While obesity is not rightly a disease, it is a condition that relates to emotional pain and disease. Let us try to understand some of its major causes, so that we may make headway on the correction of these disorders. Obesity is a complex condition with no one cause but a multiplicity that often have their roots in childhood. When this is the case, the basis for obesity is much more difficult to discover and control. This fact should be an incentive to young people to estab-

lish eating habits for themselves and their children that will prevent this problem. Here it is true that "An ounce of prevention is worth a pound of cure."

The immediate cause is eating more food with higher calorie content than the body needs or can use. The excess is laid down as adipose tissue or plain fat. But saying that is like telling an alcoholic that he drinks more liquor than he needs or can handle. We must look at the interrelating causes.

Genetic role

The genetic or hereditary role has been investigated in depth by Dr. Jean Mayer and others. They have found obesity genes in the dog, the mouse, and the chicken. The expert knows that the Aberdeen Angus cow will fatten more rapidly than the Holstein and the razorback hog is one that stays slim and is valued for its lean hams and bacon. While this factor has not been studied in

table 20–2   Mortality of Excessive Over-
            weights in Relation to
            Disease**

DISEASE	MORTALITY-MEN Percent	MORTALITY-WOMEN Percent
HEART DISEASE	43	51
CEREBRAL HEMORRHAGE	53	29
DIABETES	133	83
DIGESTIVE SYSTEM DISEASES	68	39
MALIGNANT NEOPLASMS (CANCER)	16	13

**Metropolitan Life Insurance Company, "Overweight—Its Significance and Prevention" (from *The Build and Blood Pressure Study,* Society of Actuaries, 1959).

man as extensively as in animals, Mayer thinks it may be one factor that contributes to obesity in human beings.

In a Boston study, it was found that about 40 percent of the children who had one obese parent were also obese, as compared with 80 percent among children who had two obese parents. Only 8 to 9 percent of the children with parents of normal weight were obese. On the other hand, if you have read case histories of persons who have lost from 100 to 180 pounds in one year, they invariably reveal a gluttonous intake of food from early childhood.

Appetite and glands

Appetite and glands are factors on which we need more research. A favorite excuse given for over-

Will this baby grow up to be obese? Possibly, if both parents are. Probably not, if both parents have normal weight. His food habits will be the deciding factor.

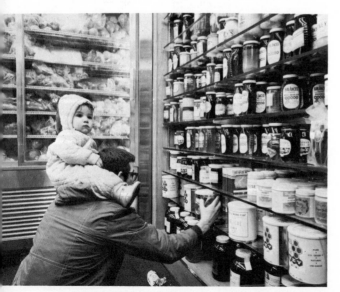

weight is improperly functioning glands. In less than 1 percent of the cases are hormones concerned with overweight, it has been found. When glandular malfunction is responsible, it is the underactivity of the thyroid that is blamed. However, it is the sex gland estrogen that makes poultry and animals fat, and castrated animals also fatten more quickly.

The appetite increases at puberty, pregnancy, and the menopause. Frequently, the latter two are periods of decreased physical activity which, added to the increased food intake, results in excessive weight gain. These three are periods of glandular change. The wise procedure, then, is to watch the diet and the scales and increase exercise at these periods of life.

Studies show that the hypothalamic area—a group of cell nuclei located at the base of the brain —may control appetite. In studies of the white rat, when the hypothalamus was punctured the animals ate two to three times as much food as normally and became fat. They seemed to have no signal to tell them when to stop eating. The hypothalamus has been called the *appestat*. It is believed that it may control the switch that turns the appetite off. We have all seen people who seem to have no signal to stop eating. They eat on and on and gain and gain weight.

Psychological causes of obesity

The obese in our society are often made to have a feeling of guilt, weakness, hostility, inferiority, lack of self-control, and unworthiness, as if they had not tried to rid themselves of their excess poundage and failed again and again. Such lack of understanding by family and friends and even physicians does not help them solve their problem.

The emotional climate in a family affects the dietary habits of its members. A calm, happy person tends to eat sensibly, while one who is tense may overeat.

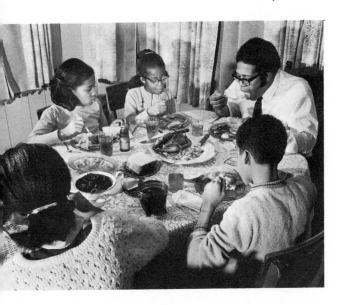

Obesity often develops as a compensation for emotional disturbances. Some people overeat because of tension, anxiety, worry, or frustration. This may occur in adults after a death in the family or of a loved one; after a disappointment in love; on separation from home; in fear of desertion; because of loneliness; or in moods of severe depression. In children, it may be because of overprotection. It also occurs in the excessively-fed child, the one who is not encouraged by his parents to engage in physical activity, or the one who is used by parents to fulfil their own emotional needs by making him overdependent on one or both of them. Such hovering attention is not really considering the child's welfare. It is a mistaken idea of parental love.

These categories are listed in a recent study of obesity:

1/Overeating when you are tense but may not know what is wrong

2/Overeating as a substitute joy in intolerable life situations

3/Overeating as a symptom of a deeper emotional illness—depression or hysteria

4/Overeating as an addiction to food (instead of an addiction to alcohol)

The millions of Americans who become fat need intelligent help in casting off their burden. Some are psychologically adjusted. Most are not.

Age and activity factors

Food intake and age

Age and activity relate to overweight. This is illustrated by the variation in the recommended food intake for different age levels. Thus in the table of Recommended Daily Dietary Allowances on pages 446–447, we see that for a girl aged 14 to 16, 2400 calories daily are recommended, but for a woman aged 55 or older, only 1700; for a young man of 14 to 18, 3000 calories, and for a man aged 55 or older, 2400. This is significant to remember. Those who do not follow this recommendation are often overweight. As we get older, our metabolic rate slows down. We don't burn up as many calories, but in many people the appetite remains the same. If we eat when we are older as we did when we were growing, we get fat.

Value of exercise

Exercise is a key factor in helping prevent and control obesity. It is not enough to be concerned with caloric intake. We must be equally concerned with energy output. Dr. Jean Mayer points out that it is a harmful myth to believe that exercise expends very little energy. He also states that the facts overwhelmingly demonstrate that exercise

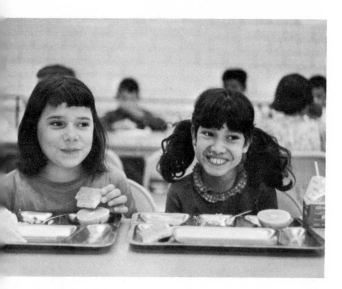

The school lunch program is helping these girls establish good eating habits. Why is it important for them to begin now on a regular exercise program?

doesn't necessarily increase food intake. Anyone who walks three to four miles a day knows by his own experience that Mayer's thesis is true. This has been demonstrated with animals and people.

Too many are misled by such charts of calorie expenditure as that in Table 20–3. It seems so little to the layman. But regular exercise adds up collectively to wide benefits. For example, speeding up the circulation through exercise achieves the following:

1/It burns up fat piled up in the bloodstream and may help prevent heart disease.

2/It eliminates waste products from cell tissues and the body.

3/It carries nutrients and oxygen to cell tissues more vigorously.

4/It strengthens all muscle tissue and may build new muscles.

5/It lessens fatigue and yields a longer span of physical endurance.

6/It promotes a buoyant feeling of emotional well-being that clears the mind and lifts the spirit. What is more, these benefits can be enjoyed by one who maintains regular activity at any age, from 2 to the 80's and 90's.

table 20–3   Energy Used and Calories Burned for Normal Activities*

ACTIVITY	CALORIES Per Kg Per Hr	CALORIES Per Lb Per Hr
Asleep	0.9	0.4
Lying still, awake	1.2	0.5
Eating, writing	1.5	0.7
Reading aloud, sewing	1.5	0.7
Standing relaxed	1.7	0.8
Dressing, undressing	1.9	0.9
Driving an automobile	2.1	1.0
Dishwashing, ironing	2.2	1.0
Typing rapidly	2.2	1.0
Piano playing, moderately	2.6	1.2
Walking 3 miles per hour	3.3	1.5
Bicycling, moderately	3.8	1.7
Walking 4 miles per hour	4.9	2.2
Dancing, moderately	5.2	2.4
Playing Ping-Pong	5.9	2.7
Running	8.8	4.0
Swimming	9.8	4.5

*Adapted from Clara Mae Taylor and Orrea Florence Pye, *Foundations of Nutrition*, 6th ed. (New York: The Macmillan Company, 1966.) Reprinted by permission of the publishers.

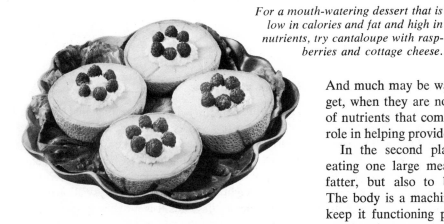

For a mouth-watering dessert that is low in calories and fat and high in nutrients, try cantaloupe with raspberries and cottage cheese.

Roughly, we burn about 1 calorie per hour per pound of body weight for ordinary activities. It requires more energy and burns more calories to swim than it does for most other activities, and the least to sleep. A girl who weighs 120 pounds and walks three miles in an hour burns 180 calories for the walk. But if she swam the crawl for only 15 minutes, she would burn about 133 calories.

Meal skipping, snacks, and coffee breaks

Meal skipping

Meal skipping, snacks, and coffee breaks can contribute to overweight. The misinformed skip breakfast and often lunch—or eat a poor meal—thinking it will help them lose weight. It doesn't work. It defeats their goal in two ways. They don't lose weight, but usually gain more—a fact repeatedly found in studies of human beings, as well as animals. Many of these people take multiple vitamin pills and think it doesn't matter what or when they eat. This is a reprehensible form of self-deception. Vitamins are not a substitute for a meal. They do not provide protein, fat, and carbohydrate that the body needs at regular intervals.

And much may be wasted of the vitamins they do get, when they are not used in balance on a team of nutrients that come from food, for that is their role in helping provide a good diet.

In the second place, skipping of meals and eating one large meal leads not only to getting fatter, but also to becoming poorly nourished. The body is a machine that needs regular fuel to keep it functioning properly. The skipped meals mean that for that period of time the body is operating without the nutrients it requires to keep it going. Then the large meal overloads the system, causing fat to store up. This undermines the basis of health and peak appearance.

Snacks and coffee breaks

Snacks and coffee breaks are chiefly social in value. But when they become a substitute for a missed breakfast or a poor one, a skipped lunch or a poor one, they are a health hazard. Indeed, some people don't eat even one well-balanced meal a day, but snack their way through from morning to bedtime. This is a factor of importance in the lowered nutritional condition of the affluent, as well as those in lower income levels, for snacks are too often high in calories and low in needed nutrients.

On the other hand, the snack or coffee break can contribute to the total nutrients in a well-balanced diet for the day. One way to improve the situation would be to serve two choices of balanced breakfasts on the job for working people or school children a half-hour before work or school begins. Some schools do not allow candy bars or soft-drink machines. Instead, they provide vending machines with fresh fruit, fruit drinks, and milk. See Table 2–4 on page 28 for a list of nutritious snacks for any age.

Pitfalls of
the crash reducing diet

It is possible to lose weight on a crash reducing diet, but not to maintain the weight loss. The constant parade of new reducing diets placed before us in all the news media is eloquent testimony to their failure and to our ignorance of the deeper causes of excessive weight. The new diets usually have only a new name for an old concept that has falsely attracted millions, to their disillusionment, in the past. Take the "Drinking Man's Diet," for example. What is it? Simply the high-fat, low-carbohydrate diet that has appeared as the so-called Mayo Clinic Diet, the DuPont Diet, and others. All have had misleading and scientifically unsound suggestions. Dr. Jean Mayer suggests that any low-carbohydrate, high-fat diet causes an immediate weight loss because of partial dehydration, but is of no lasting significance. He further links this type of diet to possible heart disease: "A diet high in fat, where calories and alcohol can be consumed at will—and some nonnutritionists have urged exactly that—not only tends to make the one who uses it fat and inebriated, but it may increase serum cholesterol and precipitate atherosclerosis."

Another fad approach to diet is that in *Calories Don't Count*, which we discussed in Chapter 17. This is one of many ridiculous fad diets that advocate eating, snacking, drinking, or chewing your way right into that desired weight. The good results—loss of weight—are temporary, for the basis is not sound. There is no re-education of poor eating or drinking habits. The grapefruit diet keeps reappearing in various forms, as do the banana and buttermilk, lamb chop and pineapple, and yogurt diets—all consisting of good foods, if eaten as part of a balanced diet.

Formula diets

The formula diets help achieve the goal of lost weight for a few weeks. But any diet of only 900 calories a day would do that. They, too, disregard the fact that a reducing diet, to be of permanent benefit, must help the user learn how to keep the desired weight by eating food, not swallowing a formula like a pill. Thus it is a delaying tactic that postpones meeting the real problem and solving it by acquiring the knowledge to eat wisely on a life-long diet that will control weight.

Formula (or liquid prepared) diets are advertised as having all the nutrients you need and as being "a painless, permanent, perfectly safe way of losing and controlling weight." But both diar-

Crash reducing diets don't effect permanent weight loss. Why is a vegetable platter valuable in a reducing diet? What is needed to complete the meal?

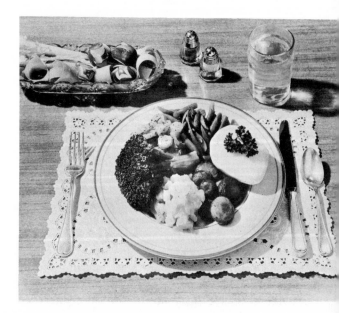

Why is fish a good food for those with weight problems?

rhea and constipation have been reported by users. As Philip L. White, secretary of the Foods and Nutrition Council, points out, "The formula per se is certainly not a panacea for obesity. . . . When weight reduction must be considered a long-term procedure, education of the individual to the faults of his past dietary practices is essential. Only the dietary program which results in permanent weight loss and lifetime control of weight will be a satisfactory one."

Reducing drugs and pills

Drugs and pills for reducing, often purchased over the counter by the user, but more seriously prescribed by the unscrupulous physician, are the most dangerous dieting abuses. You may recall the U. S. Senate Judiciary Antitrust and Monopoly Subcommittee's hearing on the subject. An Associated Press release dated February 1, 1968 reports testimony from the Illinois Coroners' Association in which 14 deaths in that state were suspected of being caused by diet pills. Most of those affected had been young and had died suddenly and unexpectedly, their autopsies showing no anatomical cause of death. Senator Philip A. Hart of the committee said, "It is clear there is great danger in this kind of obesity treatment." Dr. Albert Kaptus, Professor of Medicine at the University of California at Los Angeles, testified, "This is a pernicious type of medical practice," and added, "It is really highly unscrupulous to operate in that way."

Dr. E. S. Mary, a heart specialist and chairman of the Dade County (Florida) Medical Association's Committee on Quackery, noted that the public needs to be alerted to "the dangers inherent in attempting to shortcut weight loss" and warned of "illness and even death" from taking drugs in the combinations found in the popularly used weight-reducing pills.

In June, 1965 in Brooklyn Federal Court an advertising agency was fined $50,000 "for fraudulently promoting worthless regimen diet pills." The company manufacturing the pills was fined $53,000 and the corporation's president fined $50,000 and sentenced to 18 months in jail. This trial represents the results of vigilance by the Food and Drug Administration. However, such convictions are usually appealed. While many in industry cooperate with the Food and Drug Administration, others spend great sums of money to fight it. The consumer must always be alert to possible abuses and actively support the agencies working to protect his interests.

"Spurious Heart Disease Induced by Reducing Pills" is the title of an article appearing in the *Nutrition Reviews* of June, 1969. The article shows that in persons taking reducing pills such changes occurred in the heart that, when an electrocardiogram (i lek trō kärd′ ē ə gram) was made, heart disease was incorrectly diagnosed.

Another report deals with the reprehensible use of the drug digitalis by physicians in treating "unsuspecting patients who were trying to lose

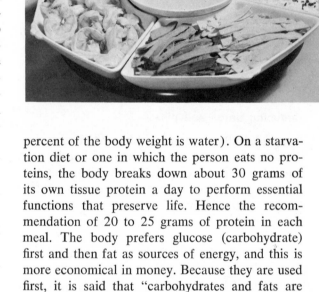

Fasting is dangerous. For weight loss with sparkling well-being, a lunch like this tomato aspic and "Slimline Lazy Susan" is ideal: low in calories, satisfying, and healthful.

weight." The study, conducted by Drs. A. A. Kattus, Jr., B. W. Biscoe, A. M. Dashe, and N. H. Davis, was of six patients who were suspected of having heart disease. They were of both sexes and ranged in age from 20 to 50 years. The investigation was initiated because a healthy, vigorous, athletic 20-year-old girl was denied a job as airline hostess because of an abnormal electrocardiogram. It was found that she and the five other patients had been taking various combinations of reducing pills containing digitalis, diuretics, thyroid, amphetamine, and cathartics. All these drugs are being prescribed in weight-reducing regimens by physicians.

The investigators point out that this is "potentially extremely dangerous" and "life threatening," and add that "It is especially dangerous when practiced by members of the medical profession in whom there is public trust. It is hoped that means may be devised to inform the public of these dangerous practices. It would also be hoped that physicians who are engaged in this type of practice will be exposed."

Fasting

Fasting has become a popular way of losing weight when all efforts of the physician and patient have failed. So much has been written about this "successful" method for excessively overweight persons that many try it without medical supervision. This is a highly dangerous procedure, for it amounts to starvation and can cause death, unless directed and closely guided by an alert physician.

There is no doubt that sensational results have been obtained through fasting, but the persons involved are hospitalized during the fast. What the layman does not know is that much of the weight loss comes from water, not fat (55 to 65

percent of the body weight is water). On a starvation diet or one in which the person eats no proteins, the body breaks down about 30 grams of its own tissue protein a day to perform essential functions that preserve life. Hence the recommendation of 20 to 25 grams of protein in each meal. The body prefers glucose (carbohydrate) first and then fat as sources of energy, and this is more economical in money. Because they are used first, it is said that "carbohydrates and fats are protein sparers." Remember that the reserve supply of carbohydrate (glycogen) is used up in 24 to 48 hours. Then fat is burned as energy.

Physiologists find that, without protein or fat, the carbohydrate reserve would be used up in 13 hours and that, with 15 percent body fat at the beginning of a fast, all the fat is used up in five to six weeks. Then protein is broken down to use as energy. Since this depletes body cells, death usually follows quickly, for the cells can't perform their duties. They are starved. Another factor is that the reserve of B vitamins and vitamin C is used up in about a week and this hastens deficiencies and total destruction.

The important point to remember about total fasting as a method of reducing weight is that it

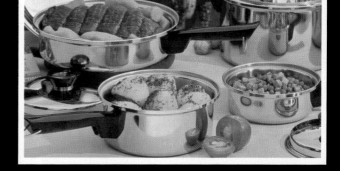

Stainless steel cookware is popular because it is easy to keep clean and shining. (below) *The modern homemaker stores much food in plastic containers. This keeps it fresh and free from contamination and outside odors.*

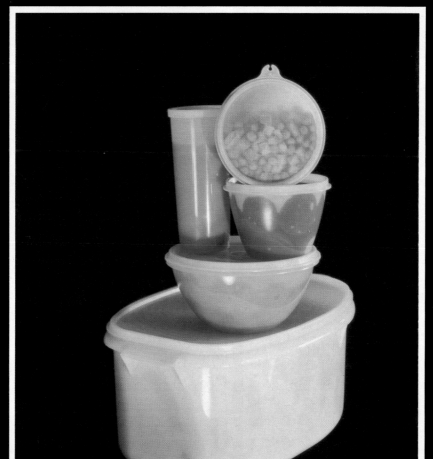

(right) *Copper utensils are attractive and give quick, even heat.* *(below, left)* *Practical, economical aluminum has achieved new glamour with its brightly colored baked-on finish.* *(below, right)* *Work counters and appliances should be at a comfortable level, to prevent fatigue.*

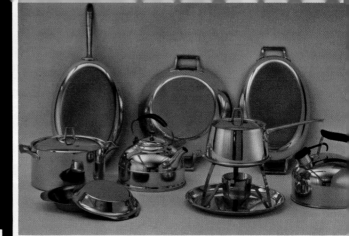

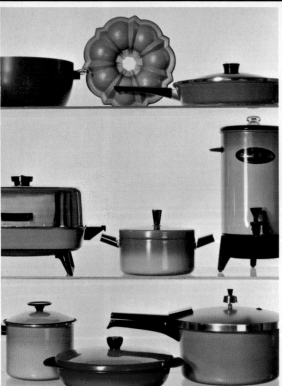

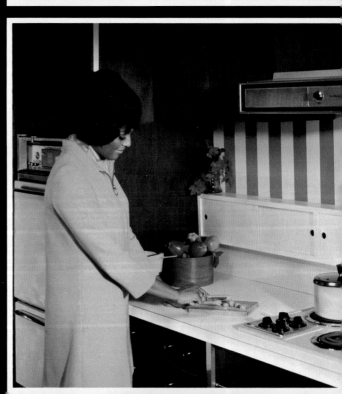

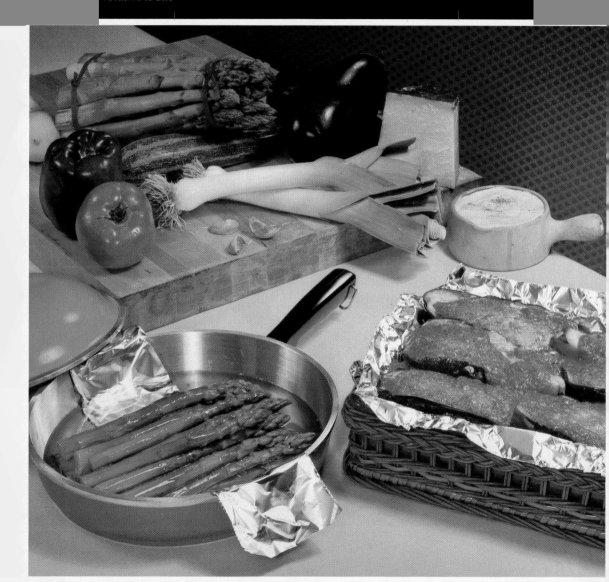

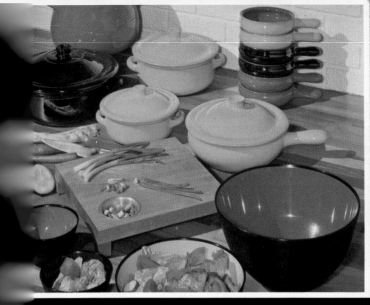

(left) *The kitchen has becon[e] picturesque and gay since col[or has] been introduced to cooking u[tensils.] Enamelware and pottery add [to the] appeal and may be used for b[oth] cooking and serving. (below[)] Stoves, refrigerators, and oth[er appli]ances also come in attractive c[olors] and help make the kitchen a p[leasant] place to work in.*

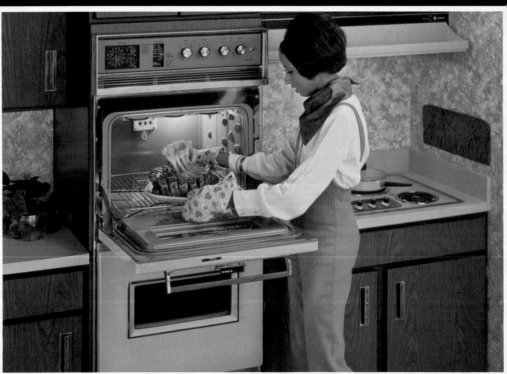

Sample menus

Guides for Low-Fat, Low-Cholesterol Balanced Reducing and Maintenance Diets

	No. 1 1200-CALORIE REDUCING DIET		No. 2 1800-CALORIE REDUCING OR MAINTENANCE DIET	
		Approximate Calories		
BREAKFAST	½ grapefruit	50	65	1 whole orange
	1 oz. shredded wheat	90	164	1 egg scrambled with ¼ c. low-fat cottage cheese and ½ t. vegetable oil
	1 slice whole wheat bread	60		
	1 t. safflower oil soft margarine	33		
	1 8 oz. glass skim milk	90	45	1 4-oz. glass skim milk
	Coffee or tea	0	60	1 slice whole-grain toast
	Total	323	33	1 t. soft special margarine
			18	1 t. jam or marmalade
			0	Coffee or tea
			385	Total
LUNCH	Tuna fish salad (1 tomato, 2 t. mayonnaise, lettuce, diced celery, parsley,		165	Lean ham sandwich (fat-trimmed) on
			60	1 slice whole wheat or rye bread
	2 oz. drained tuna)	153	95	¾ c. coleslaw with 2 t. each safflower oil and vinegar
	1 slice rye bread	60		
	1 apple	70	90	1 8-oz. glass skim milk or buttermilk
	1 8-oz. glass skim milk	90	60	½ cantaloupe
	Coffee or tea	0	0	Coffee or tea
	Total	373	470	Total
DINNER	½ broiled chicken breast	155	160	4 oz. baked fish fillet
	1 ear corn, 1 t. soft margarine	103	90	1 medium baked potato
	½ c. broccoli, seasoned with ½ t.		33	1 t. soft special margarine
	vegetable oil, onion flakes, celery salt, salt, pepper	41	40	½ c. diced carrots with ½ t. margarine
	1 4-oz. glass skim milk or buttermilk	45	60	Tossed salad with ½ t. vegetable oil, 1½ t. lemon juice, seasoning to taste
	Coffee or tea	0		
	Total	344	178	¾ c. low-fat yogurt, ¼ c. frozen strawberries
			0	Coffee or tea
			570	Total
	Total calories for day	1040	1425	
SNACKS	Carrot sticks, celery, raw pepper strips, other raw vegetables of choice, or nonfat milk			

should be used only under the supervision of a trustworthy and capable physician, preferably with the patient hospitalized. It is dangerous as a self-directed crash reducing diet.

How to attain desirable weight you can maintain

Safe dieting

The safest and most permanently effective method to reduce weight is on a miniature well-balanced diet, eating three meals a day and skipping none. The 1200-calorie menu for a day illustrates how this can be done. A balanced diet contains no less than 14 percent protein and no more than 30 percent fat. This leaves 56 percent of the calories from carbohydrate, most of which should come from starches and not ordinary sugar. This emphasizes vegetables, fruits, cereal-bread, and the natural sugar in whole or skimmed sweet milk and cheese. Great variety may be found within this division of your calories among different nutrients.

When reducing on a balanced diet that is low in total calories, you are educating yourself into sound eating habits that can help you maintain normal weight on a healthy diet—the highest goal of reducing. This is the one method that does not fail.

Motivation

Examine your reasons or motives for reducing. They must be strong, if you are to succeed. When you decide the goal is worth the effort, stay with your decision and you will win. You might use the same approach as the Weight Watchers organ-ization, which is similar to that of Alcoholics Anonymous: eat what you need today and no more, one day at a time, and don't worry about tomorrow. The tomorrows fall properly in place when you keep your routine resolutely today.

Safeguarding Health

Have a physical examination by a competent physician before you begin, to find out exactly what your general health situation is. If your weight is excessive, you may need medical guidance. You may also need to work with a nutritionist to whom he may refer you. These two often work together.

When you attain normal weight, maintain it for at least two years without any relapses. Research shows that this is basic to maintaining normal weight once it is achieved. It gives you confidence and assures you of future success, if you maintain the same eating habits and expenditure of energy.

Adults should aim at losing two pounds per week and young people no more than one pound. This is a goal you can attain and maintain on a balanced diet.

The total calories on the 1200-calorie diet add up to 1040, leaving only 160 for you to use in other foods in meals or snacks. In the 1800-calorie diet you have a leeway of 375 calories. Also observe that the calories in each diet are about equally divided among the three meals. The protein in Breakfast No. 1 adds up to only 16 grams, which can be boosted by 6 grams with the addition of an ounce of lean ham, or by 6 grams with an egg, or by 8½ grams with a quarter-cup of cottage cheese, meeting the recommended allowance. The day's meals more than meet the protein requirement, with 38 grams for lunch and 35 for dinner on the 1200-calorie diet, for a total of 89 grams for the day; and on the 1800-calorie diet 23 grams of protein at breakfast, 24 grams at lunch, and 33 grams at dinner, totaling 80 grams for the day.

The loss of weight on such a diet is so gradual that it does not result in looseness of skin, wrinkles, or undue risk to health and appearance. Since it takes 3500 calories to produce a pound of fat on the body, 500 fewer calories a day than your normal needed diet will drop off the recommended pound a week for a young person and 1000 calories fewer per day will reduce an adult's weight by two pounds, as recommended for optimum health. This adds up to 52 pounds lost in a year by a teen-ager and 104 by an adult. This is an

Seafood and salad are a filling, appetizing combination of particular value for those who wish to control their weight.

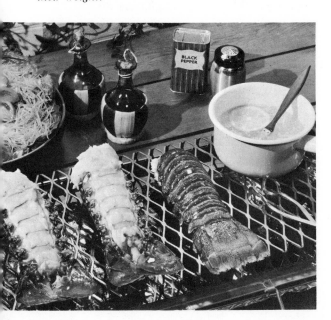

enormous incentive. It is important to take a long-term view and not allow yourself to get in a hurry and seek a crash shortcut.

Research shows that once fat cells are made by the body they do not go away. They collapse when you reduce the fat out of them, but they are right there, ready to fill up again when you consume more calories daily than you expend in energy.

Dieting hints

Depend on raw and cooked vegetables and fruits in each meal to fill up the bulk and help you feel full and satisfied. Use no sugar on fruit; instead, depend on its natural sugar. Use little fat in seasoning vegetables, and make that fat vegetable oil or soft safflower margarine, high in linoleic acid. Use the amount of cereal-bread recommended in the balanced diet, unless you use more vegetables and fruits. Use nonfat milk in some form in each meal and for a bedtime snack in the form of nonfat yogurt or milk, if you need a snack and it fits into your total calorie allowance.

Eat an egg a day for its wide variety of nutrients, unless your physician disapproves. Follow the suggestions for preparing food in Part I and also in Chapter 21. These will help you in diet control and also in prevention of heart disease.

Snacks are permitted if planned as part of the total calories and nutrients for the day. Fill up on raw vegetables for a snack or use nonfat milk or low-sugar fruits.

Stop eating before you feel full. If you are to have dessert, make yourself feel a little hungry by eating less in the main meal.

When you have reached normal weight and can maintain it, allow yourself small servings of your favorite foods at intervals. Remember that you need not give up favorite foods completely, but eat only small amounts of them if they are rich and fattening.

Weigh yourself before breakfast every four days and keep a record of your weight. If you have gained, take the excess weight off at once.

To put off until tomorrow is to head for defeat. Your aim is success and you can achieve it. Watch your diet. Watch your scales. Watch your mirror. Decide on exercise you can maintain each day or varied activities you enjoy. Remember that, if you cheat, it is yourself you are cheating.

Meaningful words

appestat
beltline test
castrated animals
electrocardiogram
endocrinologist
genetic
hypothalamus
medical frauds
menopause
obesity
overweight

Thinking and evaluating

1. On the basis of this study, do you consider yourself overweight? Obese? If so, list the different things you have tried to do about it. Are they sound? Do you think you need a new plan for improvement?

2. Why are the latest height-weight tables a better guide for weight than those of the past?

3. Explain why obesity and overweight are undesirable.

4. What are the causes of overweight and obesity? Why is it so important to understand these causes?

5. Why is it so necessary to be concerned about energy output as well as calorie intake? Do you think you get sufficient exercise every day? Can you make a plan to improve?

6. Give your evaluation of meal skipping, snacks, and coffee breaks on the basis of latest medical findings and also your own experience and observation. What plan would you make for one who is overweight to improve in these respects?

7. What are the pitfalls of crash reducing diets? Which crash diets have you tried, if any? Did you get the permanent results you sought? Why do most crash diets fail? Why are most of them dangerous? How would you evaluate a diet scheme that you read about in a popular magazine or newspaper or heard described on television or radio?

8. Explain how to attain desirable weight on a diet you can maintain the rest of your life. What are the advantages of this plan?

Applying and sharing

1. In your library, find out what is available in the literature on reducing and weight control. Be prepared to report to the class on your findings. Evaluate your findings.

2. For a two-week period, note down all advertising of products for weight reduction on T.V. and radio and in newspapers and magazines you have access to. What are the products advertised? The prices? The psychology used to persuade you to use the products? How has this study helped you evaluate such advertising? How would you help a friend understand the waste of money and danger to health in what is presented?

3. Plan a week's menus that would meet your nutritional needs and at the same time enable you to reduce one to two pounds of weight per week, if you need to do so. Do the same for a young man 21 years old. What is the difference between these menus and the normal well-balanced diet of those who are not reducing?

4. Plan well-balanced menus for a family including a young wife, a young husband, and a three-year-old child, that would be enjoyable to eat and would help each maintain normal weight.

5. Cooking:
   a. Prepare one breakfast, lunch, and dinner with the menus you planned above and serve each to your family.
   b. Prepare snacks for a child and an adult that fit in with what you have learned about weight control.

preventing and controlling heart-circulatory disease

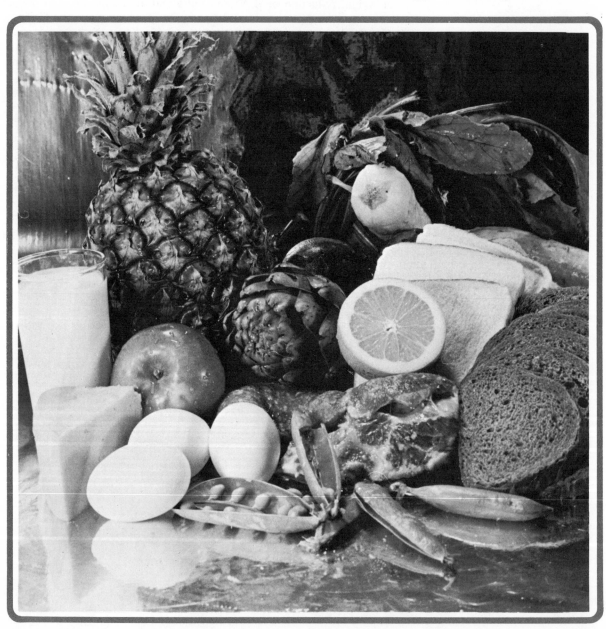

Heart disease and youth

Until recently, most young people thought of heart disease as for the "aged." While it is true that the larger proportion of those suffering from cardiovascular diseases (those affecting the heart and blood vessels) is among the middle-aged and older group, there is a growing body of research showing that the young are not immune. This is illustrated in Table 21–1, which shows that arteriosclerosis (är tir ē ō sklə rō′ səs) is fatal to all age groups. Arteriosclerosis is an abnormal thickening of the inside wall of the arteries. It can begin in infancy and that is why such hope is pinned on helping young people understand this before they start their own families.

A shocking number of our young men who fell in the Korean and Vietnam wars showed on autopsy advanced arteriosclerotic disease, though no outward symptoms were present. Studies show that when a young man has a heart attack, it is usually more serious than when an older person does. The young today are asking, "What can I do to prevent hardening of the arteries and heart attacks?" Not only are they concerned for their lives, but also for their professional usefulness and the freedom to live a full life.

Physicians tell us that man-hours lost from work because of atherosclerosis (the plugging of an artery by fatty deposits) make man-hours lost by strikes and work stoppage seem insignificant. In 1966, for instance, 69 million man-hours of work were lost because of heart-circulatory disease. These were not just old men ready to retire. Many were in the most vigorous and productive years of life. For men between 30 and 34 years of age, the mortality rate from this disease is almost four times as great as that for the 25 to 29 age group.

Since heart disease and cerebral hemorrhage are the chief causes of death in our country, affecting over a million persons per year and disabling many more, let us in this chapter consider some causes contributing to this disease. What role does food play in preventing and controlling it?

What is coronary atherosclerosis?

Coronary atherosclerosis underlies most heart attacks, yet many people who have them don't understand what it means. Stated simply, it means that the arteries which supply the heart with blood to provide oxygen and nourishment become hardened because of the buildup of fatty plaques.

Role of plaques in heart attacks

Segments of coronary arteries of persons autopsied after heart attacks were examined under the microscope by a team of San Francisco scientists recently. The studies, conducted by Meyer Friedman, a cardiologist, and G. J. Vanden Bokenkamp, a physiologist, of the Harold Brunn Institute at Mount Zion Medical Center, in cooperation with pathologists in hospitals near San Francisco, have produced a clue as to how plaques are formed. This is indicated in Figure 21–1.

You will note that when the artery is normally healthy the wall, which is made of an inner layer of tissue, a layer of muscle, and an outer covering, is smooth. Hence the blood flows normally. In Part 2, fatty plaques have formed inside the artery. In Part 3, this is more advanced. It has ruptured, resulting in a clot which blocks the passage of the blood. A coronary occlusion, or heart attack, occurs.

fig. 21-1 : *Development of a heart attack: (1) cross section of a normal artery; (2) atherosclerotic deposits formed in inner lining; (3) the narrowed channel is blocked by a blood clot.*

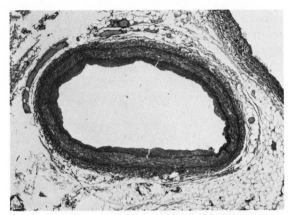

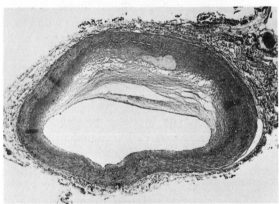

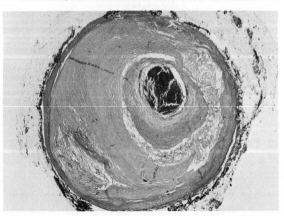

table 21-1 *Death Rate Per 100,000 Population from Arteriosclerosis**
Ages from Birth to Over 82, 1963

AGE	MALE	FEMALE
Birth–1 yr.	0.3	0.2
1–4	0.1	0.0**
5–9	0.1	0.0***
10–14	0.1	0.1
15–19	0.4	0.2
20–24	1.4	0.6
25–29	4.7	2.0
30–34	17.3	4.8
35–39	53.6	11.1
40–44	126.0	25.8
45–49	257.1	50.8
50–54	449.4	104.4
55–59	725.5	202.3
60–64	1099.2	399.8
65–69	1702.8	714.5
70–74	2322.2	1218.5
75–79	3237.1	2018.7
80–84	4729.1	3458.1
85 and over	7754.0	6736.1

*SOURCE: *Facts on the Major Killing and Crippling Diseases in the United States Today* (New York: National Health Education Committee, Inc.), 1966.
**0.0 = less than 0.05 percent per 100,000 population.
***0.0 = zero rate: that is, no deaths.

These researchers discovered that the mass in the plaque is composed of waxy, fatty cholesterol and calcium. They found that 39 of the 40 cases examined had ruptured and the debris was not pus, as in an abscess, but chalky fat.

When the artery is plugged by a clot, it deprives the heart of oxygen and nutrients. Great progress

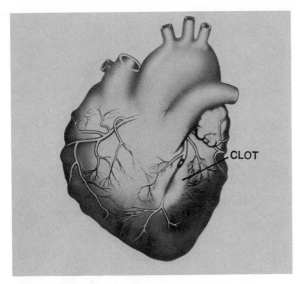

fig. 21–2: *Four days after the attack—white cells are clearing away the dead tissue. Scar tissue is beginning to form.*

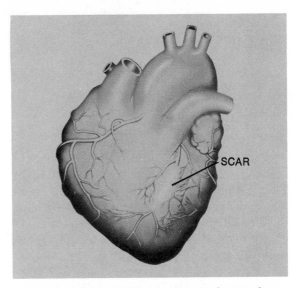

fig. 21–3: *Eight weeks after the attack—tough scar tissue has formed.*

can be made today in relieving this condition, if a competent heart specialist sees the patient immediately. When the patient survives the attack, a scar is formed, as seen in Figure 21–3. When the heart is strong, the person can resume a normal life, within limits.

Medically, other names for heart attacks are coronary thrombosis (blood clot within a blood vessel) and myocardial infarction (death of localized tissue in the heart, caused by blockage of blood vessels by a blood clot). If the clot forms in the brain, it is a stroke, and if in a limb (usually a leg), it is called phlebitis.

The physiologist A. C. Guyton reports that "almost half of all human beings die of arteriosclerosis; approximately two-thirds of the deaths are caused by thrombosis or hemorrhage of vessels in other organs of the body—especially the brain, kidneys, liver, gastrointestinal tract, limbs, and so forth."

Factors contributing to heart-circulatory disease

Cholesterol was the first factor that attracted attention to diet as a cause of heart attacks. Many who are not familiar with the new research still consider it to be the chief villain. But this is not the case. Further research shows that when there is a low functioning of the thyroid gland or severe diabetes, great quantities of cholesterol are deposited on artery walls. Studies show that large amounts are made in the artery walls of animals. This needs further investigation, as heart attacks occur in some persons with low serum cholesterol and don't occur in others with high serum cholesterol. Nor does their serum cholesterol necessarily relate to the intake in the diet.

Studies on fat

Fat studies provide a real breakthrough in solving this riddle. To cite one example: In Oslo, Norway, a cardiologist made a five-year study of 412 persons who had suffered a myocardial infarction. The group was divided equally, one unit serving as a control and eating as usual, while the other, the experimental unit of 206 people, ate a strictly supervised diet. Their total fat intake was slightly over 40 percent of the total calories, which is considered high by the American Heart Association and others. But their saturated fat was quite low and the linoleic acid quite high. The experimental unit was given little red meat and removed all visible fat from what it did eat. Red meat was replaced with poultry, fish, shellfish, and whale. They had one egg a week. No whole milk, cream, butter, margarine, lard, hydrogenized shortening, or olive oil was allowed. The fat they used was chiefly soybean oil. The experimental diet added up to 92 grams of protein a day (368 calories), 104 grams of fat (936 calories), and 269 grams of carbohydrate (1076 calories). The diet was supervised in the homes by dieticians. What was the result? The experimental group had only 80 relapses or sudden death, as compared with 120 in the group who ate as they pleased.

Dr. Jean Mayer of the Harvard University Department of Nutrition suggests that "Such diets may be equally as valuable in preventing heart attacks as in treating them." This study supports the recent dietary concept that a lowering of saturated fat in the diet and an increase in polyunsaturated fats high in linoleic acid has a beneficial effect in lowering blood serum cholesterol.

Heredity

Heredity is a factor in producing heart disease in some families, studies reveal. In some people, there seems to be an inborn tendency to high blood serum cholesterol, despite low amounts in the diet. A. C. Guyton points out that, since this trait is sometimes carried in the dominant gene, "once the trait enters the family, a high incidence of the disease occurs among the offspring."

Overweight

Overweight is an established factor contributing to cardiovascular disease. Overweight persons have twice the mortality from coronary disease as those with normal weight.

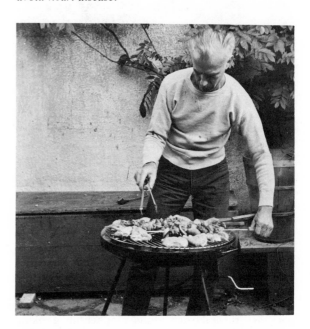

Avoiding stress and tension helps us avoid heart disease.

Age

Age is a factor in heart disease, as Table 21–1 indicates. While no age is immune from this disease, as we now know, the mortality rate is higher as we get older, especially at middle age and later.

Sex

Sex is a factor, as all statistics show. Men are affected earlier in life, more severely, and in greater numbers than are women, except during and after menopause. At that stage of life, women are quite vulnerable because of the decrease in female hormones. It is thought that the male hormone may accelerate the deposit of plaques inside the arteries, whereas the female hormone protects against their formation.

Exercise

Insufficient regular exercise seems to be a factor in the abnormal clotting of blood. Fat can pile up in the bloodstream following a fat-rich meal and exercise helps burn up the fat, thus helping prevent the formation of plaques. After a heart attack, scar tissue forms which is called dead tissue. Exercise helps the heart muscle build corollary arteries to take over a part of the work once done by the healthy artery and its tinier branches—another example of how wonderfully we are made. It is significant that exercise helps strengthen the whole heart muscle and all other body tissues. It improves a person's ability to relax and sleep normally and adds to the sense of well-being.

Stress and tension

Stress and tension seem to be factors leading to heart disease for some. We live in a swift-moving world filled with competition, pressures, and anxiety. Each person must learn to cope with the stresses and strains that surround him in our society and in his family. It is thought that when the blood vessels constrict under emotional stress, this presents a condition within the arteries that is favorable to the formation of plaques.

On the other hand, soothing the emotions enables the blood vessels to relax and they become more elastic, instead of tight. Here is a paradox: those who smoke claim emotional satisfaction that is relaxing, yet physiologists find that smoking makes the blood vessels constrict, favoring plaques.

Tables 21–2 and 21–3 show how the recommendations made by the American Heart Association to the public in 1968 can be practically applied. The limit on eggs applies to yolks only.

Preparing meals for the low-fat, low-cholesterol, low-calorie diet

In preparing meals for the heart patient, your basic aim is to follow the physician's recommendations, for he knows the person's overall condition. As a young person, your basic aim is:

1/To establish a meal pattern and develop eating habits that provide the balance of nutrients you need daily—protein, vitamins, minerals, fat, and carbohydrates—for the growth of new cells and repair of old ones

2/To establish a calorie level daily which can include the nutrients you need and can enable you at the same time to maintain desirable weight

3/To lower your total intake of fat in the diet to below 40 percent of the calories (preferably to 30 to 35 percent)

4/To increase the amount of polyunsaturated fat in the diet and lower the amount of saturated fat

5/To learn to prepare balanced meals and good snacks that you and your family and friends enjoy eating

Here are a few practical suggestions that may help you.

Fats

To increase the amount of polyunsaturated fat in the daily diet, allow two to four tablespoons of fat per person, depending on the age and condition of each person. This should come primarily from vegetable oils high in linoleic acid and/or margarines and salad dressings high in linoleic. Safflower oil is about 38 percent higher in linoleic acid than corn, cottonseed, and soybean oil. This means that two tablespoons of safflower oil pro-

Poultry and brown rice are low in saturated fats and calories—and first-rate in nutrients.

vide the same amount of linoleic acid as three tablespoons of the other oils mentioned. It has the advantage of doing this with 125 fewer calories from fat. Learn to use spreads that are high in linoleic acid. Soft margarine made with safflower oil is the highest (see Table 11–2, page 210). Be sure that the first ingredient on the label is liquid safflower oil, corn oil, or another oil high in linoleic acid, indicating it is in the largest amount. For practical suggestions on how to achieve a balance of fat in the diet, reread Chapter 11.

Meat, poultry, fish, eggs, legumes, and nuts

These are key foods in a well-balanced diet, whether we have heart disease or merely wish to prevent it. Chicken, turkey, fish, and veal are the meats lowest in saturated fat and total fat. A food from the meat group should be included in each meal.

RED MEATS. Beef, lamb, pork, and proc-essed foods made from them are quite high in saturated fat. Therefore, the American Heart Association recommends that a heart patient choose these meats for only five meals during the week, counting three to four ounces, cooked, as a serving. These should be trimmed of fat before cooking, and all visible fat removed as you eat. Broil, roast, bake, or cook these meats with moist heat, skimming off the fat. You may eat all the egg white you wish, as it contains no cholesterol or fat, but the American Heart Association rec-ommends only about three whole eggs per week for heart patients.

LEGUMES. Since some legumes cause gas for some people and this is undesirable for heart patients, the individual can determine the kind and amount of foods in this group that he can tolerate. Among the nuts, the plain dry-roasted (without oil) are best and the walnut is highest in linoleic acid.

EGGS, ORGAN MEATS, SHELLFISH, AND VEAL. Eggs, liver, other organ meats, shellfish, and veal are the common foods which are high in cholesterol, egg yolks and liver being highest. Per-sons who do not eat eggs or organ meats may keep the cholesterol intake from food as low as 200 to 300 milligrams per day.

The liver makes most of the cholesterol, and this is made in proportion to the body's need. More is produced when the diet is low in it, and less when the cholesterol intake is higher. For the normal healthy person, it is a fallacy to omit eggs from the daily diet or liver once weekly, on the premise that this will lower the cholesterol metabolism. Research shows that the saturated fat in large amounts in the food is the key to high cholesterol in the blood, not cholesterol per se, and that low-saturated fat with twice as much linoleic acid in the diet has a lowering effect on blood cholesterol.

Research is under way in our country and in Denmark to produce, through selective breeding, animals with less fat and more meat, and with fat content that is higher in linoleic acid and lower in saturated fat.

In the preparation of foods for heart patients, Part I of this book will be helpful. Remember that the four food groups are interrelated in their use in meals, as are also fats and sugars.

table 21–2 Daily Meal Plans for Fat-Controlled Diets*

FOODS FOR THE DAY	1200 CALORIES	1800 CALORIES	2000–2200 CALORIES	2400–2600 CALORIES
SKIMMED MILK	1 pint	1 pint	1 pint	3 cups
VEGETABLES (at least one serving of yellow or leafy green vegetables)	3 or more servings	4 or more servings	ad lib (4 or more servings)[1]	ad lib (4 or more servings)[1]
FRUITS (at least one serving of citrus fruit or juice)	3 servings	3 servings	ad lib (5–6 servings)[1]	ad lib (6 servings)[1]
BREADS AND CEREALS	4 servings	7 servings[4]	ad lib (8–10 servings)[1]	ad lib (10–12 servings)[1]
MEAT, FISH, OR POULTRY	6 ounces	6 ounces	6–8 ounces	6–8 ounces
EGGS	3 or less per week	3 or less per week	3 or less per week	3 or less per week
FATS AND OILS	1⅔ tablespoons	3 tablespoons	3 tablespoons or more[3]	4 tablespoons or more[3]
SPECIAL MARGARINE	1 teaspoon	1 tablespoon	1 tablespoon or more	1 tablespoon or more
SUGARS AND SWEETS	none	2 tablespoons[2]	ad lib (4 tablespoons)[2]	ad lib (5 tablespoons)[2]

*American Heart Association, Note to the Physician (New York: American Heart Association, 1968).
[1]Number of servings following ad lib were used to calculate diet plans.
[2]If simple sugars are to be restricted, substitute breads and cereals.
[3]One additional tablespoon of oil will yield a diet containing 35% calories from fat and 13% calories from linoleic fatty acids.
[4]Some nutritionists prefer extra servings of vegetables, fruits, and skim milk, rather than so much bread-cereal.

table 21–3 Nutrient Composition of Fat-Controlled Diets at Four Calorie Levels*

NUTRIENTS		CALORIC LEVELS			
		1200	1800	2000–2200	2400–2600
CARBOHYDRATE	grams	120	200	270	335
PROTEIN	grams	75	85	95	110
FAT	grams	42	68	70	84
SATURATED FATTY ACID	grams	7	10	11	12
LINOLEIC FATTY ACID	grams	14	26	26	33
CHOLESTEROL	milligrams	258	258	279	286
IRON	milligrams	12	14	17	19
PERCENT CALORIES FROM CARBOHYDRATE		40	45	51	52
PERCENT CALORIES FROM PROTEIN		26	20	18	17
PERCENT CALORIES FROM FAT		32	35	30	30
PERCENT CALORIES FROM SATURATED FATTY ACID		5	5	4	4
PERCENT CALORIES FROM LINOLEIC FATTY ACID		10	13	11	11
P:S RATIO[5]		2:1	2.6:1	2.4:1	2.8:1

*American Heart Association, Note to the Physician.
[5]P:S is the ratio of linoleic to saturated fatty acids.

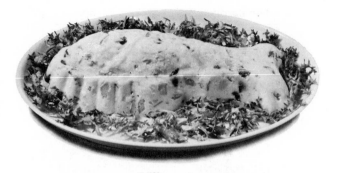

Nonfat dry milk is a major ingredient in this nutritious low-fat molded tuna salad.

NUTS. Plain nonhydrogenated peanut butter contains more linoleic acid than the usual hydrogenated form. The former is in your market or may be obtained by request. Also, plain peanuts and nuts not cooked in oil are better for us than those roasted or toasted in oil. Walnuts are highest in linoleic acid, with one-fourth cup yielding 162 calories, 144 of which are fat and 90 of these in the form of linoleic acid. By comparison, one-fourth cup of peanuts, roasted and salted, yields 210 calories, with 162 from fat and only about 47 of these in the form of linoleic acid.

FAT AND VITAMIN E. In research on animals, it has been found that a high intake of polyunsaturated fat increases the need for vitamin E. In human beings this is no problem, if they eat whole-grain breads and cereals, liver, eggs, milk, oils from seeds, green leafy vegetables, fruits, and wheat germ, in which vitamin E is found—another encouraging reason to eat a balanced diet both when we are young and as we grow older. A good diet is highly important for the heart patient. Because of the restrictions in calories, fat, and cholesterol, too often the diet of heart patients is inadequate for good nutrition.

Milk and milk products

MILK. Serve milk and milk products that are low in dairy fat, according to the listings by age in the Recommended Daily Dietary Allowances, pages 446–447. In a fat-controlled, low-choles-terol meal plan, the American Heart Association in its pamphlet *The Way to a Man's Heart*, published in 1968, recommended that all age groups, including children, use nonfat milk fortified with vitamins A and D. If this is not available in your market, use regular nonfat milk and ask your physician for a supplement of these vitamins.

CHEESE AND ICE CREAM. Use cheeses made from nonfat milk or low-fat milk, such as cottage cheese, mozzarella, farmer cheese, ricotta, baker's cheese, or sapsago. When you make your own ice cream for a heart patient, you can put in it what is needed and know what you are getting. Variety in flavor is achieved by a topping of fresh or frozen fruit. Make your own nonfat yogurt by using nonfat dry milk. This is a highly desirable food, for which a taste can be cultivated.

Vegetables and fruits

Vegetables and fruits contain no cholesterol. With the exception of coconuts, olives, and avocados, they are low in fat. Thus they are first-rate foods for each meal. They help prevent and control cardiovascular disease. A rich source of vitamin C in every meal helps maintain the tensile strength of blood vessels, as well as holding cells together. The heart patient especially needs the benefit of generous amounts of vitamins C and A, found in deep green leafy vegetables and the yellow vegetables and fruits, citrus fruits, and others of this group.

Not a small contribution is the great amount of soft bulk that these foods contribute to help elimination of wastes, an important function for heart patients. Along with milk, they are key foods in helping the body maintain its acid-alkaline balance naturally. Many families eat four or more vegetables and fruits at one meal.

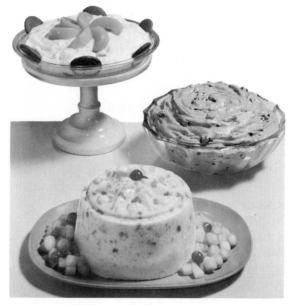

The heart patient need not go without dessert. These luscious fruit chiffon desserts are made with unflavored gelatin and whipped nonfat dry milk.

Bread-cereal

Bread-cereal in its natural state contains no cholesterol and the cereal grains are high in linoleic acid. But foods prepared from grain products and flour—such as pastries, cakes, cookies, sweet breads, casseroles, doughnuts, and other fried foods—may be quite high in saturated fats. When you make your own bread and baked sweets or pastries, you can control all ingredients that go into them. When buying such products, be sure to read the label carefully. Most mixes and ready-to-eat products are not for the heart patient. Buy nonfat commercial bread and add your favorite spread, preferably one high in polyunsaturated fats.

When you eat dry cereal for breakfast, mix a half-cup of nonfat dry milk with about two-thirds of a cup of water to provide 12 grams of protein. Add one to two teaspoons of vegetable oil high in linoleic acid. Remember that breads, cereals, and starchy vegetables are a much healthier form of carbohydrate for you than sugars and sweets.

Snacks, desserts, beverages, herbs, and spices

Contrary to common opinion, the heart patient may need to eat four or five small meals a day or three small meals and a snack or two to get the good nourishment he needs. Your aim is never to overeat or drink at one meal or in one day. This is not difficult for one who understands good nutrition. Most commercially prepared snacks and tidbits are "off limits." They are usually loaded with saturated fat and calories. The snacks suggested for the overweight in the preceding chapter are good choices in helping prevent and control heart-circulatory disease, especially fresh fruits, unsweetened canned fruits, and raw vegetables.

Snacks and desserts to avoid, with an occasional exception, are those that are made with saturated fat and that are high in cholesterol. These include cream, whole milk, cheese, regular ice cream, butter, shellfish (except occasionally shrimp, crab, lobster, and oysters), fish roe, caviar, canned meats, frankfurters, sausages, cold cuts, bacon, high-fat meat (highly marbled), goose, duck, chicken or turkey skin, commercially made quick breads, pastries, cakes (except angel food), pies, rolls and products made from them, whipped cream desserts, chocolate, coconut, commercial popcorn, coffee cream substitutes, commercially fried foods, frozen and packaged dinners, creamed soups, creamed casseroles, sauces, and gravy, unless the fat is skimmed off.

Since alcohol causes a rise in blood cholesterol and yields high calories which may contribute to overweight or poor nutrition, or both, follow the guidance of your physician in its use. The American Heart Association recommends moderation in the use of alcohol, sweets, ice milk (imitation ice cream), sherbet, and bottled drinks. Tea and coffee or Sanka should be used without milk or cream. Nonfat milk is a desirable beverage. Evaporated nonfat milk may be used in beverages as a substitute for cream.

In Part I and in the next chapter you will find many ways to use spices, herbs, and combinations of foods to excite the appetite of those on a low-fat diet. Another fallacy that research has exploded is that spices are not good for you. Enjoy yourself with these additional enhancers of flavor.

Good eating habits

If you are about to establish your home as a young wife and mother or husband and provider, one of the best things you can do for yourself and

Fresh melon, berries, prepared cereal, and skim milk add up to a refreshing, healthful breakfast for all ages.

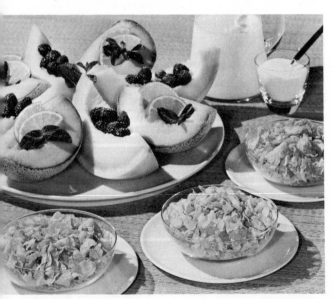

your children is to establish eating habits that can help you prevent heart-circulatory disease. Many of us are inclined to delude ourselves and think, "It can't happen to me." Under the combination of certain circumstances, as we have seen, it can happen to anyone.

The good eating habits and pattern for a well-balanced diet is built on the best research we have in this field today. You have noted that **a good diet for a heart patient varies only slightly from a good diet for anyone**—lower total fat, lower saturated fat with about twice as much linoleic acid as saturated fat in the diet. Remember, it is not just heart disease that a good diet can help prevent or control, but many other ailments as well. It is well known that those who are poorly nourished have low resistance to infections and contagious diseases.

Dr. Charles G. King, discoverer of vitamin C, expressed it this way: "We live in a strange world, when we are overproud of our food supply without knowing or caring much about how to use it. When the topmost four causes of death in the United States are cogently related to abuse of our food supply, the situation is not trivial. . . . We are only on the threshold of reaching levels of health available to us, on the basis of a more intelligently selected and enjoyable food supply."*

While diet is only one factor, it is becoming increasingly clear that the earlier we establish a good food pattern, the better for us in helping prevent and control heart-circulatory disease. You are the first generation that has known this! What are you going to do about it?

---

*Charles G. King, *Significance of Recent Advances in Nutrition Research*, paper presented at dinner meeting, National Food and Nutrition Institute, Agriculture Handbook No. 56 (Washington, D.C.: USDA).

Meaningful words

arteriosclerotic disease
cardiovascular (heart-
  circulatory) disease
cerebral hemorrhage
coronary athero-
  sclerosis
coronary occlusion
coronary thrombosis
myocardial infarction
phlebitis
stroke

Thinking and evaluating

1. What is the best time in life to develop eating habits that can help you prevent some types of cardiovascular disease? Up to this moment, do you think you have these habits? In what ways should you change?

2. Why is it important for the husband and children that the wife and mother understand how to plan and prepare balanced menus that can help protect them from heart-circulatory disease? What age groups are affected by it?

3. Name the factors that contribute to cardiovascular disease. What can you and your family do about these factors, other than diet planning?

4. In view of what you learned in Part I of this book, explain the different ways in which foods play an important role in helping prevent or control heart-circulatory disease.

5. How would you modify and prepare a low-fat diet high in linoleic acid for a member of your family, to help prevent or control this disease? What foods would you avoid?

Applying and sharing

1. Share with your family what you have learned in this chapter. What do you think will help them most now? Later? In what ways?

2. Has the study of the preceding parts of this book helped you understand this chapter better? If so, in what ways? How can you start applying this information now?

3. Write down the food you ate at meals and between meals yesterday and analyze it as to whether it would be a good, fair, or poor diet for prevention of heart-circulatory disease from this point in your life. How do you rate your diet?

4. Suppose you were married to a young man whose physician told him to take precautionary measures to prevent the development of heart disease and that, first of all, he must lose 20 pounds and maintain that loss. Make a plan of menus for one week showing how to provide a balanced diet of 1200 calories per day, that is low in saturated fat and high in linoleic acid, with only 25 to 30 percent of the total calories from fat. In what other ways could you participate with him in developing good habits to prevent heart disease?

gourmet meals in your future

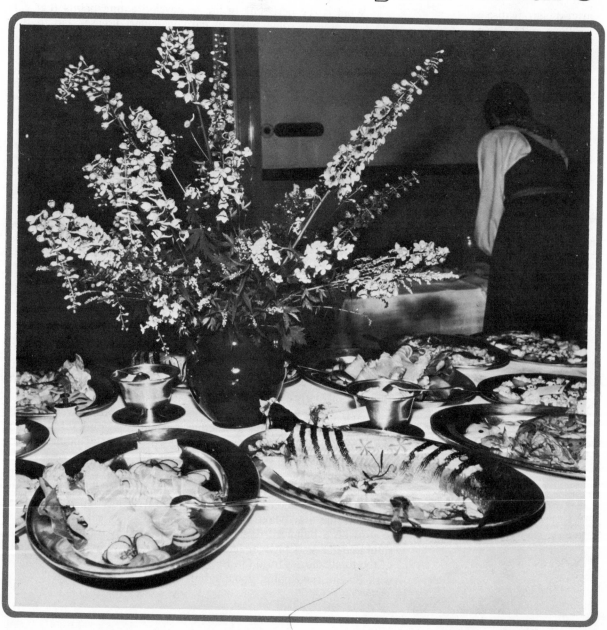

Brillat-Savarin, the noted French nineteenth-century writer, politician, and gourmet, defined a gourmet as "one who can make the delectable most out of amazingly little." Today, as then, the gourmet has a heightened appreciation of good food prepared with taste and imagination.

Young Americans are awakening to the unending possibilities of the gourmet style in meal preparation. We are a nation made up of people who came from other lands. Each group brought its food traditions and its best recipes and adapted them in the new homeland. This has given us a broader appreciation of food because of the intermingling of our mixed national ancestry.

Then, too, in the twentieth century many of us have traveled and lived abroad. We have eaten the foods of other lands, liked them, learned how to prepare or adapt them, and often created new and tastier dishes for our own families and friends.

The meaning of *gourmet*

The modern gourmet holds firmly to the importance of palatability and artistic excellence in a dish or a meal, but adds a third dimension: The meal must contain a variety of food to provide the balance of nutrients we need. **The modern gourmet is interested in keeping his figure and his health while he enjoys delicately flavored and beautiful meals.**

The future you are entering with food has unlimited horizons. You can acquire the excellence in cooking that has been learned from many nations. At the same time, you have access to all of the splendid research which is showing us how to use food more wisely for longer life and life with greater vitality to the very end. This is a more sophisticated concept than the original one that placed emphasis only on the appearance and palatability of food.

Today the men in the family are taking to the kitchen with enthusiasm to prepare "gourmet" meals and are masters of outdoor cooking. Groups of all ages form gourmet clubs that prepare meals in turn in their homes at a fixed price per couple, or as alternating hosts.

Contrary to the suspicion held by some, a gourmet is neither a snob who wishes to impress others with exotic, rare, and expensive food nor a glutton who overstuffs himself, though a few may be found who are. There are a few who wish to show off and prove that they understand the best in the art of fine cooking and dining. The modern gourmet has a delicate appreciation of the fine flavors and subtle distinctions that can be created with amazingly little money. He is imaginative, creative, flexible, and a good manager. He selects and prepares food artistically so that the whole meal blends in flavor and each dish is a harmonious part of the whole, all having a captivating feeling of excellence. A gourmet is experimental. He will taste any new dish and enjoys analyzing the flavors with the discriminating appreciation one might have for a poem or a piece of fine music, for he is an artist with food—or wishes to become one.

Although the French have held the reputation of world leaders in good cooking and dining, other nations dispute this today, for both excellent and poor meals are found in the homes and eating places of all nations.

The gourmet as a reflection of a culture

It is not surprising that the United States should be among the world's leading nations in gourmet cooking and dining. Cookbooks are written by the

It is easy to make fish into a gourmet treat with a tangy marinade.

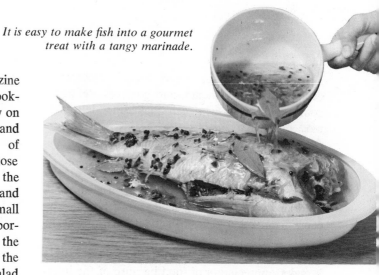

dozen on this subject; newspaper and magazine editors fill their pages with examples of fine cooking. A great deal of money is being spent today on eating out and in searching for the "good" and "authentic" restaurant that serves the food of other nations as it is prepared and served in those countries. We need not travel abroad to taste the finest in worldwide dining. In our country and elsewhere, the best food is often found in small restaurants, located in less expensive neighborhoods. The emphasis is not on the decor or the expensive outfits of the waitresses, or even the view. If the meat is tough and fibrous, the salad limp and tasteless, the vegetables overcooked from standing on a steam table for hours, fancy decor does not compensate for poorly prepared food or

Chefs in a fine Parisian restaurant prepare a meal.

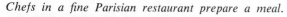

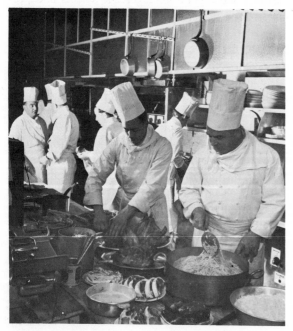

menus. No amount of fancy swirls on the pastry can make up for a tart that is largely dough with a dab of fruit and a mound of whipped cream. We want to taste the flavor of the real food behind the elaborate trappings. To paraphrase Craig Claiborne, food editor of *The New York Times*, "It is food, not napery, that maketh the meal!"

The organizer of the first hotel school at Cornell University was once asked, "Where do you get your standard for the best cooking and style of serving meals, at the Waldorf?" "No," he replied, "The Waldorf and all other fine hotels get their highest standards from the best of dining in the homes of this country and abroad." It is the homemaker, then, who sets the standard for the best in cooking and dining style.

The gourmet style can be learned. You simply need to be awakened to the exciting flavors that can be created with simple foods. You can find your own "special" style with practice. You need a desire to experiment and improve, and you can create "the delectable most out of amazingly little." Table 22–1 gives you a list of herbs and spices and shows how they may be used imaginatively to produce gourmet dishes and gourmet meals.

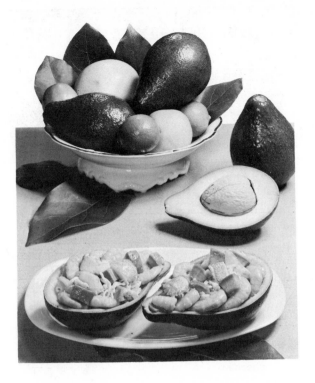

Avocado, once considered a luxury fruit, is now used in moderate and low-cost menus for special occasions. Stuffed with seafood, it makes an elegant, tasty appetizer or entree.

American specialties

We have had many gourmets in our history, from our founding fathers to this day. Mark Twain was one of our most dramatic gourmets. He left his excitement over good food strewn among his writings like the golden October leaves blown by the wind, to enchant those who follow. Writing of the watermelon, for instance, he said, "It is the chief of this world's luxuries. . . . When one has tasted it, he knows what angels eat. It was not a Southern watermelon that Eve took; we know it because she repented." This illustrates the fact that delicacies can be simple and that exciting food does not have to be laboriously prepared.

Each section of our country can boast of its special culinary adventures. Here are a few examples of dishes that imaginative homemakers have prepared first for their families. These dishes have proved so successful that many have spread the length and breadth of our land and to other countries. To survive over the years and spread to other parts of the world is a good test for the gourmet style with food, as it is with classics in literature and music.

Some American food specialties

Hot biscuits	Harvard beets
Hot yeast bread	Scalloped potatoes
Hot crackling corn bread	Mashed sweet potatoes
Hot cakes	Angel food cake
Spoon bread	Upside-down cake
Beaten biscuits	Baked Alaska
Blueberry muffins	Strawberry shortcake
Manhattan clam chowder	Molasses cake
New England clam chowder	Pecan pie
New Orleans chicken gumbo	Pumpkin pie
Fruit cup	Barbecued spareribs
Fruit juice cocktail	Hamburgers
Cranberry sauce	Lobster Newburg
Watermelon pickle	Deviled crabs
Roast turkey	Planked shad
Southern fried chicken	Virginia baked ham
Chicken à la king	Coleslaw
Chicken and dumplings	Waldorf salad
Boston baked beans	Shrimp salad
Stuffed baked potatoes	Crabmeat salad
Succotash	Chef's salad
Hominy	Stuffed tomato salad
Corn on the cob	Avocado salad
Corn pudding	Chicken salad
Green beans and bacon	Chiffon pie
Green leafy vegetable with bacon	Apple pie à la mode
	Coconut custard pie
	Cantaloupe à la mode
	Cold watermelon
	Parfait
	Ice cream sundae with fruit, nuts, or sweet sauce

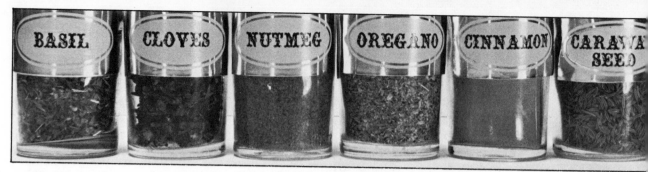

table 22–1 **Gourmet Variations for Meats, Poultry, Fish, and Eggs with Herbs and Spices**

SPICE OR HERB	RED MEAT	POULTRY	FISH	EGGS
ALLSPICE	Pot roast, stew, patties, loaf, glaze on roast	Stew, pie, fricassee	Poached	Eggnog
ANISE	Stew	Braised, roast, pilaf		
BASIL	Lamb, beef, or veal roast, stew, chops, pies, balls	Fried, boiled	Broiled, baked, poached	Deviled, sandwich, scrambled, soufflé
BAY LEAF	Lamb, beef, or veal stews, pot roast, soup, organ meats	Fricassee, stew, soup	Shellfish, bisque, poached	
CARAWAY SEEDS	Roast, stew, sauer-braten	Goose	Broiled, poached, stuffed	Scrambled, omelet, spread
CARDAMOM SEED	Curry	Curry	Curry	
CAYENNE	Curry, croquettes, soup, sausage	Curry, barbecued, broiled	Curry, broiled, soufflé	Deviled, omelet, soufflé
CELERY SEED CELERY SALT	Pot roast, loaf, stew, broiled, soup	Roast, fricassee, stew	Chowder, baked, broiled	Omelet, soufflé, sandwich
CHILI POWDER	Chill con carne, stew, loaf, pie, meatballs	Casserole, barbe-cued, broiled, fried	Broiled, baked, poached, chowder	Omelet, soufflé, deviled, sandwich, scrambled
CINNAMON	Stew, sauerbraten, glaze on roast			
CLOVES	Corned beef, stew tongue, ham			
CURRY POWDER	Curry, meatballs, loaf, broiled	Curry, broiled, stuffing	Curry, shellfish, salad, soufflé	Scrambled, omelet, soufflé, deviled
DILL	Chops, stew, roast	Creamed, pilaf	Broiled, pilaf	Deviled, spread
MACE	Meat loaf, veal	Fricassee	Bisque	
MARJORAM	Lamb, beef, or veal roast, stew, pot roast, loaf	Roast, fried, fricassee, stuffing	Poached, salad	Scrambled, omelet, soufflé

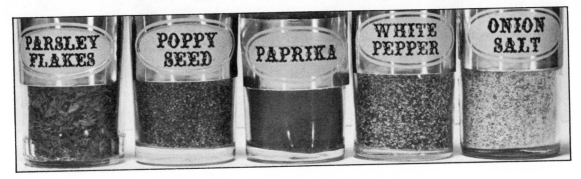

SPICE OR HERB	RED MEAT	POULTRY	FISH	EGGS
MINT	Lamb stew, sauce			
MUSTARD	Pork, loaf, meatballs			Sandwich, deviled
NUTMEG	Pot roast, stew, patties, loaf, glaze on roast	Stew, pie, fricassee	Poached	Eggnog
PARSLEY	Beef, veal, or lamb, hamburgers, loaf, meatballs, stew, soup	Fricassee, salad, pie, soup, stuffing	Garnish, soup, poached, stuffing, creamed	Creamed, omelet, scrambled, deviled
PEPPER PAPRIKA	All kinds	All kinds	All kinds	All kinds
POULTRY SEASONING	Casserole, stew, stuffing	All dishes	Broiled, baked, stew, stuffing	
ROSEMARY	Liver, lamb, shish kabob, pot roast	Broiled, roast, stew, casserole, salad, stuffing	Loaf, salad, croquettes, stuffing	Loaf, salad, croquettes, stuffing
SAGE	Pork, sausage	Roast, casserole, fried, stuffing	Chowder, stuffing, baked, broiled	
SAVORY	All roasts, pies, loaf, meatballs	All dishes	Broiled, stuffing	Omelet, scrambled
SESAME	Garnish	Broiled, roast, fried	Fried, roast, broiled	Scrambled
TARRAGON	All lamb and veal	Fricassee, fried, stew	Salad, broiled	Scrambled, all dishes
THYME	All roasts, stew, loaf, croquettes, liver, organs	Roast, broiled, fried, stew, stuffing	All dishes	Scrambled, shirred, deviled

GARNISHES FOR MEATS

FOR ANY MEAT	Parsley, watercress, lettuce, green or red pepper rings
FOR LAMB	Mint, radish roses, pickled peaches or pears
FOR FRESH OR CURED PORK	Baked apples, crabapples, apricots, pineapple
FOR POULTRY	Sliced oranges, cherry tomatoes, watercress, fresh greens
FOR FISH	Lemon or lime slices, cherry tomatoes, watercress

Some American family special-occasion menus

THANKSGIVING DINNER

GRAPEFRUIT HALF, CHERRY GARNISH
CELERY, RADISHES, OLIVES
ROAST TURKEY, GIBLET GRAVY
CHESTNUT DRESSING
CORN BREAD-WHEAT BREAD STUFFING
SWEET POTATO-PINEAPPLE CASSEROLE
CRANBERRY SAUCE   BRUSSELS SPROUTS
HOT ROLLS   BUTTER OR MARGARINE
PUMPKIN PIE
COFFEE   CIDER

NEW YEAR'S EVE BUFFET SUPPER

HOT WELSH RAREBIT IN CHAFING DISH
CUBES OF FRENCH BREAD
SLICED COLD BAKED HAM   PICKLES
SMALL HOT ROLLS
ASSORTED FINGER VEGETABLE TRAY
ASSORTED FRUIT KABOB TRAY
CHRISTMAS COOKIES AND FRUITCAKE
COFFEE

NEW ENGLAND BAKED BEAN SUPPER

HOT CLAM-AND-TOMATO JUICE
BAKED BEANS WITH PORK
CABBAGE AND PINEAPPLE SALAD
BROWN BREAD OR CORN STICKS
BUTTER OR MARGARINE
APPLE PIE   SHARP CHEESE
COFFEE   MILK

BRIDAL SHOWER REFRESHMENTS #1

MERINGUE SHELLS FILLED WITH CRUSHED
STRAWBERRIES, TOPPED WITH
VANILLA-FLAVORED SOUR CREAM
ASSORTED NUTS   MINTS
COFFEE

CHRISTMAS DINNER

HONEYDEW MELON, LIME SLICE GARNISH
CARROT STICKS, RADISH ROSES, CELERY, PICKLES
ROAST TURKEY, CHICKEN, OR CORNISH HEN
MUSHROOM-BROWN RICE STUFFING
GIBLET GRAVY
BAKED WINTER SQUASH
SWEET-SOUR RED CABBAGE
HOMEMADE WHOLE WHEAT YEAST BREAD
RAW CRANBERRY-ORANGE RELISH
APPLESAUCE FRUITCAKE
COFFEE   MILK

BIRTHDAY DINNER

MANHATTAN CLAM CHOWDER
ROAST LOIN OF PORK
BAKED STUFFED POTATOES
CHOPPED KALE WITH BROWN PORK DRIPPINGS
WALDORF SALAD
LADY BALTIMORE CAKE   STRAWBERRIES
COFFEE   MILK

JULY FOURTH OUTDOOR PARTY

POPCORN   CHEESE CUBES
SOUTHERN FRIED CHICKEN
CORN ON THE COB   BUTTER OR MARGARINE
SLICED TOMATOES, CUCUMBERS, NEW ONIONS
ASSORTED BREADS
COLD WATERMELON SLICES
HOT COFFEE   ICED TEA   MILK

BRIDAL SHOWER REFRESHMENTS #2

CHICKEN SALAD IN TOMATO CUP
HOT HOME-BAKED YEAST ROLLS
BUTTER OR MARGARINE
BAKED ALASKA
COFFEE   TEA

For family celebrations, a gourmet meal may be eaten at home or in good restaurant.

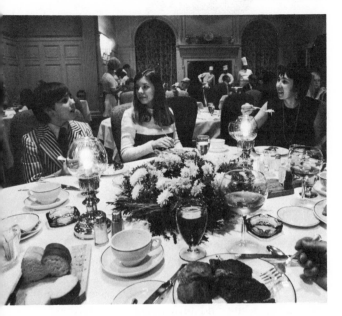

their meals and day's diet nutritionally adequate. This was illustrated by Dr. M. J. Keilling, director of France's Institute of Biology Applied to Nutrition and Food, who reported to the delegates at the Eleventh International Congress of Home Economics at the University of Bristol, England, in 1968 that there is not enough milk in France and other European countries for all the people to have an adequate amount. He added that France has decided to sacrifice the old people and give the milk to the young.

While France lacks sufficient milk, she does have a good growing climate, a good soil, and thousands of little farms that grow many fresh vegetables, small fruits, and poultry; and the seas that touch her shores abound with fish. The people

Decorating a platter of exquisitely prepared food is a special pride of a good chef.

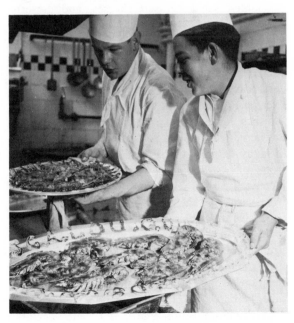

France and the art of gourmet cooking

It is said that Napoleon's cook during the Russian campaign had his skill and ingenuity taxed to the utmost, when food supplies were so low and monotonous, to find new ways of making the few dishes in a meal varied and flavorful for the general. He was so successful in cooking well with so little that he received a citation for his skill and art in cooking!

The story illustrates the ability of the French with food. They take pride in making the same old ordinary food taste extraordinary. The word "gourmet" comes from the French language and eating, to the French, is more than satisfying hunger. It is an aesthetic and intellectual part of life.

French leaders in nutrition are now trying to add a new dimension to their cooking: to make

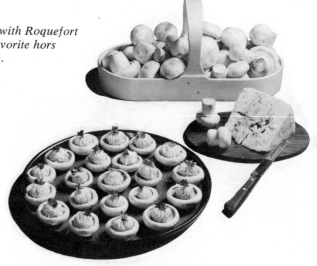

Mushroom caps stuffed with Roquefort cheese are among the favorite hors d'oeuvres of the French.

make much of their milk into cheese. The Institute, working with home economists, hopes to bring the French homemaker into the twentieth century through an understanding of all the nutritional values of foods. She will then be able not only to plan and prepare tasty dishes in a meal, but also to make the meal and the diet more adequate for health. Leaders in nutrition there and in other countries are aware that the future belongs to young people who are strong, healthy, and wise enough to assume their responsibilities.

Specialties in French cooking

There are many specialties in French cooking. These include hors d'oeuvres (a French expression that means something that is not part of the regular meal, thus a side dish or appetizer), soups, meats, vegetables, salads, dessert cheeses, and desserts.

HORS D'OEUVRES. Among the favorites in France are black and green olives, paper-thin slices of smoked salmon on pumpernickel bread, cucumbers, asparagus, artichokes, eggplant, deviled eggs, caviar, canapés, pâté de foie gras (goose liver pâté) served with warm crusty French bread, radishes, mushrooms, peppers, celery, cheese, and chicken in tiny stuffed rolls. These foods are used in many different ways. Most are expensive, aside from a few vegetables. If you wish to use hors d'oeuvres wisely, select one or two, rather than a wide variety of the expensive items, and use less expensive vegetables with them.

SEASONING. Seasoning is most important in French cooking. It is delicately used to bring out the best in any dish. The *bouquet garni* is a combination of bay leaf, thyme, rosemary, parsley, or other herbs, tied in cheesecloth and added to meats cooked with moisture, soups, and some vegetable

combinations. The French use all members of the onion family—leeks, shallots, chives, and garlic, as well as regular yellow onions. In addition, fennel, chervil, mustard, tarragon, pepper, orange and lemon peel and juices, nutmeg, cloves, various types of vinegar, wine, butter, cream, bacon, olive oil, cheese, white and brown sauces, watercress, and other vegetables are used as seasoning.

SOUPS. Several French soups are used internationally: onion, vichyssoise served hot or cold, consommé, consommé Madrilène, and lobster bisque. The pot-au-feu (literally, pot on the fire) is a mainstay for soup stock in most French homes. Traditionally, every scrap of unused food that many throw away (such as the bones of meat, fish, and fowl; the outside leaves of lettuce and cabbage and all imperfect leafy vegetables; the peelings of all root vegetables; and the hulls and pods of peas and beans) is tossed into this kettle and simmered. The soft remains are pushed through a strainer, to go into the soup or another mixture. Naturally, many of the vitamins are lost in this process, but minerals and other nutrients remain.

Another soup that is well-prepared in France, Spain, Italy, and other Mediterranean countries is bouillabaisse. This soup is also well-prepared in many parts of our country, especially where fish abound. It is made of a combination of shellfish and fish fillets cut in bite sizes, with a fine assortment of vegetables, herbs, and seasonings. Such a soup is the main dish of the meal and it becomes a well-balanced meal when served with a tossed green salad, warm crisp French bread, and fresh fruit or cheese for dessert.

Soup is so important to the French that children who take their lunch to school traditionally carry a jar of soup. Working people do the same.

VEGETABLES. Vegetables are usually garden-fresh in the villages, and often in Paris and other cities they are brought into the city fresh every day. There is also an increasing number of canned and frozen foods in the markets of the cities of Europe, including Paris.

Usually, vegetables are quickly cooked and simply seasoned with salt, pepper, and a fat. The long green bean that is split in half is a "French-style" bean—the oblique lengthwise cut is for artistic effect. Tiny onions are cooked with new peas. Young peas are cooked in the pod. Mushrooms are a favorite vegetable and may be served alone or with another vegetable, meat, or poultry. Artichokes and asparagus are widely grown and considered a delicacy in many homes throughout Europe. Dried beans are used in many ways and provide a fair share of the protein. The potato, spurned when introduced from America by the first explorers, is now used as "French fries" around the world, as well as in potato salad, soups, and many other dishes. More turnips and rutabagas are used in European meals than we use. These vegetables are usually included in many types of soups.

SALADS. Salads are so respected that they are usually served as a separate course, after the main dish. They consist chiefly of green leaves of lettuce with simple French dressing.

MEATS. Meats are so well-prepared that the toughest grade and lowest cut can be prepared to the delight of a gourmet. This is done by slow cooking at low temperatures and using liquid, usually a wine, as part of a sauce.

Poultry. Some famous chicken dishes include Chicken Marengo, *coq au vin, poulet au vin blanc*, chicken *à la Bourgogne*, breast of chicken with grapes, chicken legs with mustard, and *poulet à la Valencienne*. All of these are cooked with moist heat, using either chicken stock or wine, or both, as the liquid and different seasonings for variety of flavor. Another favorite is duck or duckling with orange sauce. It is in the use of various seasonings and accompaniments that the skill and artistry of the gourmet are shown.

Veal cutlets become gourmet fare when served with olive sauce.

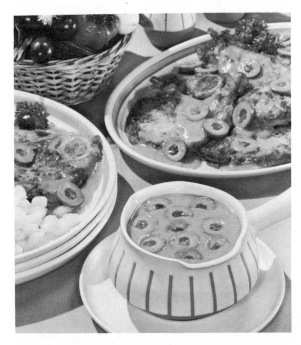

Red Meats. Red meats are not as plentiful or as widely used in France as in our country. *Boeuf à la mode* may sound like a dessert, but it is the Frenchman's favorite pot roast. The French brown the roast first on all sides in hot butter, add vegetables and wine, and simmer the meat until it is tender. *Boeuf Bourgignon* is a variation on the same theme of pot roast. *Steak au poivre*, or steak with pepper, is a favorite. *Langue de boeuf froide*, or cold beef tongue, makes a tasty cold cut for lunches. Liver pâté made with pork liver and truffles is superb in flavor and highly nutritional. *Porc au Maréchal* is a favorite pork chop served with an orange-and-wine sauce. Lamb stew is made from neck or shoulder of lamb with vegetables, wine, and seasonings. Veal, a favorite meat, is served as stew, soup, or cutlets.

Fish. Fish is another food that the French prepare particularly well. They are famous for lobster thermidor and cook sole in many different and delicious ways, such as *sole Mornay, sole meunière, sole Marguerite*, and *sole Normandie*. Frequently, a province gives its name to a dish (Normandie, Bourgogne, and so on). Fish is also used in custard in France, as in the Scandinavian countries. Frogs' legs, snails, eels, and mussels are fare for the gourmet and are served in homes throughout France. Smoked oysters on the half shell are served as a first course or as hors d'oeuvres.

FRENCH BREAD. The bread most generally used is a long, slender, crusty loaf, though there are rolls and the flaky croissants and brioches, which are served for breakfast. We serve all these breads. The French loaf is popular around the world and quite tasty when sliced to the bottom crust, spread with garlic butter, and heated for serving at dinner or lunch.

MILK AND CHEESE. Milk is not a major part of the diet for any but small children in France.

A great deal of cheese is used as dessert, accompanied by fresh fruit; in soufflés; as hot rarebit; and in other ways. Coffee is served at breakfast as *café au lait*, or coffee composed of equal amounts of hot milk and coffee.

EGGS. Eggs are used more at supper or lunch. The French omelet is a world-famous dish, as are also eggs scrambled in meat drippings—a custom our ancestors adopted, using ham juice. As more is learned about nutrition in France, more eggs are being eaten at breakfast. They form an important part of the many *soufflés* made in the country.

Oriental cooks are famous for their skill. Shrimp and other seafood are served in many delectable forms. Fresh chopped spinach and a mushroom sauce make this dish memorable.

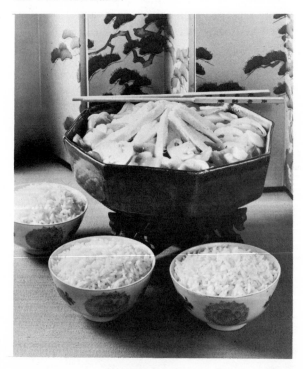

DESSERTS. Desserts range from *petits fours, meringues,* fruit tarts, puff pastry, *mousses,* ices, custards, *crêpes Suzette,* and *soufflés* to cheese and fresh fruit.

Gourmet style with food—recurrent themes in different countries

We have used our own country and France to illustrate how the gourmet style develops in a nation. It is usually in the home where an imaginative homemaker cares a great deal about "making the delectable most out of amazingly little."

Great cooks are not born, but made. You can read all the books about the values in foods and cooking, and own the latest cookbooks, but the learning comes when you get in the kitchen with the food and your pots and pans! You must try out your ideas until they are perfected.

One person may have more sensitivity for flavor with food than another, but even this can be developed. The writer may take the courses in writing, but this alone will not make him a great writer. First, he must be overflowing with his subject, and have many ideas arising from a background thoroughly assimilated and understood. But ideas are of no value until he sits down to the typewriter to put his thoughts into words, into organized and readable form. Even then, he throws away far more pages of writing than he keeps. So it is with the "born" cook. She will try out recipes again and again, until she succeeds in producing perfect results.

After you have mastered the basic principles of simple, nutritious cooking, you develop a few

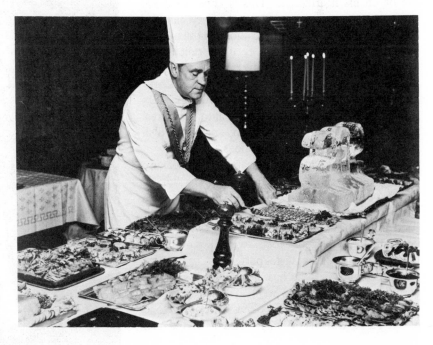

The artistry and inventiveness of the Scandinavian chef are evident in this Smörgasbord arrangement.

food specialties for which you become noted. When your family and friends come, they will want your specialties. One may be a hot loaf of bread served from oven to table, for example.

It is always a good idea when you go to a new restaurant to ask what the specialty of the house is. Order it. In France, this is called *plat maison*.

Most homemakers throughout the world begin with the same basic foods. The creative spirit asserts itself in transforming basic foods into delicious dishes with a special character of their own. While the foods are the same, there is a difference each country may develop in what is done with these foods. Take the potato, for example. In many countries, potatoes are boiled in the skin— and there is no more nutritious way to prepare them, except baking them in the skins, as the early American did in the hot ashes over a campfire or on his hearthstone. This is considered the tastiest way to cook potatoes by many families around the world today. The most popular item on many restaurant menus is the French-fried potato, which is served all over the world. The distinct twist that the Germans and other Europeans gave to the potato was to grate it raw, mix it with flour and eggs, and make it into pancakes. Remember that wide use doesn't make a dish gourmet, but having distinction does.

The true gourmet doesn't eat merely because he is hungry or drink merely because he is thirsty. He savors each bite of food to feel the pleasure of its taste in his mouth. Eating is mingled with good friendship and good conversation. It cannot be rushed. With good food, well-prepared, the most inexpensive meal tastes perfect.

The woman of India has an admirable concept of her role in preparing food. Traditionally, the Indian people believe the cooking of food is "one of God's revelations to man" and a divine art.

Thus the homemaker approaches cooking with pleasure and devotion.

In this chapter we have considered some basic principles that may guide you in developing a gourmet style of cooking. You will now aim to bring your own creativity to full bloom in the preparation of meals. You will develop your own originality and artistry with food and, in so doing, find the fulfillment all creative people know.

This magnificent Smörgasbord table runs the full 140-foot length of the Golden Hall in the Stockholm (Sweden) City Hall. This grand ballroom is used for many festive occasions, including the Nobel Prize awards.

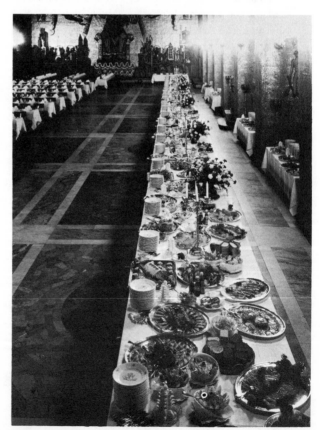

Useful food substitutes and equivalents (Approximate Measure)

1 T. = 3 t. or ½ fluid ounce
1 T. all-purpose flour = 1½ t. cornstarch, potato starch, rice starch, or arrowroot starch or
    2 t. quick-cooking tapioca
1 t. baking powder = ¼ t. baking soda + ½ c. sour milk or buttermilk or ¼–½ c. molasses
1 c. = 16 T. or 8 fluid ounces
1 c. cake flour = 1 c. less 2 T. (⅞ c.) all-purpose flour
⅓ c. instant nonfat dry milk + ¾ c. water = 1 c. skim milk
1⅓ c. instant nonfat dry milk + 3-3½ c. water = 1 qt. skim milk (See directions on package.)
1 c. whole milk = 1 c. nonfat dry milk reconstituted + 2 t. fat (this can be polyunsaturated,
    as in oil or soft margarine)
1 c. buttermilk = 1 c. milk + 1 T. lemon juice or vinegar
1 14½-oz. can evaporated milk (1⅔ c.) + 1⅔ c. water = 3⅓ c. whole milk
1 6-oz. can whole or skim evaporated milk = ⅔ c. whole or skim milk
1 15-oz. can sweetened condensed milk = 1⅓ c.
1 lb. grated cheddar cheese = 4 c.
1 lb. cottage cheese = 2 c.
1 c. butter, oleomargarine, or shortening = 1 c. less 2 T. vegetable oil or 1 c. less 2 T.
    lard + ½ t. salt
1 c. honey = 1½ c. sugar + ¼ c. liquid
1 c. corn syrup = 1 c. sugar + ¼ c. liquid
1 c. brown sugar, tightly packed = 1 c. white granulated sugar
1 oz. chocolate = 3 T. cocoa + 1 T. fat
8–10 graham crackers = 1 c. crumbs
1 c. whole large eggs (2 oz. each) = 5 eggs
1 c. egg whites = 8–9 eggs
1 c. egg yolks = 12 eggs
2 c. sifted egg powder + 2 c. water = 12 large eggs

terms

[...]erge first in
[...] a few
[...]tes, and
[...]r, as for
[...], or

[...]t or
[...] amount
[...] and
[...]r.

[...]lend
[...]oth
[...] a
[...]er.

[...]en

cut in: to mix evenly a solid mixture, such as fat, into a dry mixture, such as flour, by using knives, a pastry blender, fingertips, an electric mixer, or an electric blender.

fold in: to blend by use of a wide spoon, spatula, or wire whip by cutting down through a mixture such as beaten egg whites, bringing a portion up, and folding it over into mixture gently.

pan-broil: to cook on a hot ungreased or lightly greased skillet or griddle, pouring off fat as it accumulates.

purée: cooked food blended or pressed through a food mill or a sieve to form a smooth product.

sauté: to cook in skillet or saucepan in a small amount of hot fat until tender.

scald: to heat milk or other liquid hot (until bubbles form on sides) but not boiling.

scallop: to bake in layers with a sauce.

sieve: to press through a strainer.

simmer: to cook in a liquid just below the boiling point.

Meaningful words

boeuf à la mode
bouillabaisse
bouquet garni
cafe au lait
gourmet
hors d'oeuvres
petits fours
pot-au-feu
shish kabob
soufflé
vichyssoise

Thinking and evaluating

1. What is meant by the "gourmet style with foods"? What is the difference between the modern concept of a gourmet and the one mistakenly held by some? Explain why anyone who wishes to do so may become accomplished in the gourmet style with food.

2. Why have the French received so much credit for gourmet cooking? What is the secret of their success? In what ways could you improve on it?

3. What have you learned in this chapter that can stimulate you to a wider exploration of the food other nations eat? How can this help you later? What aims do you have for yourself in developing a gourmet style with food?

4. Why is meal preparation considered at the top of feminine accomplishments by so many nations?

5. How would you rate American homemakers in the gourmet style of meal preparation? Explain your answer.

Applying and sharing

1. Use a notebook for "Gourmet Style Meals and Foods," and list in this your successes and also points where you can improve when you try dishes and menus from other nations or create new ones.

2. In a bookstore, look over cookbooks that present foods of other nations. Make a list of those you might like as gifts. Put them on your gift list when you are engaged to be married.

3. Look up in your library the food customs and cultural origins of the foods of different nations in which you are interested. Explore these in your kitchen.

4. Select moderate-priced restaurants that specialize in foreign foods and try these according to your financial ability to eat out. Study their menus and the flavor of each food you eat.

5. Plan menus and prepare meals at your home typical of at least three other nations. Evaluate your results. Make a plan to improve. Repeat the best one for guests.

ruth white's low-calorie, low-fat cookbook

BASIC RECIPES WITH GOURMET VARIATIONS

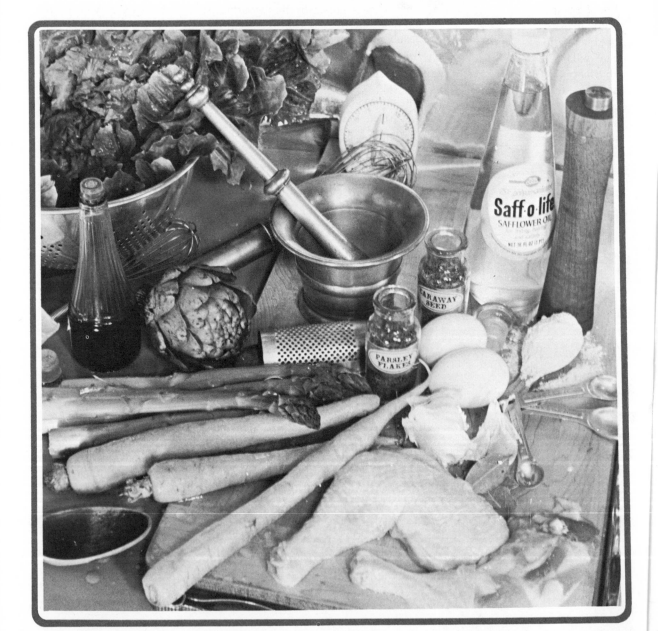

About this cookbook

The recipes in this cookbook have all been tested. They embody the principles of modern nutrition presented in the text. Their purpose is to combine the best nutrition with attractive appearance and delicious taste. Thus both the ingredients and the method of cooking them are important.

Following the latest scientific findings, these recipes are low in calories and fat. The fats recommended are those with low saturated fatty acid and high polyunsaturated (linoleic) fatty acid content. Nonfat dry milk is used wherever possible. This is economical and nutritionally valuable.

The recipes, with their suggested variations, form a foundation upon which even a beginner can develop skill and confidence. From foods, you can go on, using your imagin creativity, to produce gourmet dishes f meals, good snacks, and tasty party f

When you learn to cook and serv as part of balanced meals, you are niques that will help you enjoy enjoy a vigorous, healthy life. gratification of success—succe self and your family with we food. And you will be form foods that provide the nut health and attractive app life.

Technique of using a recipe

READ the recipe critically all the way through before you begin.

ASSEMBLE in your mixing center all the ingredients and utensils required.

DO all preliminary preparation, such as chopping nuts or onions, peeling vegetables, oiling pans, or preheating the oven, before you start.

MEASURE accurately in standard cups or spoons.

FOLLOW the recipe exactly, except in seasoning (which varies according to taste), until you are experienced in technique and understand the principles of food relationships in cooking.

NOTE any mistakes you may make. Review the recipe and your procedure. If necessary, make a plan to improve. Try the recipe again until you succeed, eliminating any previous mistakes, such as inaccurate measuring or failing to preheat the oven.

EXPERIMENT with herbs and spices to suit yo' taste. Note down what you do.

PERFECT each recipe to suit you, then broaden your experience by using others.

Read the recipe t
what you know.
you use it. Ask y

1/Does it
in the meal?

2/Is it c
of nutrit
use the
are und

3/
can
ex

Some usef

blanch: to subt
boiling water fo
seconds or minu
then in cold wat
tomatoes, peach
almonds.

braise: to cook me
vegetables in a sma
of liquid by coverin
simmering until tend

cream: to soften and
fat and sugar until smo
and light by mixing with
spoon or an electric mix

cube: to cut into small ev
pieces.

MEAT GROUP

BROILED FISH AND MEAT

BROILED FISH STEAKS WITH ALMONDS

(yield: 3 servings per pound)

SELECT fresh or thawed frozen salmon, filet of sole, halibut, haddock, red snapper, trout, shad, or other fish you prefer, boned.

WASH and dry the fish, if fresh.

RUB the fish on each side with the Self-Basting Marinade (recipe page 411), omitting the Kitchen Bouquet sauce in the recipe if desired.

SPRINKLE with slivered almonds.

BROIL in a preheated broiler until the fish is lightly browned and flakes tenderly (7–10 minutes, depending on thickness).

SERVE hot at once, garnishing with sliced lemon, lime, tomato, or greens. Complete the meal with brown rice, stewed tomatoes, okra and onion, cabbage salad, and café au lait, plus any dessert you prefer.

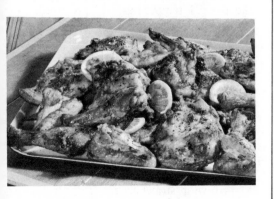

BROILED HERBED STEAK

(yield: 4–6 servings)

3–4 lbs. high-quality steak
  or tenderized round or rump
¼ t. crushed tarragon leaves
1 crushed clove garlic
¼ t. celery salt
½ t. coarsely ground black pepper
¼ c. soft margarine

TRIM the surplus fat from the outside of the steaks and wipe them with a clean damp cloth.

PLACE on a slightly oiled, preheated broiler rack and broil on each side 5–8 minutes, according to the thickness of the meat and the degree of rareness desired.

MIX the herbs with the margarine and spread the mixture over each serving as it is served (on a hot plate).

BROILED CHICKEN, TURKEY, OR CORNISH HEN

SPLIT broilers, chicken or turkey breasts or joints, or Cornish hens to make serving-size pieces. Wash and dry the meat.

RUB all sides with Self-Basting Marinade (recipe page 411) or herbed seasoning used for steak.

PLACE in a lightly oiled shallow oblong baking pan, skin side up, in a preheated broiler.

BROIL on one side 20–30 minutes and turn, brushing the top with marinade. Broil until done (flesh is tender and no pink is showing).

SERVE with a potato or alternate, a green or yellow vegetable, green salad, milk, and Fruit Cocktail Cake (recipe page 441).

ROASTS

ROAST BEEF

Standing rib, rolled sirloin,
sirloin tip or rib eye of beef
Salt and pepper to taste
Herbs and spices to taste

WIPE the meat carefully with a clean damp cloth or a paper towel.

SEASON it with salt, pepper, and other seasonings before, during, or after cooking. Seasoning penetrates only ¼ inch.

PLACE the meat on a rack in a shallow pan with the fat side up. Add no liquid.

INSERT a meat thermometer in the center of the meat, not touching the fat or bone.

ROAST at 200°–300°F for tender, even, juicy meat. Use the lower temperature for a large roast or one of lower grade or cut.

COOK until the desired doneness is reached, as indicated by the thermometer.

REMOVE the meat from the oven 15–20 minutes before serving, for better cutting, and at a temperature 10° lower than desired. Meat continues cooking for a few minutes out of the oven.

SERVE hot with brown juice drippings (but not fat) on a hot platter.

Variations

1/LAMB OR VEAL ROAST

USE the leg, loin or shoulder and follow above directions.

2/FRESH PORK ROAST

USE the loin, shoulder, ham, or picnic shoulder.

3/CURED PORK ROAST

USE cured ham or picnic shoulder.

ROAST LAMB, TURKISH STYLE

(yield: 2–3 servings per pound)

1 boned leg lamb
½ c. vegetable oil
¼ c. lemon juice
4 crushed garlic cloves
2 crushed bay leaves
2 t. fresh ground pepper
salt to taste

HAVE your butcher bone the lamb. Trim off the fat.

WIPE the meat with a clean damp cloth and place it in a flat pan.

MIX the remaining ingredients and rub them well into the lamb on all sides.

MARINATE it in the refrigerator overnight, spooning the liquid over the meat at intervals. Three hours before roasting, remove the meat from the marinade and allow it to dry.

PLACE on a rack in a shallow pan.

INSERT a meat thermometer in the center of the thickest part.

ROAST in a preheated oven at 300°F or 325°F, until the thermometer reaches the desired temperature. If preferred, reduce the heat to 200°F after one-half hour and cook until the meat thermometer registers the desired degree of doneness. The lower temperature takes about one and one-half times the cooking time, or more, but yields the best flavor, has the least loss of nutrients and juices, and has the least shrinkage.

SERVE, for a gourmet Turkish meal, with pilaf, eggplant, or squash, rye bread, lettuce-and-tomato salad, yogurt topped with strawberries, fresh fruit, and coffee.

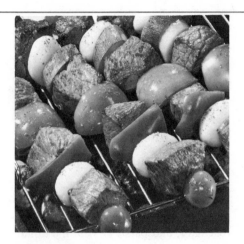

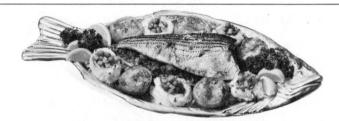

SELF-BASTING MARINADE OR SEASONING PASTE FOR POULTRY OR FISH

½ c. flour	1 t. crushed thyme leaves
¼ c. lemon juice	1 T. salt
¼ c. vegetable oil	½ t. black pepper
2 T. grated onion	1 T. paprika
2 crushed cloves garlic	½ t. Kitchen Bouquet

BLEND all ingredients and rub the poultry or fish, either whole or in pieces, on all sides just before baking, placing the sauce more thickly over the breast of poultry. Needs no basting.

BASTE with the juices that run off, just before serving, for a beautiful, appetizing effect. This gives a juicy, tender, flavorful roast when cooked at low temperature. *For a thicker sauce*, use more flour; for a thinner one, less flour.

Variations

1/SHISH KABOB

HAVE the lamb cut in 1-inch cubes and marinate as for roast (or use tender beef, if you prefer).

PLACE the meat on individual skewers, alternating with two or more of these vegetables: eggplant, summer squash, mushrooms, bell peppers, onions, cherry tomatoes.

ROAST or broil until done.

SERVE hot as part of a balanced meal.

2/HAM KABOB WITH PINEAPPLE

CUT precooked or canned ham in 1-inch cubes.

PLACE them on skewers, alternating with pineapple.

ROAST or broil until done.

SERVE hot with hot brown rice and scrambled eggs for breakfast or brunch, preceded by fresh fruit or juice. A good company dish for supper, too, accompanied by a salad and a caramel baked custard for dessert.

BAKED STUFFED FISH

1 fish, 3–4 lbs., or
2 large fillets
Self-Basting Marinade
Stuffing

CLEAN and prepare the fresh fish.

SEASON it inside and out and place stuffing in the cavity or the center of one fillet, laying the other on top and tying it lightly around each end and the center. Cover with Self-Basting Marinade (recipe above).

BAKE it in a preheated oven at 325°F, until it is done. (If a deeper brown color is desired, flash it under the broiler for a few minutes, being careful not to let it burn.)

SERVE it hot at once as part of a balanced meal.

BRAISED MEAT

POT ROAST WITH VEGETABLES (yield: 6 servings)

3–4 lbs. lean meat*	2 t. salt
⅓ cup flour	2 bay leaves
2 T. oil	1 crushed clove garlic
½ c. diced onion	1 c. diced celery
½ c. water or vegetable juice	4 quartered large potatoes
½ t. black pepper	6 small onions
¼ t. celery seed	8 quartered carrots

WIPE the meat with a damp cloth, then dry and dredge it in flour.

PLACE the oil in a thick-bottomed pan, such as a Dutch oven or chicken fryer, and brown the meat on all sides.

ADD the desired herbs or spices and the liquid. Cover tightly and allow to simmer until done, or cook in a pressure saucepan at 15 pounds pressure for 12–15 minutes.

REMOVE the meat and dip off the excess fat, but not the drippings.

ADD the vegetables and cook them until just tender. If the pan is large enough, cook the vegetables with the meat the last 20 minutes (or in the pressure cooker about 3–5 minutes).

SERVE the meat hot in the center of a hot platter, surrounded by vegetables and covered with the nonfat drippings. Garnish with parsley or chopped green onions.

ACCOMPANY with bread, milk, green salad, and molasses cake or gingerbread.

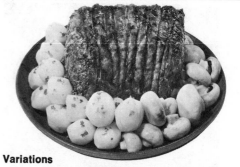

Variations

1/BOEUF A LA MODE (French)

ADD bouquet garni (bay leaf, thyme, rosemary, and parsley) with the liquid, following basic directions for pot roast. Omit the carrots.

ADD 1 cup sliced mushrooms with other vegetables.

SERVE with warm French bread, green salad, small pastry, fresh fruit, and cheese.

2/IRISH STEW

USE lean meat in 1-inch cubes and omit the celery. Proceed as in the basic recipe.

SERVE with milk, bread, spread, fresh onions, and deep-dish apple pie.

3/MEXICAN STEW

USE 2 cloves garlic, 2 crushed dried chili peppers, 1 cup tomato paste; omit carrots.

FOLLOW the basic method for braising.

SERVE with tortillas, milk, and a whole orange.

*See text pages 74–75 for types of meat suitable for braising.

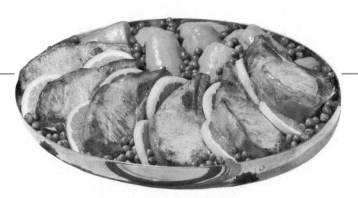

NIGERIAN GROUNDNUT (PEANUT) STEW

(yield: 8 servings)

2 T. vegetable oil
1 c. finely diced onion
2 crushed cloves garlic
1–3 dry crushed red chili peppers
   or 1–3 t. chili powder
½ t. nutmeg
2 c. cubed eggplant
4 c. cubed cooked chicken
3 c. chicken broth
2 6-oz. cans tomato paste
¾ c. crushed peanuts
2 t. salt
6 c. hot cooked brown rice

Toppings

Chopped peanuts
Diced orange, pineapple, papaya
Thin slices or small wedges of tomato
Finely sliced green onions
Diced green pepper
Grated coconut
Chutney or watermelon pickle

HEAT the first six ingredients in a 4-quart pan until crisp-tender, stirring to prevent sticking.

ADD the next five ingredients and mix.

BRING to a boil, cover, and let simmer 3–5 minutes.

SERVE hot over hot rice, using the toppings you prefer.

ACCOMPANY with milk or café au lait and white coconut cake. Stew made the day before and stored in the refrigerator overnight has a better flavor. It also saves time for a busy hostess on the day of a party. Heat only till bubbling hot and serve.

PANFRIED OR SAUTÉED MEATS

SOUTHERN FRIED PORK CHOPS AND YAMS

(yield: 4 servings)

4 thick pork chops
2 large yams
¼ c. flour
salt and pepper
1 T. vegetable oil
1 c. skim milk

TRIM the fat from the pork chops and dredge them in the seasoned flour.

BROWN the chops on both sides over moderate heat in a hot, lightly oiled thick skillet or Dutch oven.

REMOVE them from the pan.

REMOVE any excess fat from the pan and add 2 tablespoons flour, stirring until it is brown.

ADD the skim milk, season to taste, and stir until smooth. Return the pork chops to the gravy.

PEEL and split the yams, making four servings, and lay them on top of the chops.

COVER tightly and cook at a simmer or bake in a moderate oven until the chops and yams are tender.

SERVE hot with collards, turnip greens, or another green leafy vegetable, corn bread, margarine, milk, fresh green onions, and applesauce. A nourishing and delicious meal!

Variation
PORK CHOPS HAWAIIAN

ADD pineapple chunks and ½ cup pineapple juice the last 2 minutes of cooking.

STEAK AU POIVRE (French steak with pepper)
(yield: 4–6 servings)

2 lbs. tender boneless steak
  (1″–1½″ thick)
1 t. coarsely ground pepper
1 t. salt
2 T. vegetable oil
¼ c. cognac or
¼ c. boiling water and 2 bouillon
  cubes

WIPE the steak with a slightly damp paper towel. Trim off the fat and cut the meat in serving pieces.

RUB the meat on both sides with the salt and pepper, pressing the pepper well into the meat.

HEAT the oil in a thick-bottomed skillet until hot, but not smoking.

BROWN the steak on one side, turn and brown it on the other side quickly.

LOWER the heat and cook the meat to the desired degree of doneness.

HOLD in a low oven until the sauce is ready. Pour off the fat, then add the cognac or the water and bouillon cubes, stirring so that all the brown drippings in the pan are absorbed into the sauce. Pour the hot sauce over the meat and serve on a hot platter or individual plates. The superb flavor of this dish accounts for its popularity all over the world, especially in Europe. Excellent when served with baked or mashed potatoes, green peas and baby onions, romaine lettuce salad, and yogurt topped with fruit.

Variations

1/ MEXICAN STEAK OR VEAL

ADD to the browned meat drippings after the meat is removed: ½ cup tomato paste, 3 fresh peppers (red or green), seeded and cut in strips, 1 teaspoon chili pepper.

ADD 3 tablespoons lemon juice.

HEAT to boiling point and spoon over the meat.

SERVE with seasoned seashell macaroni topped with Parmesan cheese, green salad, zucchini squash, and fresh fruit and cheese.

2/ BOMBAY STEAK OR VEAL

ADD to the basic recipe another clove of garlic, ½ teaspoon curry powder, and ½ cup seedless raisins. Proceed according to the basic recipe.

SERVE with rice and a cooked vegetable, and yogurt with orange or papaya slices for dessert.

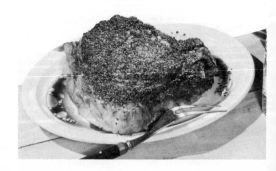

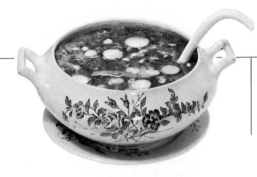

VEAL CORDON BLEU

(yield: 4 servings)

1 lb. thinly sliced veal
4 thin slices cooked ham
4 slices Emmenthaler (Swiss) or sharp
  cheddar cheese
salt and pepper to taste
3 T. oil
1 egg
bread crumbs
flour
2 t. lemon juice

FLATTEN the veal, pounding it with a meat cleaver, a heavy knife, or a meat hammer. Season it with salt, pepper, and lemon juice.

CUT the veal in four pieces.

PLACE a slice of ham and a slice of cheese in the center of each piece of veal.

ROLL the veal and fasten it with a toothpick. Roll it in flour.

DIP the meat into the seasoned beaten egg and then roll it in the bread crumbs.

SAUTÉ slowly in the hot fat in a large skillet until it is brown on both sides.

DRAIN on doubled paper towels and keep warm in a flat pan in a slow oven (175°F).

SERVE hot with brown rice or noodles, broccoli, tomato and cucumber salad, whole wheat French bread, café au lait, and vanilla cream pie or pudding.

SOUPS

BASIC BEEF-VEGETABLE SOUP

(yield: 8–10 servings)

1 split marrowbone	1 c. diced potatoes
2 lbs. lean meat, in 1-inch cubes	1 c. sliced carrots
	1 c. sliced celery
3 c. water	1 c. diced turnips
1 T. salt	1 c. diced onion
¼ t. black pepper	1 c. minced parsley
1 crushed dried chili pepper (optional)	1 c. thinly sliced okra (optional)
1 whole onion	3 c. canned tomatoes
	1 crushed clove garlic

COMBINE the first seven ingredients in a large kettle or pressure pan and cook until the meat is tender.

REMOVE the meat and the bone from the pot and set it aside. Skim off the fat.

COOK the vegetables in the liquid until just tender and season to taste, if necessary. Add boiling water to the desired thickness (about 4 cups).

RETURN all the meat to the pot with the vegetables. Bring the soup to the boiling point, but do not boil.

SERVE hot with crackers or corn sticks as the main dish in the meal, together with tossed lettuce salad, milk, and lemon fluff pie (recipe page 431). Good enough for guests!

STORE one meal of leftover soup in the refrigerator. Freeze the remainder. Tastes even better the second time it is used. One way to introduce new vegetables is in soup.

Variations

1/MEXICAN VEGETABLE SOUP

OMIT the potatoes and turnips.

ADD 1 cup each of fresh or canned kernel corn and red beans, 2 cloves of garlic, and 1 tablespoon chili pepper.

(For more variations see page 416.)

Soup variations

2/*FISH CHOWDER*

HAVE 2 pounds of fresh or frozen fish skinned and boned. Wash and cut it into 1-inch cubes.

ADD 3 tablespoons of lemon juice and proceed as in the basic recipe, simmering the fish until tender (about 5 minutes). If a thickened soup is desired, blend ½ cup flour with 1 cup water until smooth and add the mixture to the soup, stirring until it is slightly thickened.

RETURN the fish to the chowder and add 4 cups of liquid nonfat milk, heating until boiling hot, but do not boil.

SERVE as the main dish in a balanced meal, garnished with a slice of lemon or lime. This is a low-fat, low-calorie, highly nourishing soup that is also very tasty.

3/*HAM AND BEAN SOUP*

USE a ham bone or hock with about 2 cups of cubed lean ham, instead of the beef.

ADD 2 tablespoons vegetable oil, 2 whole cloves, and 2 whole allspice.

WASH 1 cup of dried beans (any type), split peas, black-eyed peas, or lentils and add to the meat with 7 cups of water (5 cups for pressure cooking), 2 teaspoons dry mustard, and seasonings to taste.

BOIL for 2 minutes. Turn off the heat and let the mixture soak for at least 2 hours. This tenderizes the meat, cuts down the cooking time, and makes the beans hold their shape better.

COOK about 2½ hours, or until tender. If using a pressure saucepan, remove the bone and bring the pressure to 15 pounds. With the exception of navy and pinto beans (which require only 10 minutes' cooking time), all beans, peas, and lentils should be cooked for 5 minutes at 15 pounds pressure. Let the pressure return to normal, then add boiling water until the soup is the desired thickness.

SERVE as the main dish in a balanced meal, garnishing with diced fresh green pepper or onions, or both.

EGGS IN MEALS

QUICHE LORRAINE
(yield: 6 servings)

1 9-inch pastry or biscuit
  dough shell, unbaked
6 strips bacon, fried crisp
  and crumbled
1½ c. grated Swiss or sharp
  cheddar cheese
4 large eggs
salt and pepper to taste
½ c. yogurt or milk
2 T. flour
½ t. dry mustard
⅛ t. nutmeg
½ c. drained mushrooms

BEAT the eggs until foamy and blend in the remaining ingredients, except the bacon.

SPRINKLE half the bacon over the shell and pour the egg mixture into the shell.

BAKE in a preheated oven at 375°F until the custard is firm (about 30 minutes).

GARNISH the top with the remaining bacon crumbs.

SERVE hot as the main dish for lunch, supper, breakfast, or brunch. For a gourmet luncheon or Sunday night supper, serve this as the main dish, preceded by French onion soup and accompanied by fresh spinach and tomato salad, plain white cake (recipe page 440) topped with fresh or thawed frozen strawberries, and café au lait.

MILK GROUP

BASIC MERINGUES

2 egg whites, large	½ t. cream of tartar
⅔ c. fine sugar	½ t. almond extract
¼ t. salt	½ t. vanilla

PLACE the egg whites in a mixing bowl. Add the salt, cream of tartar, and flavorings and beat until foam begins to form.

ADD the sugar, 1 tablespoon at a time, and beat until thoroughly dissolved and the whites are in moist, shiny peaks.

SHAPE the meringues in shell form or drop by teaspoonfuls onto a lightly oiled cookie sheet (preferably nonstick), about 2 inches apart.

BAKE at 250°F for about 50 minutes. While warm, remove the meringues with a pancake turner or spatula, being careful not to break them.

FILL the meringues with fresh or frozen peaches, strawberries, or other berries; with chocolate, vanilla, or lemon sauce; or with fruited ice cream.

TOP with whipped cream or sweetened yogurt, if desired. Garnish with one whole fresh berry or other fruit. The meringues may be baked as cookies.

Variation
NUT CHOCOLATE CHIP MERINGUES

ADD 1 cup each of semisweet chocolate chips and broken walnut meats.

DROP by teaspoonfuls onto a lightly oiled cookie sheet and bake at 350°F for 50 minutes. Makes 40–50 delicious cookies.

HORS D'OEUVRES (Appetizers)

COTTAGE CHEESE CLAM DIP
(make the day before)

1½ c. low-fat cottage cheese	⅔ c. drained minced clams
1 T. grated onion	(7½ oz. can)
1 T. minced parsley	¼ t. salt
1 T. lemon juice	dash hot sauce
1 T. horseradish	paprika

BLEND all the ingredients, except the paprika, until smooth.

ADD clam juice to give the desired consistency.

PLACE in a covered container in the refrigerator overnight.

BRING to room temperature when ready to use.

SERVE at once in a pretty bowl, garnished with paprika and accompanied by thin, crisp crackers.

QUICK COTTAGE CHEESE PIZZA

OIL split English muffins lightly and brown in the broiler.

SPREAD each half with low-fat cottage cheese.

SPREAD about 1 tablespoon of canned pizza sauce over the cottage cheese.

ADD chili pepper, if desired.

TOP with finely diced chives or green onion tops and a generous sprinkling of grated Parmesan or sharp cheddar cheese.

GARNISH with 6 slices of stuffed olive and heat under the broiler until the cheese melts.

SERVE hot as the main dish for lunch or cut each muffin in six wedges and serve as an hors d'oeuvre at a party.

SOUPS AND MAIN DISHES

CREAM OF VEGETABLE SOUP*

(yield: 5–6 servings)

1 c. vegetable purée
1 T. grated onion
2 c. thin white sauce
3–6 chicken bouillon cubes
⅛ t. celery salt
⅛ t. garlic salt
salt and pepper to taste

MIX all the ingredients in a thick-bottomed 2-quart pan and heat until boiling hot; then simmer 1 minute.

SEASON to taste.

SERVE hot in warm soup bowls or mugs, garnishing with minced parsley, chopped chives, a slice of lemon or lime, or cheese croutons.

*Foods suited to cream soups include tomato, potato, spinach, watercress, kale, broccoli, lettuce, leek, onion, peas, beans, asparagus, celery, corn, carrot, squash, pumpkin, avocado, mushroom, cauliflower, beet, rutabaga, almond, peanut, fish, ground poultry, ground meat, or a combination of some of these.

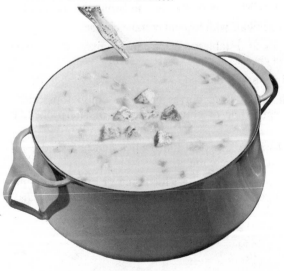

BASIC LOW-FAT, LOW-

	MILK*
THIN	1 c.
MEDIUM	1 c.
THICK	1 c.
EXTRA THICK	1 c.

BLEND to a smooth paste equal amounts of flour and milk with the oil and salt.

ADD seasonings and any additional ingredients called for by the specific recipe, such as herbs, spices, eggs, and/or sugar.

HEAT the remaining milk to scalding and add it gradually to the first mixture.

Variations

1/MEXICAN CREAM OF VEGETABLE SOUP

COMBINE corn and beans and add 1½ teaspoons chili pepper.

2/ITALIAN CREAM OF VEGETABLE SOUP

ADD 1 clove of crushed garlic, ¼ teaspoon oregano, and 2 tablespoons minced parsley.

3/INDIAN CREAM OF VEGETABLE SOUP

ADD ½ teaspoon curry powder.

CALORIE WHITE SAUCE

OIL	FLOUR	SALT
1 T.	1 T.	¼ t.
1 T.	2 T.	¼ t.
1 T.	3 T.	¼ t.
1 T.	4 T.	¼ t.

COOK in a thick-bottomed covered pan at low heat until the desired smoothness and thickness are obtained, stirring to prevent lumps. When extract is added for cream-type pies and the like, add it after the cooking is completed.

*For low-cost nonfat milk, use ½ cup nonfat dry milk and 1 cup water per cup of liquid milk in the sauce.

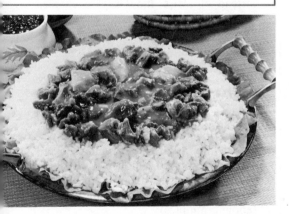

TROPICAL CHICKEN

(quick top-of-stove guest or family main dish)

(yield: 10–12 servings)

3 c. diced cooked chicken or turkey	2 T. oil
6 chicken bouillon cubes	1 large green pepper
3 c. thinly sliced green celery	¼ c. toasted almonds
1 crushed clove garlic	2 T. soy sauce
2½ c. medium white sauce or 2 cans cream of mushroom soup	2 T. grated onion
salt and pepper to taste	1 1-lb. can pineapple chunks, including juice
	4 c. cooked brown rice, noodles, macaroni, or bulgur

CUT the pepper in strips and heat it with the garlic, onion, and oil in a 4-quart saucepan for about a minute. Drain off excess oil.

BLEND in all the remaining ingredients, except almonds, stirring gently until well blended and boiling hot.

SERVE over hot cooked brown rice and top with toasted almonds. This may be prepared the night before, poured into a casserole, covered tightly, and refrigerated. When it is to be used, heat in a preheated oven at 375°F until it bubbles in the middle (about 25 minutes). Serve at once with a green vegetable, tossed salad, milk, and pumpkin nut bread (recipe page 432).

Variations

1/HAM AND CHICKEN CASSEROLE

USE cooked leftover ham or fresh pork, or equal amounts of pork and chicken.

2/MEXICAN CASSEROLE

ADD ½ cup diced green chili peppers, removing the seeds, 1 cup diced canned tomatoes, and 1 cup (4 ounces) grated sharp cheddar cheese; blend in.

CHEESE SOUFFLÉ (Swiss type)

(yield: 4 servings)

½ c. flour
2 T. vegetable oil
1 t. salt
dash nutmeg
⅛ t. white pepper
1 c. (4 oz.) grated Gruyère cheese
1 c. (4 oz.) grated Swiss cheese
2 c. skim milk or 1 c. nonfat dry milk
    + 2 c. water
5 eggs, separated

PREPARE a *thick* white sauce by placing the flour, oil, dry milk, and water (or skim milk) in a heavy-bottomed 3-quart saucepan, stirring vigorously until smooth.

COOK the sauce until it is thick and smooth, stirring to prevent lumps.

ADD the slightly beaten egg yolks, grated cheese, nutmeg, and pepper and blend into the sauce.

BEAT the egg whites and salt in a 4-quart mixing bowl until moist, firm peaks are formed.

FOLD the hot cheese mixture gradually into the egg whites, turning gently with a wide spoon, over and under, until blended.

POUR into a buttered 1½-quart casserole or small individual casseroles.

BAKE in a preheated oven at 350°F until done (about 45–50 minutes).

SERVE hot at once with cucumber, lettuce, and tomato salad, hot green beans, and warm French garlic bread, using fruit in season for dessert. This may be a main dish for any meal. Excellent for guest luncheon or supper.

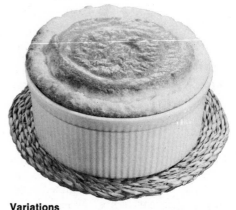

Variations

1/AMERICAN CHEESE SOUFFLÉ

ADD a dash of cayenne pepper, 1 teaspoon dry mustard, and 1 tablespoon grated onion to the white sauce.

USE ½ lb. grated sharp cheddar cheese instead of Swiss and Gruyère cheese.

ADD ½ teaspoon cream of tartar to the egg whites before beating, to give a firmer texture.

2/SCANDINAVIAN CHEESE SOUFFLÉ

POACH 1 pound of boneless fish with ½ teaspoon each of fresh black pepper and thyme, a dash of cayenne pepper, 1 teaspoon grated lemon peel, 1 tablespoon lemon juice, and ¼ cup of boiling water. Cover and cook until tender (about 5 minutes).

MASH the fish fine and add it to the cheese, using the broth in which it is cooked as part of the liquid in making the sauce with nonfat dry milk.

PROCEED as in the basic recipe. Serves 6–8.

3/FRENCH CHEESE SOUFFLÉ

SERVE with a thin mushroom sauce, using ½ cup sliced cooked mushrooms per cup of thin white sauce.

4/MEXICAN CHEESE SOUFFLÉ

PREPARE the soufflé as the American version, but serve with a medium tomato sauce, using tomato juice instead of the milk and adding 1 diced green pepper, 2 tablespoons diced onion, and 1½ teaspoons chili peppers. If desired, ½ cup of diced green chili peppers may be added for each 2 cups of sauce.

5/CHICKEN OR TURKEY SOUFFLÉ

ADD 2 cups of diced cooked chicken or turkey to the American variation.

SERVE hot at once, with a mushroom sauce, as the main dish in a balanced meal.

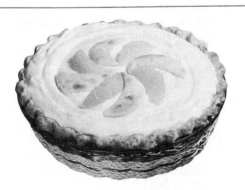

DESSERTS

VANILLA CREAM PIE

(yield: 1 pie)

½ c. packed brown sugar
4 T. flour
1 c. nonfat dry milk
2 c. water
1 T. soft margarine
3 eggs, separated
1 t. vanilla
¼ t. cream of tartar
¼ t. salt
7 T. white sugar (for meringue)
1 9-in. precooked pastry shell for pie

MIX in a thick-bottomed 2-quart saucepan the dry milk, brown sugar, flour, fat, and ½ cup of the water, to form a smooth paste.

ADD the remaining water and the egg yolks, lightly beaten.

COOK until the mixture is smooth and thickened, stirring to prevent lumps.

REMOVE from the heat and blend in the vanilla.

PREPARE a meringue: Beat the egg whites with the salt and cream of tartar until they start to foam, then beat in the white sugar, 2 tablespoons at a time, until all is dissolved and the meringue stands in firm, moist, glazed peaks.

POUR the hot filling into the baked crust.

SPREAD the meringue over the top of the pie to the edge of the outer crust (this helps the meringue hold to the crust), swirling for an attractive design.

BAKE in a preheated oven at 450°F until golden brown (7–10 minutes). Remove.

COOL and serve as dessert in a balanced meal.

(For variations, see page 422.)

Variations on cream pie
1/OTHER CREAM PIES

Most cream pies may be made from this recipe. Fillings may be served as pudding without a crust, over cake or topped with fruit, nuts, semisweet chocolate, sweetened yogurt, or whipped cream.

2/VANILLA PUDDING

FOLD the beaten egg whites (without adding the white sugar) into the hot filling at once.

COVER and let stand until the egg whites have had time to cook. Do not place the pudding on the stove.

POUR into sherbet glasses or a large bowl.

TOP with desired garnish and serve.

3/PINEAPPLE CREAM PIE OR PUDDING

ADD 1 cup well-drained crushed pineapple just before the mixture is removed from the heat.

4/BANANA CREAM PIE OR PUDDING

ADD a thick layer of sliced ripe bananas over the pie crust before pouring in the cream filling.

5/COCONUT CREAM PIE OR PUDDING

ADD ¼ cup shredded coconut to the cream filling.

SPRINKLE ¼ cup of shredded coconut over the meringue before baking.

6/CHOCOLATE CREAM PIE OR PUDDING

MIX 5 tablespoons cocoa with ¼ cup sugar and blend in at the first step.

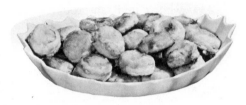

CHEESE SCONES

(adaptation of British recipe)

2 c. all-purpose flour
2 t. double-action baking powder
½ t. salt
½ t. baking soda
¼ c. sugar
1 egg
½ c. grated sharp cheddar cheese
1 c. yogurt or buttermilk
¼ c. vegetable oil

SIFT the dry ingredients together thoroughly into a mixing bowl.

BEAT the egg slightly.

MAKE a hole in the middle of the dry ingredients and add all the remaining ingredients, mixing lightly.

ROLL or pat on wax paper to ¾-inch thickness and cut scones with a 2-inch cookie cutter.

PLACE the scones, well apart, on a lightly oiled cookie sheet.

BAKE in a preheated oven at 450°F until golden brown (about 12 minutes).

SERVE hot at once with soft margarine and jam or honey.

VEGETABLE-FRUIT GROUP

HORS D'OEUVRES

BROILED STUFFED MUSHROOMS

SAUTÉ fresh or canned mushrooms in a small amount of soft margarine, with salt and pepper to taste.

REMOVE the stems and save them for a soup or a creamed dish.

STUFF the inverted mushrooms with chicken or potted ham spread.

BROIL and serve hot on circles of bread or crackers or on toothpicks.

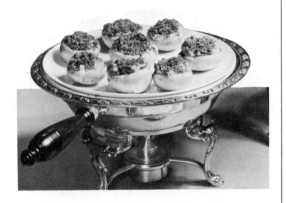

SICILIAN CAPONATA (EGGPLANT ANTIPASTO)

(yield: 5 cups or about 20 servings)

1 large eggplant	¼ c. wine vinegar
⅓ c. vegetable oil	½ c. diced black olives
1½ c. finely diced celery	2 T. sugar
1½ c. finely diced onion	1 t. salt
1 c. (8 oz.) thick tomato paste	¼ t. coarse black pepper
2 T. capers	¼ c. coarsely chopped walnut meats

HEAT the oil in a large, thick-bottomed skillet and brown the peeled cubes of eggplant in it. Remove the cooked eggplant and drain on a paper towel.

SAUTÉ the onion and celery in the skillet, stirring about 2 minutes.

DRAIN off the excess fat.

ADD all the remaining ingredients and the eggplant.

COVER and cook over low heat until thick (about 20 minutes), stirring to prevent sticking. Taste and adjust the seasoning according to your preference.

STORE in a covered refrigerator dish. This will keep well for 10 days.

SERVE at room temperature with warm French garlic bread as a first course.

GUACAMOLE   (yield: 2 cups)

2 mashed ripe avocados
1 crushed clove garlic
2 T. lemon or lime juice
1 T. grated onion
½ t. chili pepper
¼ t. salt

COMBINE all the ingredients in a mixing bowl and blend thoroughly.

SERVE in a pretty bowl as a dip with raw vegetables or crackers or as a salad dressing.

SALADS

CHEF'S SALAD (yield: 4 servings)

1 qt. bite-size torn green lettuce (bib, Boston, bronze-tipped, Romaine)
1½ c. cubes or strips of any one of the following or a combination: chicken, turkey, ham, fish, or shellfish
1½ c. thin strips of Swiss or sharp cheddar cheese or 1½ c. cottage cheese
2 sliced tomatoes
½ c. sliced cucumber and/or green pepper strips
½ c. diced celery
2 finely sliced onions
¼ c. French dressing

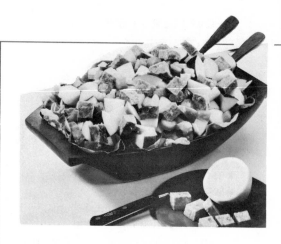

TOSS all the ingredients lightly, except the tomatoes and cottage cheese, and arrange attractively in a salad bowl or individual bowls or plates. If cottage cheese is used, use a small mound for each serving and place the vegetables around it.

GARNISH with the tomato slices.

SERVE as the main dish for lunch, preceded by a hot bouillon or lentil soup and accompanied by popovers, hot muffins, hot rolls, or nut bread. For dessert, serve floating island or hot bread with jam.

Variations

1/TOSSED SALAD

OMIT the meat and cheese.

USE a combination of any fresh or cooked vegetables you like.

GARNISH with watercress, radish roses, sliced hard-cooked eggs, avocado slices, or pepper strips, and any dressing you prefer.

2/CITRUS–AVOCADO SALAD

TOSS bite-size lettuce pieces with dressing and place on individual salad plates.

ARRANGE alternate sections of citrus fruit, apple slices, avocado slices, and/or pear slices over the lettuce.

PLACE a mound of cottage cheese (⅓ to ½ cup) in the center of each salad.

TOP with a cherry tomato or a strawberry. When strawberries are in season, make a circle of fresh berries around the outside of the salad.

SERVE, preceded by a French onion soup or split pea soup and accompanied by hot bread and café au lait. A beautiful luncheon or supper main dish.

CABBAGE, CARROT, AND PINEAPPLE MOLD

(yield: 6–8 servings)

¼ c. water
1½ pkg. (1½ T.) unflavored gelatin
¼ c. lemon juice
1 c. crushed pineapple
¼ c. sugar
½ t. salt
1 c. pineapple juice (including amount drained from crushed pineapple)
1 c. grated cabbage
1 c. grated carrots
¼ c. mayonnaise
Sour cream
Mayonnaise
¼ c. chopped walnuts

SOFTEN the gelatin in the cold water, then add it to the scalding hot pineapple juice, stirring until it is dissolved.

ADD the salt and sugar and stir until dissolved. Cool.

ADD all but the last three ingredients, mixing thoroughly.

RINSE a 1½-quart mold with cold water and pour the salad into it. Chill until firm.

UNMOLD by setting the mold into hot water for 10 seconds and turning it upside-down on a flat plate.

SURROUND the mold with chicory and green lettuce.

MIX equal parts of sour cream and mayonnaise, add the chopped walnuts, and place the mixture in the center hole of the mold. If preferred, use individual small molds. Delicious and nutritious.

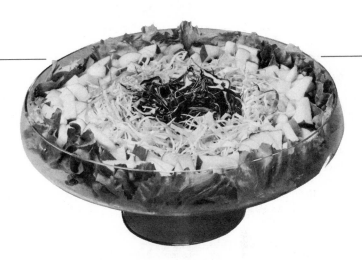

CABBAGE SALAD COMBINATIONS

(yield: 4–6 servings)

1/CABBAGE-FRUIT SALAD

TOSS lightly 2 cups shredded cabbage, 1 cup diced oranges, 1 cup pineapple chunks with your favorite dressing. This may also be used as a molded salad, omitting the dressing and adding the ingredients to 1 package of orange-flavored gelatin prepared according to the package directions.

2/CABBAGE-TOMATO-ONION SALAD

TOSS 1 quart shredded cabbage, 2 tomatoes cut in wedges, 1 green onion sliced thin, and oil-and-vinegar dressing.

3/CABBAGE-APPLE SALAD

MIX 3 cups shredded cabbage, 1 cup diced apples, ½ cup peanuts, 1 cup diced celery, and just enough mayonnaise to moisten.

4/CABBAGE-CARROT-ORANGE SALAD

MIX 2 cups shredded cabbage, 1 cup coarsely grated carrots, 1 cup orange cubes, and mayonnaise.

SOUPS

WINTER FRUIT SOUP (Scandinavian-type)

(yield: 12 servings)

4 c. water
1 c. seedless raisins
1 c. pitted prunes
3 c. sliced apples
2 c. (1-lb. can) sliced peaches
2 T. lemon juice
¼ t. cloves
¼ t. nutmeg
1 t. cinnamon
2 c. pineapple juice
sugar to taste
1 orange, sliced, with peel
¼ c. quick-cooking tapioca

PLACE uncooked fruits, spices, sliced orange, and 2 cups boiling water in a 4-quart pressure saucepan; cook at 15 pounds pressure 1 minute, allowing the pressure to return to normal (or cook in a covered saucepan until tender).

MIX the tapioca in the remaining water and add it to the hot fruit.

COOK until slightly thickened.

ADD pineapple juice and sugar to taste (not more than ¼ cup).

SERVE hot or cold as dessert, garnishing with a slice of lime or orange or a cherry. Easy, tasty, nutritious.

COOKED VEGETABLES

SUKIYAKI (Japan)

(yield: 4–6 servings)

1½ lbs. lean round steak
1 T. vegetable oil
3 T. soy sauce (this is salty)
½ c. water
2 chicken bouillon cubes
1½ c. celery, sliced
   diagonally
salt and pepper to taste
1½ c. sliced green onions
1 c. sliced mushrooms
1 lb. finely cut fresh spinach
   or 1 10-oz. pkg. frozen
   chopped spinach, thawed
1 5-oz. can bamboo shoots,
   drained and sliced
4–6 c. hot cooked brown
   rice, with ginger to taste

TRIM all fat from the meat and cut it in ¼″ x 2″ diagonal strips. Brown in hot oil.

PUSH the meat to one side and add all the remaining ingredients, except the spinach and rice.

STIR and simmer, uncovered, until the vegetables are tender, adding a small amount of liquid as needed. Add the spinach and cook until tender (about 1 minute).

SERVE the meat-vegetable mixture hot over hot rice, at once. If the sukiyaki is cooked at the table, serve melon or citrus fruit as the first course and lemon cookies or meringues (recipe page 417) as dessert, with tea.

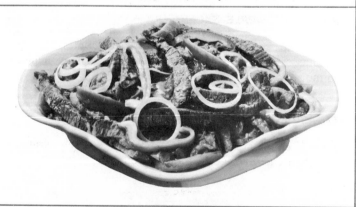

YELLOW WINTER SQUASH CASSEROLE

(yield: 6–8 servings)

4 c. cooked mashed squash
   (butternut, Hubbard, acorn,
   banana, others)
2 T. soft margarine
½ c. nonfat dry milk
½ c. brown sugar
1 t. grated lemon peel
1 t. grated orange peel
½ c. orange juice
½ t. nutmeg
½ t. mace
½ t. salt

COMBINE all ingredients thoroughly and turn into a 1½-quart casserole.

BAKE in a preheated oven at 375°F until bubbly and slightly brown.

SERVE hot as a potato alternate. This blends well with any meat, vegetable, or salad as part of a balanced meal.

Variation

SWEET POTATO OR YAM CASSEROLE

USE either sweet potatoes or yams and follow the above recipe.

TOP with marshmallows for the last few minutes of baking, if desired, for a party dish.

SOUTHERN COOKED COLLARD GREENS

(yield: 4–6 servings)

2 lbs. fresh greens or
   2 pkg. frozen greens
1 red dried pepper
1 ham bone with meat or
   4 chopped slices bacon
salt to taste (about 1 t.)
1 med. chopped onion
⅓ c. boiling water or brown
   pork drippings (not fat)

REMOVE all tough stems and damaged parts from fresh greens.

WASH thoroughly and chop.

SAUTÉ the crumbled red pepper and the chopped onion with chopped bacon or ham fat in a 4-quart saucepan or pressure cooker until it is soft, but not brown.

ADD all the remaining ingredients plus ¼ cup boiling water (if using a pressure saucepan) or ½ cup (if using a regular saucepan), using the brown pork drippings as part of the liquid. Bring the pressure to 15 pounds and cook 2–4 minutes (or boil until tender in a regular saucepan).

BOIL down the liquor and serve it with greens. Add vinegar to the greens at the table for a tangy flavor.

GARNISH with sliced hard-cooked egg, if desired.

SERVE with hot skillet corn bread, ham, black-eyed peas, sliced tomatoes, green onions, and cold milk or buttermilk. A good dessert with this meal is nut pie or pudding.

Variation

MIXED GREENS

MIX equal amounts of two or more of these greens for a delicious flavor: collards, Savoy cabbage, outer leaves of green or red cabbage, broccoli, turnip greens, kale, mustard greens, dandelion greens, Swiss chard, beet tops, endive, or spinach. These may also be cooked alone as above. Remember that spinach or Swiss chard should be cooked only about 1 minute at boiling temperature. When mixing greens, add the spinach last.

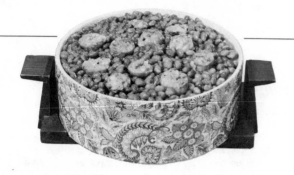

BAKED BEANS

(shortcut top-of-stove method)

(yield: 8–9 servings)

1 lb. (2¼ c.) dried pea beans
1 c. chopped onion
2 strips bacon, diced
⅔ c. dark molasses
1 T. salt
1 T. oil
1 t. dry mustard
⅛–¼ t. red pepper or 2 dried chili
   peppers
2 T. lemon juice or vinegar
2 c. water
1½ c. tomato juice

PRECOOK the beans with the water, tomato juice, and vegetable oil for 2 minutes at 15 pounds pressure (or boil them in a covered pot for at least 2 minutes) and then let the beans stand, covered, to soak for at least 2 hours.

ADD all the remaining ingredients and cook in a pressure saucepan at 15 pounds pressure for 5 minutes, letting the pressure return to normal gradually. (Boiling in a regular pan requires 2½–3 hours.) If desired, pour the beans into a casserole and brown under the broiler before serving.

SERVE as a meat alternate with corn sticks, spinach-cheese casserole (recipe this page), sliced onion and orange salad, apple pie, and milk.

SPINACH AND CHEESE CASSEROLE

(Italian type)

(yield: 6–8 servings)

1 c. thick white sauce (recipe pages
   418–419)
2 10-oz. pkgs. frozen chopped spinach
   or 2 lbs. fresh spinach
¾ c. low-fat cottage cheese
3 eggs
½ c. nonfat dry milk
½ t. salt
¼ t. coarsely ground pepper
⅛ t. nutmeg
¼ t. marjoram
¾ c. grated Parmesan or sharp
   cheddar cheese
¼ c. slivered almonds or walnuts
1 t. soft margarine

COOK the spinach in the soft margarine until dry and just tender. (Do not add liquid, as water clings to both frozen and fresh washed spinach.) Stir to prevent burning.

BEAT the eggs slightly in a mixing bowl and add all the remaining ingredients, except ½ cup of grated cheese and the slivered almonds.

MIX thoroughly and pour into a 1½-quart casserole.

SPRINKLE the top with the reserved cheese and the slivered almonds.

BAKE in a preheated oven at 350°F until the casserole is firm and bubbly and the cheese is golden brown.

SERVE hot at once with baked potato, raw finger vegetables, roast fresh picnic ham, fresh fruit and cheese, and café au lait.

Variations

1/SPINACH AND CHEESE SOUFFLÉ

SEPARATE the eggs. Use the yolks in the mixture and beat the whites to stiff, moist peaks. Before pouring the mixture into the casserole, fold in the egg whites.

BAKE as above. Serve hot at once.

2/BROCCOLI AND CHEESE CASSEROLE OR SOUFFLÉ

USE chopped broccoli instead of spinach for a casserole or a soufflé.

COOK the broccoli in ¼ cup water and use the water as part of the liquid for the sauce. Proceed as above.

SUCCOTASH MEXICAN STYLE

(yield: 4–6 servings)

HEAT in a thick-bottomed pan 1 cup each of fresh, frozen, or canned corn, baby lima beans, and chopped tomatoes.

ADD ¼ cup diced onion, 1 crushed clove of garlic, 1 teaspoon salt, 1 teaspoon chili pepper, ¼ teaspoon black pepper, and 1 tablespoon vegetable oil or soft margarine.

BRING to a boil and simmer until the vegetables are just tender.

SERVE hot with brown rice, meat loaf, fish, or liver, surrounded by yogurt salad, green onions; carrot sticks; with pineapple upside-down cake (recipe page 440) for dessert.

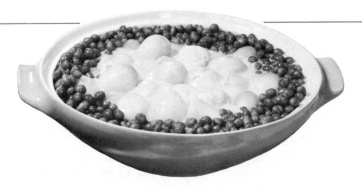

CREAMED PEAS, CARROTS, AND ONIONS

(yield: 4–6 servings)

1¼ c. fresh peas or 1 10-oz. pkg. frozen peas
1 c. sliced carrots
1 c. baby onions
1 t. sugar
salt and pepper to taste
1 c. medium white sauce (recipe pages 418–419)

COOK the carrots and onions, if raw, with ¼ cup water for 2 minutes in the pressure saucepan at 15 pounds pressure or boil gently until tender.

ADD the peas and white sauce and cook until tender.

ADD the sugar and salt and pepper.

SERVE hot as part of a balanced meal.

Variations

1/OTHER CREAMED VEGETABLES

CREAM any of the following vegetables (fresh, frozen, or canned): new potatoes, asparagus, cabbage, broccoli, spinach, cauliflower, lima beans, green or snap beans, turnips, rutabagas, or celery. Use 2 cups of vegetables to 1 cup of medium white sauce.

ADD seasonings to taste (see Table 22–1 for herbs and spices appropriate for this purpose).

(For further variations, see page 430.)

Creamed vegetable variations

2/VEGETABLE AU GRATIN

USE any of the cooked vegetables suitable to creaming and place in a casserole.

ADD ½ cup grated cheese to the white sauce and top the casserole with strips of cheddar, Swiss, or processed cheese.

SPRINKLE with paprika and bread crumbs, if desired, and bake at 350°F until the cheese topping is melted and the vegetable hot and bubbly.

SERVE hot at once as part of a balanced meal.

3/SCALLOPED POTATOES

ALTERNATE layers of thinly sliced potatoes with thin white sauce to within 1 inch of the top of a casserole. Add sliced onion at the middle, if desired.

BAKE in a preheated oven at 350°F until done. Any vegetable suitable for creaming may be scalloped.

4/POTATOES AND HAM

ADD either slices of ham or pork chops to the top of the scalloped potato casserole and bake until done.

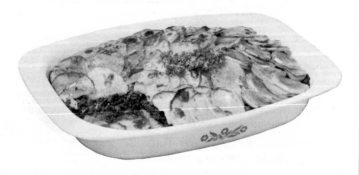

PANNED VEGETABLES (Oriental)

SHRED finely any of the mixed greens (page 427) or slice thinly on the diagonal asparagus, cauliflower, any summer squash, green or snap beans, onions, Brussels sprouts, or broccoli.

MEASURE the vegetable after shredding and use 1 cup of raw greens or ¾ cup of the other vegetables per serving.

HEAT 1 teaspoon of vegetable oil per serving in a heavy skillet with a tight cover.

ADD the vegetable, stirring until all of it is covered with oil.

SALT lightly and add other seasonings to taste. (See Table 22–1 for suggestions on herbs and seasonings to use.)

STIR thoroughly. Cover the pan.

LOWER the heat and stir at intervals to prevent scorching and to allow the acids that turn green vegetables an olive color to escape.

COOK until just tender and serve at once as part of a balanced meal. Sauces may be added to panned vegetables as desired, but they are delicious and lower in calories when cooked and served simply.

DESSERTS

LIME PIE

1 15-oz. can sweetened condensed
   milk
½ c. nonfat dry milk
3 egg yolks
1 t. grated lime rind or lemon rind
¾ c. lime juice

3 egg whites
¼ t. salt
¼ t. cream of tartar
7½ T. sugar

1 t. vanilla

graham cracker crust (recipe page
   438)

MIX the first five ingredients thoroughly.

BEAT the egg whites for a meringue (see the recipe on page 417).

POUR the filling into the crust and top it with the meringue.

BAKE in a preheated oven at 400°F for 10 minutes. Turn off the heat and leave the pie in the oven for 30 minutes.

COOL. Cut and remove the wedges carefully with a pancake turner.

SERVE as part of a balanced meal.

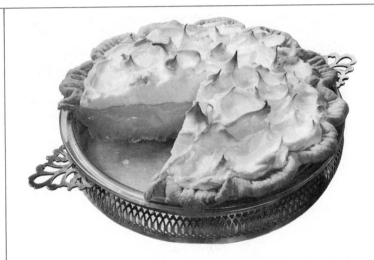

Variations

1/ *LIME FLUFF PIE*

BEAT the egg whites, omitting the sugar, and fold the custard into the stiffly beaten egg whites, with a gentle over and under movement.

POUR into the crust and proceed as above. When ready to serve, cover each piece with a thin layer of sweetened and flavored yogurt or sour cream.

TOP with fresh or thawed frozen berries or orange sections. If there is more filling than the crust will hold, cook it separately in a custard cup. This is tastier and has fewer calories than lime pie.

2/ *LEMON FLUFF PIE*

SUBSTITUTE lemon juice for the lime juice and proceed for either type of pie.

3/ *ORANGE FLUFF PIE*

SUBSTITUTE orange juice for lime juice and proceed as above.

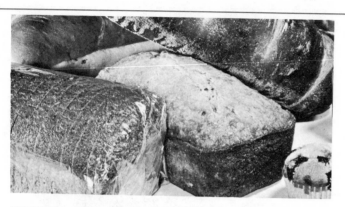

PUMPKIN NUT BREAD

(yield: 1 large or 2 small loaves)

⅓ c. nonfat dry milk
1⅔ c. sifted all-purpose flour
2 t. baking powder
½ t. salt
½ t. cinnamon
½ t. nutmeg
½ t. vanilla
½ t. ginger
1 T. grated orange rind
⅓ c. vegetable oil
1⅓ c. packed brown sugar
3 eggs
1 c. fresh or canned mashed pumpkin
⅓ c. milk
½ c. broken walnut meats

SIFT together the first three ingredients.

MIX the other ingredients thoroughly in another mixing bowl.

ADD these ingredients to the first mixture and blend until smooth.

SPOON into a nonstick loaf pan (9" x 5" x 3") or an oiled and floured one.

BAKE in a preheated oven at 350°F until the loaf springs back when gently touched in the center (about 1 hour).

SLICE and serve warm at room temperature for breakfast or for dessert at other meals. (May be frozen and reheated, if desired.)

BREAD-CEREAL GROUP

BREADS

WHOLE WHEAT YEAST BREAD

(yield: 2 1-lb. loaves)

2 eggs
2 pkgs. dry or compressed yeast
⅓ c. dark molasses
1 c. nonfat dry milk
2 c. warm water (110°–115°F)
2½ t. salt
2 c. sifted enriched white all-purpose flour
3½–4 c. sifted whole wheat flour
1 T. oil

BEAT the eggs slightly in a large bowl and add the next five ingredients, mixing until smooth.

ADD the white flour and beat by hand or in a mixer at medium speed until it is elastic.

ADD the oil, then whole wheat flour, one cup at a time, until 3 cups are added, beating after each addition. The dough should now pull away from the sides of the bowl.

COVER and let "rest" about 10 minutes, if time permits, to "firm up."

SPRINKLE the remaining half-cup of whole wheat flour on a bread board and shape the dough in the center. Knead lightly—bring the far edge of the dough toward you, fold over, and press with the heels of your hands. Turn the dough and repeat the kneading process until a *soft* elastic ball forms.

PLACE the dough in an oiled mixing bowl, oiling the top.

COVER and set in a warm place, out of a draft, and allow the dough to rise until it is double in bulk (about an hour). If time permits, punch the dough down and let it rise again until it is double in bulk.

SHAPE the dough into a firm, elastic ball and lay it on the mixing board.

CUT it in half and shape it to fit an oiled pan 9″ x 5″ x 3″.

PLACE the dough seam side down and brush the top with oil. Cover the bread lightly with wax paper and set it in a warm place, out of a draft, to rise until double in bulk.

BAKE in a preheated oven at 400°F for 15 minutes. Reduce the heat to 350°F and bake until done (the bread will spring back when touched in the center).

REMOVE the bread from the oven and let it stand in the pan for 2 minutes to loosen.

RUN a spatula around the edges and remove the bread to a cake rack.

RUB the crust lightly with soft margarine.

SERVE hot for best flavor, as part of a balanced meal. Cut warm bread with a knife, using a light sawing motion without pressure. If only one loaf is baked, oil the outside of the remaining dough, place it in a bowl, cover, and store it in the refrigerator until you are ready to shape it, let it rise to double bulk, and bake it. Fresh-baked bread may be frozen in airtight wrapping and then reheated in a slow oven until hot. It is like fresh-baked bread.

Variations

1/ BRAN BREAD

If whole wheat flour is not available, ask your store to get it for you. You can substitute 1 cup of 100 percent bran cereal and ½ cup wheat germ for 1½ cups of the whole wheat flour and use enriched white flour for the remaining flour in the recipe. Proceed as above.

2/ WHITE BREAD

USE all enriched white flour and substitute ½ cup brown sugar for the dark molasses. Proceed according to the basic method.

3/ FRENCH-TYPE BREAD

DIVIDE the dough (whole wheat or white) after the first rising, to form two loaves 14 inches long and 2 inches wide, tapering at the ends.

OIL the loaves all over the outside and place them on a cookie sheet.

CUT seven diagonal slashes ⅛ inch deep across the tops of the loaves.

SPRINKLE the tops with cornmeal or sesame seed and let the loaves rise in a warm place until they are double in bulk.

BAKE at 425°F for 20 minutes, then reduce the heat to 350°F and bake until done (5–10 minutes). Serve warm. Cut through the gashes for thick slices. If desired, use a spread made of soft margarine with a crushed clove of garlic blended into it. Garlic bread is especially tasty when warmed in the oven.

4/ RAISIN BREAD

ADD 1½ cups seedless raisins with the warm milk and proceed according to the basic recipe.

(For further variations, see page 434.)

Bread variations

5/ROLLS

SHAPE the basic dough (when it is ready to bake) into rolls of any desired shape. *Cloverleaf rolls* are made by shaping three small balls of dough into half the depth of a muffin tin. For *Parkerhouse rolls*, the dough is rolled ¼ inch thick, cut in circles with a biscuit or cookie cutter, and one half folded over the other, with the edges pressed together. For *crescent rolls*, the dough is rolled ¼ inch thick and cut in pie-shaped wedges, which are then rolled, beginning at the wide end, until the corner is at the top; the edges are then curved in slightly.

PLACE the rolls on an oiled pan so that they touch one another.

BRUSH the tops with melted soft margarine. Proceed as with the basic recipe, but bake at 425°F for about 12–15 minutes or until golden brown.

6/LOW-CHOLESTEROL BREAD

OMIT the egg yolks from the basic recipe and add 4 egg whites, beaten until they begin to foam.

PROCEED with the recipe. This may be used with all variations.

7/PIZZA

DIVIDE the basic dough into four equal parts. Then take one part and divide it in two.

ROLL each part to fit a 12-inch pizza pan with a rim to stand above the pan.

PLACE the dough in the pan and fill it with your favorite pizza filling.

BAKE at 350°F 30 to 35 minutes, or until done.

CUT into pie-shaped slices and serve warm for lunch with a glass of milk and a fresh fruit.

MUSHROOM-ONION-CHEESE PIZZA FILLING

SAUTÉ 1 cup finely chopped onions with 2 tablespoons vegetable oil, 1 teaspoon salt, 1 teaspoon crushed oregano leaves, and 1 teaspoon paprika until the onions are tender.

ADD 3 ounces of drained sliced mushrooms (canned) and sauté about 1 minute.

SPREAD over the pizza. Sprinkle the top with 1 cup (4 ounces) grated sharp cheddar cheese or cheddar cheese. Then sprinkle ⅓ cup pizza sauce and paprika over the top. Garnish with sliced olives, if desired.

BAKE at 350°F 30–35 minutes or until done.

SERVE at once.

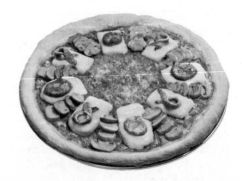

HOMEMADE QUICK BREAD MIX

10 c. all-purpose flour (2½ lbs.)
1¾ c. powdered sugar (½ lb.)
¼ c. double-action baking powder
  (2 oz.)
1½ T. salt (¾ oz.)
2 c. dry milk solids
1 c. soft margarine (8 oz.)

MEASURE and sift all dry ingredients into a large pan or bowl, 6-quart size.

MIX thoroughly with a pastry blender or in an electric mixer.

ADD the fat and blend the mixture to the consistency of coarse meal.

STORE in a *cool, dry place* in jars or cans with airtight lids.

Using the mix

1/PANCAKES

BEAT 1 egg in mixing bowl.

ADD 1 cup cold water (dry milk is in the mix).

ADD 1 cup mix all at once and blend until smooth. Makes 8–10 thin pancakes. Serve hot.

2/MUFFINS

BEAT 1 egg in a mixing bowl.

STIR in ¾ cup water.

ADD 2 cups dry mix and blend only until wet—about 15 strokes.

FILL oiled and floured muffin pans two-thirds full.

BAKE at 425°F (hot) about 20–25 minutes. Makes 12 muffins, 2-inch diameter.

3/WAFFLES

SEPARATE 3 eggs and beat the whites until they stand in stiff but moist peaks. In another mixing bowl, beat together the egg yolks and 1 c. water.

ADD about 1¼ cup mix, according to the thickness desired, and stir until smooth.

FOLD the mixture into the beaten whites (over and under), with a wide wooden spoon. *Do not beat.*

BAKE at once on a moderately hot waffle iron until golden brown. Serve hot, at once.

4/BISCUITS

MEASURE 2 c. of the mix into a bowl.

ADD 2/3–3/4 cup water, stirring to make a soft dough that will just cling together.

SPRINKLE the board with flour and fold the dough over lightly into a ball until smooth (5–10 times).

PAT OR ROLL the dough gently to the desired thickness (about ½ inch) and cut in the desired size.

BAKE on a lightly oiled cookie sheet in a preheated oven at 450°–500°F 10–12 minutes, or until the biscuits are golden brown.

SERVE hot at once.

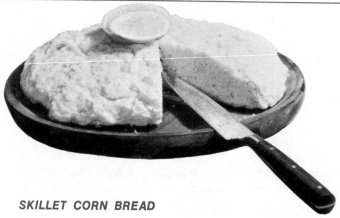

SKILLET CORN BREAD

(yield: 1 skillet of bread, 12 corn sticks, or 12 muffins)

1½ c. yellow cornmeal
½ c. sifted enriched flour
1 c. buttermilk + ½ t.
   baking soda or ½ c.
   nonfat dry milk + 1 c.
   water
3 t. baking powder
1 t. salt
1 T. sugar
2 T. vegetable oil
1 egg

BEAT the egg in a mixing bowl with the milk, sugar, and oil.

ADD the remaining ingredients at one time and mix. Do not beat.

POUR into a hot, lightly oiled and floured skillet and bake in a preheated oven at 425°F until done (about 25 minutes). Or pour into hot oiled corn stick or muffin pans and bake.

SERVE hot as part of a balanced meal.

Variations

ADD any one of the following: ¼ cup crisp cracklings, bacon crumbles, or diced ham; ½ cup chopped green chili peppers; ¼ cup grated onion; ¼ cup chopped red or green sweet pepper; 1 teaspoon poultry seasoning, chili pepper, or thyme.

HAWAIIAN QUICK FRUIT BREAD

(yield: 1 loaf)

½ c. less 1 T. vegetable oil
3 large eggs
1 c. packed brown sugar
1 c. finely diced bananas
1 c. crushed pineapple, with juice
⅓ c. orange juice
1 t. vanilla
1 T. grated orange rind
2 c. sifted enriched all-purpose flour
⅓ c. nonfat dry milk
1 T. baking powder
½ t. salt
½ c. broken nutmeats

BEAT the eggs in a mixing bowl until they are foamy.

ADD all the ingredients except the last five.

SIFT the last five ingredients together and blend them into the liquid mixture.

POUR into an oiled and floured or non-stick loaf pan (9″ x 5″ x 3″) and bake in a preheated oven at 350°F for about 1–1¼ hours, or until done. (Or bake in an oblong pan 13″ x 9″ x 2″ until done—about 35–40 minutes.)

LET the loaf stand in the pan 15 minutes to loosen, then remove to a cake rack to cool. (Or leave the cake in the oblong pan and cut in squares to serve.)

SERVE as dessert at lunch or dinner, as a breakfast bread, or for teas and parties.

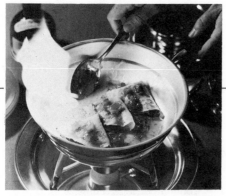

HIGH-NUTRIENT CREPES (pancakes)

(yield: 2 servings)

3 eggs, separated
¾ c. cottage cheese
⅓ c. nonfat dry milk
⅓ c. lime or lemon juice
1 t. grated orange rind or extract
1 T. vegetable oil
1 T. sugar
¼ t. salt
¼ t. cream of tartar
¼ c. buckwheat pancake mix

BEAT the first seven ingredients in the blender.

COVER and store in the refrigerator overnight.

BRING the separated egg whites to room temperature, add the salt and the cream of tartar, and beat until the egg whites stand in moist, firm peaks.

BLEND the pancake mix into the egg yolk mixture.

POUR this over the beaten egg whites in three stages, folding after each addition.

BAKE on a slightly oiled nonstick griddle at moderate heat in small-sized cakes.

TURN gently when bubbly (they are tender and break easily) and brown on the other side.

SERVE hot with orange marmalade or heated syrup to which some marmalade has been added. Delicious!

PIES

HEALTH WATCHERS' OIL PASTRY

(yield: 2 pie crusts)

2 c. sifted enriched all-purpose flour
1 t. salt
½ c. vegetable oil
4 T. cold milk

MEASURE the sifted flour and sift it together with the salt into a mixing bowl.

ADD the oil and milk at one time from the same cup.

STIR with a fork to mix quickly and form into a moist ball (more moist than the standard pastry).

DIVIDE the dough equally to form two balls.

ROLL one ball at a time between two 12-inch squares of wax paper, to form a circle.

REMOVE the top wax paper and invert the crust over a pie pan, removing the other piece of paper and shaping the crust to fit snugly.

FLUTE the edges for a single crust and prick the bottom and sides with the tines of a fork.

BAKE a single crust in a preheated oven at 475°F for 8–10 minutes. Cool.

ADD any filling you prefer (see recipes pages 421–422) or use crushed strawberries, other berries, or peaches for a shortcake. If *two-crust pie with fruit* is desired, do not prick the bottom crust, but fill it with fruit (piling high in the center) and cover it with the top crust, pricking it or cutting a design on it to let steam escape. Then flute the two edges together by pressing the dough between forefinger and thumb. Bake at 450°F until the top crust is golden brown and the fruit is cooked.

Variation

STANDARD PASTRY

USE 2/3 cup soft margarine instead of oil and work it with a pastry blender into the dry ingredients until it forms a coarse meal.

PROCEED as for oil pastry.

APPLE PIE   (yield: 1 pie)

5–6 tart apples, pared and   ¼ t. allspice
   sliced thin   1 t. cinnamon
¾ c. brown sugar   1 T. lemon juice
1 T. tapioca   2 pie crusts
¼ t. nutmeg

PREPARE two crusts of unbaked pastry, following one of the preceding recipes.

CHILL standard crust (but not oil pastry) in the refrigerator until you are ready to use it.

PLACE the sliced apples on the unbaked bottom crust, piling them high in the center.

MIX the remaining ingredients and sprinkle over the apples.

COVER with the top crust.

BAKE at 450°F for 15 minutes, then reduce the heat to 375°F and bake until the top crust is golden brown and the apples are tender—about 20–30 minutes.

Variations

1/ CHERRY PIE (2-crust)

1 1-lb. can sour cherries   1 T. soft margarine
2 T. quick-cooking tapioca   (optional)
½ t. almond extract   1 t. cinnamon
⅔ c. sugar   2 pie crusts

PREBAKE the bottom crust for 5 minutes at 450°F, with an inverted pie pan inside it.

MIX all the remaining ingredients except the almond extract in a saucepan and bring the mixture to a boil. Add the almond extract.

POUR the filling into the partially baked crust.

PLACE the top crust over the filling and flute the edge lightly, putting it slightly over the rim of the pan.

BAKE in a preheated oven at 450°F until the top crust is golden brown.

LOW-FAT GRAHAM CRACKER CRUST

1 c. graham cracker crumbs
2 T. soft margarine or safflower oil

ROLL 6 graham crackers at a time between two 12-inch squares of wax paper, until the required amount is obtained.

MIX the crumbs with the fat in the pie pan until the mixture is like coarse meal, then press it into place on the bottom and sides of the pan. If you wish, a small amount may be reserved to decorate the top of the pie when the filling is added.

BAKE in a preheated oven at 325°F for 5 minutes.

COOL the crust completely, then add the filling.

2/ FRESH PEACH PIE

PILE about 3 to 3½ cups thinly sliced peaches high on the uncooked bottom crust and proceed as for cherry pie, using only 1 tablespoon of tapioca. Do not cook the filling.

3/ BLUEBERRY PIE

USE 3 to 3½ cups of fresh blueberries.

ADD 1 tablespoon lemon juice to cherry pie recipe (total is 2), 1 teaspoon

Variations

1/ SPICY GRAHAM CRACKER CRUST

ADD 1 tablespoon of grated lemon or orange rind, ¼ teaspoon nutmeg, and ½ teaspoon cinnamon. Bake as usual.

2/ VANILLA WAFER CRUST

SUBSTITUTE vanilla wafers for graham crackers.

3/ GINGER WAFER CRUST

SUBSTITUTE ginger wafers for graham crackers. This is a good base for pumpkin or squash pie.

4/ CHOCOLATE WAFER CRUST

SUBSTITUTE chocolate wafers for graham crackers, especially for lemon or lime chiffon pie.

grated lemon rind, and ½ teaspoon cinnamon instead of apple pie seasonings.

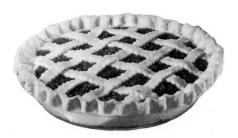

STRAWBERRY PIE OR OKLAHOMA STRAWBERRY SHORTCAKE

MIX together lightly in a saucepan 4 cups of fresh strawberries and 1/2 to 2/3 cup sugar. Let stand for 30 minutes.

REMOVE 1 cup of berries and crush the balance. Add to the crushed berries 2 tablespoons quick-cooking tapioca and boil, stirring until slightly thickened, about 1 minute.

ADD the reserved berries and mix lightly.

POUR into a prebaked pastry shell.

CUT in pie wedges and serve at once for best flavor.

TOP with sweetened yogurt, whipped cream, or ice cream, or serve plain.

Note: Fresh uncooked sweetened berries may be piled into a fresh-baked pastry shell for an easy dessert. This is a delightful pie in appearance and flavor.

STRAWBERRY-RHUBARB PIE

MIX together 2 cups young unpeeled diced rhubarb, 2 cups fresh strawberries (cleaned and hulled), 1¼–1½ cup sugar, 1 tablespoon plus 1 teaspoon quick-cooking tapioca. Let stand 15–30 minutes.

POUR into unbaked pie crust. Dot with 1 teaspoon soft margarine, if desired, and cover with lattice crust or graham cracker crust.

BAKE at 450°F for 10 minutes, reduce the heat to 375°F, and bake until the fruit is tender and the crust is golden brown.

SERVE the day it is baked. Top with sweetened yogurt or serve plain. Other berries and fruits, such as blackberry, gooseberry, raspberry, boysenberry, currant, pear, plum, and any fresh fruit in season may be substituted for the rhubarb and strawberries.

CAKES

BASIC BUTTER-TYPE CAKE USING VEGETABLE OIL

(yield: 2 9-inch layers, 12 servings, 24 cup cakes)

2 c. sifted enriched all-purpose flour
   or 2½ c. cake flour
2 t. double-action baking powder
1½ c. sugar
1 c. skim milk
1½ t. vanilla
⅓ c. vegetable oil

4 eggs, separated
½ t. salt
½ t. cream of tartar

SIFT the dry ingredients three times into a mixing bowl, using only 1 cup of sugar.

SEPARATE the eggs and beat the egg whites with the salt and cream of tartar until foamy.

ADD ½ cup sugar, 2 tablespoons at a time, beating until glossy peaks form.

MAKE a hole in the center of the bowl of dry ingredients and, using the same unwashed beater, mix in ½ cup milk, the oil, and the vanilla. Beat for 1 minute at medium speed in the electric mixer or 150 strokes by hand, scraping the sides of the bowl constantly.

ADD the egg yolks and the remaining milk and beat 1 minute more.

FOLD the batter into the meringue, using a broad spoon and mixing with an over and under movement.

POUR the batter into two oiled and floured 9-inch cake pans and bake in a preheated oven at 375°F until done—about 30 minutes. (If an oblong pan 15″ x 9″ x 2½″ is used, baking time is about 40–45 minutes; cup cakes in muffin tins require about 20–25 minutes.)

REMOVE from the oven when done and cool on a cake rack. Top with your favorite frosting and serve as dessert for family or guests.

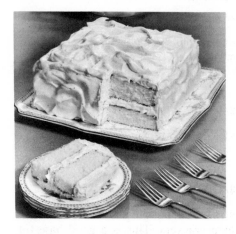

Variations

1/WHITE VELVET CAKE

(no cholesterol, polyunsaturated fat)

OMIT the egg yolks and proceed as for the basic recipe.

2/UPSIDE-DOWN CAKE

SPREAD on the bottom of an oiled oblong baking pan (15″ x 11″ x 2½″) ¾ cup tightly packed brown sugar, ¼ cup nut meats, and pineapple rings, peach halves, or other fruit. Arrange the fruit so that each serving will have some.

POUR either the basic or white cake batter evenly over the fruit and bake at 350°F until done—about 40 minutes.

CUT into squares in the pan and serve with the fruit side up.

3/*PETITS FOURS*

(French)

POUR the white cake batter into a pan 15″ x 11″ x 2½″ and bake. Cool.

CUT in 1½-inch squares and frost with glaze icing or seven-minute frosting.

ADD pink coloring, if desired.

DECORATE the top with a nut or piece of glazed fruit.

4/*FRUIT CAKE*

ADD (when mixing dry and liquid ingredients) 1 tablespoon rum flavoring, 1 cup raisins, ½ cup each nutmeats and candied pineapple, and spices for spice cake.

PROCEED as for the basic recipe.

5/*CHOCOLATE CAKE*

OMIT ½ cup flour and add ½ cup cocoa and 1 tablespoon oil at the first step.

PROCEED as for the basic recipe.

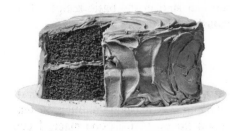

*FRUIT COCKTAIL CAKE**

(low-calorie, low-fat, low-cholesterol)

(yield: 1 9-inch square cake)

1 large egg
1 c. tightly packed brown sugar
1⅓ c. sifted enriched flour
⅓ c. nonfat dry milk
1 t. baking powder
½ t. baking soda
½ t. salt
1 1-lb. can fruit cocktail, with syrup

Baked-on Frosting

½ c. brown sugar
½ c. broken walnut meats

BEAT the egg in a mixing bowl. Add the sugar and dry milk and mix until smooth.

BLEND in the sifted dry ingredients and the syrup of the fruit cocktail.

ADD the fruit cocktail and blend (Batter is thin.)

POUR into a lightly oiled and floured pan.

SPRINKLE the top evenly with the baked-on frosting mixture.

BAKE in a preheated oven at 350°F until done (about 30–35 minutes).

CUT in squares and serve warm. (If the recipe is doubled, use drained fruit, without juice, of the second can.) This is a delicious, moist cake. Reheat leftover cake in a low oven and top with a scoop of ice milk, if desired.

---

*The only fat in this cake comes from the walnuts in the frosting. These are high in linoleic acid.

COOKIES

BASIC DROP COOKIES

(yield: 7–8 dozen)

⅓ c. orange juice	2 c. packed brown sugar
3 large eggs	4 c. sifted flour
1 c. less 2 T. vegetable oil	⅓ c. nonfat dry milk
1 T. grated orange rind	4 t. baking powder
1½ t. vanilla	1 c. broken walnut meats
½ t. salt	

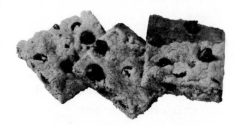

MIX the first seven ingredients thoroughly in a large bowl.

ADD the next four ingredients and blend thoroughly.

DROP from the tip of a spoon onto a lightly oiled cookie sheet, 2 inches apart.

BAKE in a preheated oven at 375°F 10–12 minutes, or until done.

REMOVE with a spatula or pancake turner to cool on a rack.

SERVE as a snack with a glass of milk or as dessert with canned, fresh, or frozen fruit.

Variations

1/ RAISIN COOKIES

COOK 1 cup of raisins in ½ cup of boiling water until plump. Drain.

ADD the drained raisins last and use ⅓ cup of raisin water instead of the orange juice.

PROCEED as for the basic recipe.

2/ OATMEAL RAISIN COOKIES

SUBSTITUTE 2 cups of quick-cooking dry oats for 2 cups of the flour and proceed as for raisin cookies. A favorite.

3/ CHOCOLATE CHIP COOKIES

ADD 2 cups of semisweet chocolate chips to the basic recipe and proceed.

4/ SESAME SEED COOKIES

TOAST 1 cup of sesame seeds and ½ cup of coconut by spreading them thinly in a large shallow pan and heating them at 300°F until lightly browned (about 20 minutes).

ADD the toasted seeds and coconut last to the basic recipe. These keep well if hidden.

5/ PEANUT BUTTER COOKIES

ADD 1 cup of chunk peanut butter at the first step in the basic recipe. Delicious!

6/ HERMITS

ADD to the basic recipe 2 teaspoons of cinnamon, ¼ teaspoon nutmeg, ¼ teaspoon cloves, ¼ teaspoon mace, 1 cup plumped raisins, 1 cup diced dates, and 1 cup glazed fruit, if desired.

7/REFRIGERATOR COOKIES

CHILL any of the above cookie doughs in the refrigerator. When ready to bake, drop from the tip of a spoon to an oiled cookie sheet. This is the best way to use the recipes. The flavors mellow as the dough stands. Will keep two weeks.

8/ROLLED COOKIES

USE a small amount of refrigerated dough at a time and roll it between two sheets of wax paper, adding a little flour on the paper if necessary.

CUT in the desired shapes and decorate, if you wish.

LIFT carefully onto the cookie sheet with a spatula or pancake turner, as this dough is quite soft, but more tasty than a dry dough.

9/MOLASSES COOKIES

OMIT the orange juice or liquid in the basic recipe, as well as the vanilla, nuts, and ½ cup of the brown sugar.

ADD 2/3 cup of dark molasses, 1 teaspoon ginger, 1 teaspoon cinnamon, ½ teaspoon cloves, ½ teaspoon mace.

PROCEED as for the basic recipe.

STORE all the baked cookies in a tightly covered jar or tin box. Reheating the cookies in a low oven before serving improves the flavor.

SIDE DISHES

IÇ PILAV   (Turkish)
(yield: 8–10 servings)

2 c. brown rice
4 c. meat or chicken stock or
   6 bouillon cubes plus water
1 c. finely chopped onion
3 T. vegetable oil
2 T. sugar
1 t. salt
½ t. coarsely ground pepper
½ t. allspice
¼ t. thyme leaves
¼ c. currants
½ c. slivered almonds
1 large tomato, chopped
½ lb. liver (calf or lamb)

HEAT the oil in a 2-quart saucepan. Cut the liver in tiny cubes, season it, and fry it in the hot oil over moderate heat.

REMOVE the liver and drain it on a paper towel. Reserve it.

SAUTÉ the onions in the same fat until golden, but not brown.

ADD the almonds, then the rice, and fry for 5 minutes, stirring constantly to prevent sticking.

DRAIN off the excess fat. Add the 4 cups of stock (or the bouillon cubes and water) and all the remaining ingredients except the liver.

BRING to a boil, then lower the heat to simmer. Cover and cook until all the liquid is absorbed and the rice is tender. Do not stir. Turn off the heat and allow the mixture to stand in a warm place 20 minutes.

ADD minced parsley and the liver and toss *gently* with two forks to mix.

SERVE in a pretty bowl with roast lamb or chicken, eggplant casserole, cucumber and lettuce salad, and yogurt topped with fresh or thawed frozen berries for dessert, followed by café au lait, demitasse, or Turkish coffee.

MAIN DISHES

TAMALE PIE

(yield: 6 servings)

Crust

1¼ c. yellow cornmeal	1 t. chili pepper
1 c. nonfat dry milk	1 T. vegetable oil
1 t. baking powder	2½ c. water
1 t. salt	

MIX all the ingredients in a 1½-quart saucepan.

BRING to a boil, stirring to prevent lumping or sticking.

SIMMER until very thick, about 3 minutes.

LINE the bottom and sides of an oiled pan 10″ x 6″ x 2″ with two-thirds of the dough, pressing to make it firm, and bake in a preheated oven at 400°F for 20 minutes, or until done.

Filling

1 lb. lean ground beef	½ t. salt
½ c. diced onion	1–3 t. chili pepper
½ c. diced black olives (optional)	1 c. (4 oz.) grated sharp cheddar cheese
2 c. canned tomatoes	2 T. diced red bell pepper or pimento
1 c. whole kernel corn	
1 crushed clove garlic	

BROWN the beef and onion in a lightly oiled skillet.

DRAIN off all the fat and add the remaining ingredients, except the cheese and the bell pepper.

POUR the hot mixture into the pan on the bottom crust.

SPOON the remaining cornmeal dough around the outer edge of the tamale filling.

SPRINKLE the top with grated cheese, then with the diced red pepper or pimento.

BAKE in a preheated oven at 350°F until the crust is brown and the tamale bubbles.

SERVE hot with sauerkraut salad or coleslaw, milk, and a bowl of fresh fruit.

CHICKEN TETRAZZINI

(yield: 4–6 servings)

2 c. cooked noodles or spaghetti
2 c. diced cooked chicken
1 c. broken walnut meats
1 c. sautéed sliced mushrooms
2 c. medium white sauce
4 chicken bouillon cubes
salt and pepper to taste
1 T. onion, grated
dash nutmeg (1/16 t.)
1 T. sherry
⅓ c. grated Parmesan cheese

MIX all the ingredients, except the cheese, in a mixing bowl and spoon into a buttered 2-quart casserole.

TOP with grated cheese and bake in a preheated oven at 375°F until golden brown and bubbly.

SERVE hot with green peas, tossed salad, milk, and pumpkin chiffon cake. (May be made ahead and refrigerated or frozen before adding cheese and baking.)

Variations

1/ *SHELLFISH TETRAZZINI*

SUBSTITUTE lobster, shrimp, crab, or tuna for the chicken.

2/ *MEXICAN CHICKEN TETRAZZINI*

ADD 1–2 chili peppers and ¼ teaspoon oregano, if desired. Substitute slivered almonds for walnuts, if preferred, with any of the above meats.

appendix

RECOMMENDED DAILY DIETARY ALLOWANCES, revised 1968

Designed for the maintenance of good nutrition of practically all healthy people in the U.S.A.

	Age[2] Years From - Up to	Weight Kg (lbs)		Height cm (in)		Kcalories	Protein gm	Fat—Soluble Vitamins Vitamin A Activity I.U.	Vitamin D I.U.	Vitamin E Activity I.U.
Infants	0 - 1/6	4	9	55	22	kg x 120	kg x 2.2[3]	1500	400	5
	1/6 - 1/2	7	15	63	25	kg x 110	kg x 2.0[3]	1500	400	5
	1/2 - 1	9	20	72	28	kg x 100	kg x 1.8[3]	1500	400	5
Children	1 - 2	12	26	81	32	1100	25	2000	400	10
	2 - 3	14	31	91	36	1250	25	2000	400	10
	3 - 4	16	35	100	39	1400	30	2500	400	10
	4 - 6	19	42	110	43	1600	30	2500	400	10
	6 - 8	23	51	121	48	2000	35	3500	400	15
	8 - 10	28	62	131	52	2200	40	3500	400	15
Males	10 - 12	35	77	140	55	2500	45	4500	400	20
	12 - 14	43	95	151	59	2700	50	5000	400	20
	14 - 18	59	130	170	67	3000	60	5000	400	25
	18 - 22	67	147	175	69	2800	60	5000	400	30
	22 - 35	70	154	175	69	2800	65	5000	—	30
	35 - 55	70	154	173	68	2600	65	5000	—	30
	55 - 75+	70	154	171	67	2400	65	5000	—	30
Females	10 - 12	35	77	142	56	2250	50	4500	400	20
	12 - 14	44	97	154	61	2300	50	5000	400	20
	14 - 16	52	114	157	62	2400	55	5000	400	25
	16 - 18	54	119	160	63	2300	55	5000	400	25
	18 - 22	58	128	163	64	2000	55	5000	400	25
	22 - 35	58	128	163	64	2000	55	5000	—	25
	35 - 55	58	128	160	63	1850	55	5000	—	25
	55 - 75+	58	128	157	62	1700	55	5000	—	25
Pregnancy						+200	65	6000	400	30
Lactation						+1000	75	8000	400	30

1. The allowance levels are intended to cover individual variations among most normal persons as they live in the United States under usual environmental stresses. The recommended allowances can be attained with a variety of common foods, providing other nutrients for which human requirements have been less well defined. See text for more detailed discussion of allowances and of nutrients not tabulated.

2. Entries on lines for age range 22-35 years represent the reference man and woman at age 22. All other entries represent allowances for the midpoint of the specified age range.

Food and Nutrition Board, National Academy of Sciences, National Research Council

	Water–Soluble Vitamins						Minerals				
Ascorbic Acid mg	Folacin[4] mg	Niacin mg equiv.[5]	Riboflavin mg	Thiamine mg	Vitamin B$_6$ mg	Vitamin B$_{12}$ μg	Calcium gm	Phosphorus gm	Iodine μg	Iron mg	Magnesium mg
35	0.05	5	0.4	0.2	0.2	1.0	0.4	0.2	25	6	40
35	0.05	7	0.5	0.4	0.3	1.5	0.5	0.4	40	10	60
35	0.1	8	0.6	0.5	0.4	2.0	0.6	0.5	45	15	70
40	0.1	8	0.6	0.6	0.5	2.0	0.7	0.7	55	15	100
40	0.2	8	0.7	0.6	0.6	2.5	0.8	0.8	60	15	150
40	0.2	9	0.8	0.7	0.7	3	0.8	0.8	70	10	200
40	0.2	11	0.9	0.8	0.9	4	0.8	0.8	80	10	200
40	0.2	13	1.1	1.0	1.0	4	0.9	0.9	100	10	250
40	0.3	15	1.2	1.1	1.2	5	1.0	1.0	110	10	250
40	0.4	17	1.3	1.3	1.4	5	1.2	1.2	125	10	300
45	0.4	18	1.4	1.4	1.6	5	1.4	1.4	135	18	350
55	0.4	20	1.5	1.5	1.8	5	1.4	1.4	150	18	400
60	0.4	18	1.6	1.4	2.0	5	0.8	0.8	140	10	400
60	0.4	18	1.7	1.4	2.0	5	0.8	0.8	140	10	350
60	0.4	17	1.7	1.3	2.0	5	0.8	0.8	125	10	350
60	0.4	14	1.7	1.2	2.0	6	0.8	0.8	110	10	350
40	0.4	15	1.3	1.1	1.4	5	1.2	1.2	110	18	300
45	0.4	15	1.4	1.2	1.6	5	1.3	1.3	115	18	350
50	0.4	16	1.4	1.2	1.8	5	1.3	1.3	120	18	350
50	0.4	15	1.5	1.2	2.0	5	1.3	1.3	115	18	350
55	0.4	13	1.5	1.0	2.0	5	0.8	0.8	100	18	350
55	0.4	13	1.5	1.0	2.0	5	0.8	0.8	100	18	300
55	0.4	13	1.5	1.0	2.0	5	0.8	0.8	90	18	300
55	0.4	13	1.5	1.0	2.0	6	0.8	0.8	80	10	300
60	0.8	15	1.8	+0.1	2.5	8	+0.4	+0.4	125	18	450
60	0.5	20	2.0	+0.5	2.5	6	+0.5	+0.5	150	18	450

3. Assumes protein equivalent to human milk. For proteins not 100 percent utilized factors should be increased proportionately.

4. The folacin allowances refer to dietary sources as determined by *Lactobacillus casei* assay. Pure forms of folacin may be effective in .doses less than ¼ of the RDA.

5. Niacin equivalents include dietary sources of the vitamin itself plus 1 mg equivalent for each 60 mg of dietary tryptophan.

Nutritive Values in Common Portions of Food*

Pct. = Percent; Cal. = Calorie; Gm. = Gram; Mg. = Milligram; I. U. = International Unit; Tr. = Trace, or an insignificant quantity; ..... = No value imputed, but possibly present

*From *Nutritive Value of Foods*, Home and Garden Bulletin 72, Revised 1970. Adapted from the more comprehensive tables in *Composition of Foods—Raw, Processed, Prepared*, Agriculture Handbook No. 8, Revised Dec. 1963. Both are for sale by the Superintendent of Documents, Washington D.C. 20402

FOOD AND APPROXIMATE MEASURE OR COMMON WEIGHT	FOOD ENERGY	PRO-TEIN	FAT	FATTY ACIDS SATU-RATED (TOTAL)	UNSATURATED OLEIC	LINOLEIC	CARBO-HYDRATE	CAL-CIUM	IRON	VITAMIN A VALUE	THIA-MINE	RIBO-FLAVIN	NIACIN VALUE	ASCOR-BIC ACID
	Cal.	Gm.	Gm.	Gm.	Gm.	Gm.	Gm.	Mg.	Mg.	I.U.	Mg.	Mg.	Mg.	Mg.
MILK AND MILK PRODUCTS														
Buttermilk, from skim milk, 1 cup	90	9	Tr.	.....	.....	.....	12	296	0.1	10	0.10	0.44	0.2	2
Milk, cow, 1 cup:														
Fluid, whole	160	9	9	5	3	Tr.	12	288	0.1	350	0.07	0.41	0.2	2
Fluid, nonfat (skim):	90	9	Tr.	.....	.....	.....	12	296	0.1	10	0.09	0.44	0.2	2
Evaporated (undiluted)	345	18	20	11	7	1	24	635	0.3	810	0.10	0.86	0.5	3
Condensed (undiluted)	980	25	27	15	9	1	166	802	0.3	1100	0.24	1.16	0.6	3
Dry (nonfat instant)	245	24	Tr.	.....	.....	.....	35	879	0.4	20	0.24	1.21	0.6	5
Yogurt (part skim)	125	8	4	2	1	Tr.	13	294	0.1	170	0.10	0.44	0.2	2
Cheese, 1 ounce:														
Cheddar, processed	115	7	9	5	3	Tr.	1	213	0.3	370	0.01	0.13	Tr.	0
Cottage, large or small curd, creamed	30	4	1	1	0.5	Tr.	1	27	0.09	48	0.01	0.07	0.03	0
uncreamed	24	5	Tr.	.....	.....	.....	1	26	0.1	3	0.01	0.08	0.03	0
Cream	106	2	11	6	4	Tr.	1	18	0.1	337	Tr.	0.07	Tr.	0
Swiss, domestic	105	8	8	4	3	Tr.	1	262	0.3	320	Tr.	0.11	Tr.	0
Cream, 1 tablespoon:														
Light	30	1	3	2	1	Tr.	1	15	Tr.	130	Tr.	0.02	Tr.	Tr.
Heavy	55	Tr.	6	3	2	Tr.	1	11	Tr.	230	Tr.	0.02	Tr.	Tr.
Beverages, 1 cup:														
Cocoa	245	10	12	7	4	Tr.	27	295	1.0	400	0.10	0.45	0.5	3
Malted milk	245	11	10	.....	.....	.....	28	317	0.7	590	0.14	0.49	0.2	2
Desserts:														
Custard, baked, 1 cup	305	14	15	7	5	1	29	297	1.1	930	0.11	0.50	0.3	1
Ice cream, plain, 1 cup	255	6	14	8	5	Tr.	28	194	0.1	590	0.05	0.28	0.1	1
Ice milk, hardened, 1 cup	200	6	7	4	2	Tr.	29	204	0.1	280	0.07	0.29	0.1	1
EGGS														
1 whole, raw, large	80	6	6	2	3	Tr.	Tr.	27	1.1	590	0.05	0.15	Tr.	0
1 white, raw, large	15	4	Tr.	.....	.....	.....	Tr.	3	Tr.	0	Tr.	0.09	Tr.	0
1 yolk, raw, large	60	3	5	2	2	Tr.	Tr.	24	0.9	580	0.04	0.07	Tr.	0

FRUITS

Food	Food energy (Cal)	Protein (g)	Fat (g)	Fatty acids: Saturated (total) (g)	Oleic (g)	Linoleic (g)	Carbohydrate (g)	Calcium (mg)	Iron (mg)	Vitamin A (I.U.)	Thiamine (mg)	Riboflavin (mg)	Niacin (mg)	Ascorbic acid (mg)
Apples, raw, 1 medium	70	Tr.	Tr.				18	8	0.4	50	0.04	0.02	0.1	3
Apple juice, fresh or canned, 1 cup	120	Tr.	Tr.				30	15	1.5	……	0.02	0.05	0.2	2
Applesauce, canned, sweetened, 1 cup	230	1	Tr.				61	10	1.3	100	0.05	0.03	0.1	3
Apricots, raw, 3	55	1	Tr.				14	18	0.5	2890	0.03	0.04	0.7	10
Dried, cooked, unsweetened, fruit and liquid, 1 cup	240	5	1				62	63	5.1	8550	0.01	0.13	2.8	8
Avocados, raw, 1/2 peeled	185	2	18	4	8	2	6	11	0.6	315	0.12	0.21	1.7	15
Bananas, raw, 1 medium	100	1	Tr.				26	10	0.8	230	0.06	0.07	0.8	12
Blackberries, raw, 1 cup	85	2	1				19	46	1.3	290	0.05	0.06	0.5	30
Blueberries, raw, 1 cup	85	1	1				21	21	1.4	140	0.04	0.08	0.6	20
Cantaloupes, raw, 1/2 melon (5 in. diam.)	60	1	Tr.				14	27	0.8	6540	0.08	0.06	1.2	63
Cherries, canned, red sour, 1 cup pitted	105	2	Tr.				26	37	0.7	1660	0.07	0.05	0.5	12
Cranberry sauce, sweetened, 1 cup	405	Tr.	1				104	17	0.6	60	0.03	0.03	0.1	6
Dates, pitted, cut, 1 cup	490	4	1				130	105	5.3	90	0.16	0.17	3.9	0
Fruit cocktail, canned, heavy syrup, solids and liquid, 1 cup	195	1	Tr.				50	23	1.0	360	0.05	0.03	1.3	5
Grapefruit, raw, 1/2, white, medium	45	1	Tr.				12	19	0.5	10	0.05	0.02	0.2	44
Grapefruit juice: Canned, unsweetened, 1 cup	100	1	Tr.				24	20	1.0	20	0.07	0.04	0.4	84
Frozen concentrate, 6-ounce can	300	4	1				72	70	0.8	60	0.29	0.12	1.4	286
Grapes, American type (slip skin), raw, 1 cup	65	1	1				15	15	0.4	100	0.05	0.03	0.2	3
Grape juice, bottled, 1 cup	165	1	Tr.				42	28	0.8	……	0.10	0.05	0.5	Tr.
Lemon juice, fresh, 1 cup	60	1	Tr.				20	17	0.5	50	0.07	0.02	0.2	112
Lime juice, fresh, 1 cup	65	1	Tr.				22	22	0.5	20	0.05	0.02	0.2	79
Oranges, 1 medium	65	1	Tr.				16	54	0.5	260	0.13	0.05	0.5	66
Orange juice: Fresh, Florida, 1 cup	110	2	1				26	27	0.5	500	0.22	0.07	1.0	124
Canned, unsweetened, 1 cup	120	2	Tr.				28	25	1.0	500	0.17	0.05	0.7	100
Frozen concentrate, 6-ounce can	360	5	Tr.				87	75	0.9	1620	0.68	0.11	2.8	360
Peaches: Raw, 1 medium	35	1	Tr.				10	9	0.5	1320	0.02	0.05	1.0	7
Canned in heavy syrup, 1 cup	200	1	Tr.				52	10	0.8	1100	0.02	0.06	1.4	7

FOOD AND APPROXIMATE MEASURE OR COMMON WEIGHT	FOOD EN-ERGY	PRO-TEIN	FAT	SATU-RATED (TOTAL)	UNSATURATED OLEIC	LINOLEIC	CARBO-HYDRATE	CAL-CIUM	IRON	VITAMIN A VALUE	THIA-MINE	RIBO-FLAVIN	NIACIN VALUE	ASCOR-BIC ACID
	Cal.	Gm.	Gm.	Gm.	Gm.	Gm.	Gm.	Mg.	Mg.	I.U.	Mg.	Mg.	Mg.	Mg.
Pears:														
Raw, 1 pear, medium	100	1	1				25	13	0.5	30	0.04	0.07	0.2	7
Canned in heavy syrup, 1 cup	195	1	1				50	13	0.5	Tr.	0.03	0.05	0.3	4
Pineapple:														
Raw, diced, 1 cup	75	1	Tr.				19	24	0.7	100	0.12	0.04	0.3	24
Canned in heavy syrup, 2 small or 1 large slice and 2 tablespoons juice	90	Tr.	Tr.				24	13	0.4	50	0.09	0.03	0.2	8
Pineapple juice, canned, 1 cup	135	1	Tr.				34	37	0.7	120	0.12	0.04	0.5	22
Plums, raw, 1	25	Tr.	Tr.				7	7	0.3	140	0.02	0.02	0.3	3
Prunes, cooked, unsweet-ened, 1 cup	295	2	1				78	60	4.5	1860	0.08	0.18	1.7	2
Prune juice, canned, 1 cup	200	1	Tr.				49	36	10.5	...	0.03	0.03	1.0	5
Raisins, 1 cup	480	4	Tr.				128	102	5.8	30	0.18	0.13	0.8	2
Raspberries, red raw, 1 cup	70	1	1				17	27	1.1	160	0.04	0.11	1.1	31
Rhubarb, cooked with sugar, 1 cup	385	1	Tr.				98	212	1.6	220	0.06	0.15	0.7	17
Strawberries:														
Raw, 1 cup	55	1	1				13	31	1.5	90	0.04	0.10	1.0	88
Frozen, 10-ounce carton	310	1	1				79	40	2.0	90	0.06	0.17	1.5	150
Tangerines, 1 medium	40	1	Tr.				10	34	0.3	360	0.05	0.02	0.1	27
Watermelons, 1 wedge	115	2	1				27	30	2.1	2510	0.13	0.13	0.7	30
CEREAL–BREAD:														
Biscuits, enriched flour, 1 biscuit	105	2	5	1	2	1	13	34	0.4	Tr.	0.06	0.06	0.1	Tr.
Bran flakes, 1 cup, 40 percent	105	4	1				28	25	12.3	0	0.14	0.06	2.2	0
Breads, 1 slice:														
Boston brown, unenriched	100	3	1				22	43	0.9	0	0.05	0.03	0.6	0
Rye (1/3 rye, 2/3 wheat)	60	2	Tr.				13	19	0.4	0	0.05	0.02	0.4	0
White, enriched, soft crumb	70	2	1				13	21	0.6	Tr.	0.06	0.05	0.6	Tr.
Whole wheat	65	3	1				14	24	0.8	Tr.	0.09	0.03	0.8	Tr.
Cakes:														
Angel food, 1/12 of 10-in. diam. cake, from mix	135	3	Tr.				32	50	0.2	0	Tr.	0.06	0.1	0
Doughnuts, cake-type, 1	125	1	6	1	4	Tr.	16	13	0.4	30	0.05	0.05	0.4	Tr.
Gingerbread, 1/9 of 8-in. square cake, from mix	175	2	4	1	2	1	32	57	1.0	Tr.	0.02	0.06	0.5	Tr.
Cupcakes, 1, from mix, with chocolate icing	130	2	5	2	2	1	21	47	0.3	60	0.01	0.04	0.1	Tr.
Sponge, 1/2 of 10-in. diam. cake	195	5	4	1	2	Tr.	36	20	0.8	300	0.03	0.09	0.1	Tr.

Food														
Cookies, sandwich, 1	50	1	2	1	1	Tr.	7	2	0.1	0	Tr.	Tr.	0.1	0
Corn muffins made with enriched, degermed corn meal, 1	125	3	4	2	2	Tr.	19	42	0.7	120	0.08	0.09	0.6	Tr.
Corn flakes, 1 cup, plain	100	2	Tr.				21	4	0.4	0	0.11	0.02	0.5	0
Crackers: Graham, 4 small or 2 medium	55	1	1				10	6	0.2	0	0.01	0.03	0.2	0
Saltines, 4	50	1	1	1	1		8	2	0.1	0	Tr.	Tr.	0.1	0
Farina, enriched, cooked, 1 cup	105	3	Tr.				22	147	0.7	0	0.12	0.07	1.0	0
Macaroni, cooked, 1 cup: Unenriched, firm	190	6	1				39	14	0.7	0	0.03	0.03	0.5	0
Enriched, firm	190	6	1				39	14	1.4	0	0.23	0.14	1.8	0
Muffins, made with enriched flour, 1	120	3	4	1	2	1	17	42	0.6	40	0.07	0.09	0.6	Tr.
Oatmeal or rolled oats, cooked, 1 cup	130	5	2				23	22	1.4	0	0.19	0.05	0.2	0
Pancakes, wheat, with enriched flour, 1 (4 in. diam.)	60	2	2	Tr.	1	Tr.	9	27	0.4	30	0.05	0.06	0.4	Tr.
Pies, 4-in. wedge (9 in. diam.): Apple	350	3	15	4	7	3	51	11	0.4	40	0.03	0.03	0.5	1
Custard	285	8	14	5	6	2	30	125	0.8	300	0.07	0.21	0.4	0
Lemon meringue	305	4	12	4	6	2	45	17	0.6	200	0.04	0.10	0.2	4
Mince	365	3	16	4	8	3	56	38	1.4	Tr.	0.09	0.05	0.5	1
Pumpkin	275	5	15	5	6	2	32	66	0.7	3210	0.04	0.13	0.7	Tr.
Pretzels, 5 med. or 10 small	10	Tr.	Tr.				2	1	Tr.	0	Tr.	Tr.	Tr.	0
Rice, enriched cooked, 1 cup: Converted, long-grain, parboiled	185	4	Tr.				41	33	1.4	0	0.19		2.1	0
Unenriched	225	4	Tr.				50	21	0.4	0	0.04	0.02	0.8	0
Rice, puffed, 1 cup	60	1	Tr.				13	3	0.3	0	0.07	0.01	0.7	0
Rolls, plain, enriched, 1 roll (12 per pound), homemade	120	3	3	1	1	1	20	16	0.7	30	0.09	0.09	0.8	Tr.
Spaghetti, enriched, cooked, 1 cup	155	5	1				32	11	1.3	0	0.2	0.11	1.5	0
Waffles, baked, with enriched flour, 1	210	7	7	2	4	1	28	85	1.3	250	0.13	0.19	1.0	Tr.
Wheat flours: Whole, 1 cup stirred	400	16	2	Tr.	1	1	85	49	4.0	0	0.66	0.14	5.2	0
All-purpose or family flour, enriched, 1 cup sifted	420	12	1				88	18	3.3	0	0.51	0.30	4.0	0
Wheat, shredded, 1 large biscuit	90	2	1				20	11	0.9	0	0.06	0.03	1.1	0

FOOD AND APPROXIMATE MEASURE OR COMMON WEIGHT	FOOD ENERGY	PRO-TEIN	FAT	FATTY ACIDS SATU-RATED (TOTAL)	UNSATURATED OLEIC	LINOLEIC	CARBO-HYDRATE	CAL-CIUM	IRON	VITAMIN A VALUE	THIA-MINE	RIBO-FLAVIN	NIACIN VALUE	ASCOR-BIC ACID
	Cal.	Gm.	Gm.	Gm.	Gm.	Gm.	Gm.	Mg.	Mg.	I.U.	Mg.	Mg.	Mg.	Mg.
VEGETABLES:														
Asparagus, cooked, 1 cup cut spears	30	3	Tr.				5	30	0.9	1310	0.23	0.26	2.0	38
Beans, lima, immature, cooked, 1 cup, fresh	190	13	1				34	80	4.3	480	0.31	0.17	2.2	29
Beans, snap, green, cooked, 1 cup	30	2	Tr.				7	63	0.8	680	0.09	0.11	0.6	15
Beets, cooked, diced, 1 cup	55	2	Tr.				12	24	0.9	30	0.05	0.07	0.5	10
Broccoli, cooked, 1 cup	40	5	1				7	136	1.2	3880	0.14	0.31	1.2	140
Brussels sprouts, cooked, 1 cup	55	7	1				10	50	1.7	810	0.12	0.22	1.2	135
Cabbage, 1 cup:														
Raw, finely shredded or chopped	20	1	Tr.				5	44	0.4	120	0.05	0.05	0.3	42
Cooked	30	2	Tr.				6	64	0.4	190	0.06	0.06	0.4	48
Carrots:														
Raw, grated, 1 cup	45	1	Tr.				11	41	0.8	12,100	0.06	0.06	0.7	9
Cooked, diced, 1 cup	45	1	Tr.				10	48	0.9	15,220	0.08	0.07	0.7	9
Cauliflower, cooked, 1 cup	25	3	Tr.				5	25	0.8	70	0.11	0.10	0.7	66
Celery, raw, diced, 1 cup	15	1	Tr.				4	39	0.3	240	0.03	0.03	0.3	9
Collards, cooked, 1 cup	55	5	1				9	289	1.1	10,260	0.27	0.37	2.4	87
Corn, sweet:														
Cooked, 1 ear	70	3	1				16	2	0.5	310	0.09	0.08	1.0	7
Canned, solids and liquid, 1 cup	170	5	2				40	10	1.0	690	0.07	0.12	2.3	13
Cucumbers, 10 ounce, raw	30	1	Tr.				7	35	0.6	Tr.	0.07	0.09	0.4	23
Endive, raw, 2 ounces	10	1	Tr.				2	46	1.0	1870	0.04	0.08	0.3	6
Kale, cooked, 1 cup	30	4	1				4	147	1.3	8140				68
Lettuce, Boston, 1 head, raw (4 in. diam.)	30	3	Tr.				6	77	4.4	2130	0.14	0.13	0.6	18
Mushrooms, canned, 1 cup	40	5	Tr.				6	15	1.2	Tr.	0.04	0.60	4.8	4
Mustard greens, cooked, 1 cup	35	3	1				6	193	2.5	8120	0.11	0.19	0.9	68
Okra, cooked, 8 pods	25	2	Tr.				5	78	0.4	420	0.11	0.15	0.8	17
Onions, raw, mature, 1	40	2	Tr.				10	30	0.6	40	0.04	0.04	0.2	11
Parsnips, cooked, 1 cup	100	2	1				23	70	0.9	50	0.11	0.12	0.2	16
Peas, cooked, 1 cup	115	9	1				19	37	2.9	860	0.44	0.17	3.7	33
Peppers, green, raw, 1 medium	15	1	Tr.				4	7	0.5	310	0.06	0.06	0.4	94
Potatoes:														
Baked, 1 medium, peeled after baking	90	3	Tr.				21	9	0.7	Tr.	0.10	0.04	1.7	20

Food														
Boiled in skin, 1 medium, peeled after boiling	105	3	Tr.	...	...	...	23	10	0.8	Tr.	0.13	0.05	2.0	22
Boiled after peeling, 1 medium	80	2	Tr.	...	...	...	18	7	0.6	Tr.	0.11	0.04	1.4	20
French-fried, 10 pieces	155	2	7	2	2	4	20	9	0.7	Tr.	0.07	0.04	1.8	12
Potato chips, 10 medium	115	1	8	2	2	4	10	8	0.4	Tr.	0.04	0.01	1.0	3
Pumpkin, canned, 1 cup	75	2	1	...	...	...	18	57	0.9	14,590	0.07	0.12	1.3	12
Radishes, raw, 4 small	5	Tr.	Tr.	...	...	...	1	12	0.4	Tr.	0.01	0.01	0.1	10
Sauerkraut, canned, drained solids, 1 cup	45	2	Tr.	...	...	...	9	85	1.2	120	0.07	0.09	0.4	33
Spinach, cooked, 1 cup	40	5	1	...	...	...	6	167	4.0	14,580	0.13	0.25	1.0	50
Squash: Summer, cooked, diced, 1 cup	30	2	Tr.	...	...	...	7	52	0.8	820	0.10	0.16	1.6	21
Winter, baked, mashed, 1 cup	130	4	1	...	...	...	32	57	1.6	8610	0.10	0.27	1.4	27
Sweet potatoes, peeled, 1 medium Baked	155	2	1	...	...	...	36	44	1.0	8910	0.10	0.07	0.7	24
Boiled	170	2	1	...	...	...	39	47	1.0	11,610	0.13	0.09	0.9	25
Tomatoes: Raw, 1 medium	40	2	Tr.	...	...	...	9	24	0.9	1640	0.11	0.07	1.3	42
Canned or cooked, 1 cup	50	2	1	...	...	...	10	14	1.2	2170	0.12	0.07	1.7	41
Tomato juice, canned, 1 cup	45	2	Tr.	...	...	...	10	17	2.2	1940	0.12	0.07	1.9	39
Turnips, cooked, diced, 1 cup	35	1	Tr.	...	...	...	8	54	0.6	Tr.	0.06	0.08	0.5	34
Turnip greens, cooked, 1 cup	30	3	Tr.	...	...	...	5	252	1.5	8270	0.15	0.33	0.7	68
MATURE BEANS AND PEAS; NUTS:														
Almonds, shelled, whole 1 cup	850	26	77	6	52	15	28	332	6.7	0	0.34	1.31	5.0	Tr.
Beans, canned or cooked, 1 cup: Kidney, red	230	15	1	...	...	...	42	74	4.6	10	0.13	0.10	1.5	...
Lima, dried, cooked	260	16	1	...	...	...	49	55	5.9	...	0.25	0.11	1.3	...
Navy or other varieties, with tomato sauce and pork	310	16	7	2	3	1	49	138	4.6	330	0.20	0.08	1.5	5
Coconut, fresh, shredded, 1 cup	450	5	46	39	3	Tr.	12	17	2.2	0	0.07	0.03	0.7	4
Peanuts, roasted, shelled, 1 cup	840	37	72	16	31	21	27	107	3.0	...	0.46	0.19	24.7	0
Peanut butter, 1 tablespoon	95	4	8	2	4	2	3	9	0.3	...	0.02	0.02	2.4	0
Peas, split, dry, cooked, 1 cup	290	20	1	...	...	...	52	28	4.2	100	0.37	0.22	2.2	...
Pecans, 1 cup halves	740	10	77	5	48	15	16	79	2.6	140	0.93	0.14	1.0	2
Walnuts, 1 cup chopped	790	26	75	4	26	36	19	Tr.	7.6	380	0.28	0.14	0.9	...

FOOD AND APPROXIMATE MEASURE OR COMMON WEIGHT	FOOD ENERGY	PRO-TEIN	FAT	FATTY ACIDS SATU-RATED (TOTAL)	UNSATURATED OLEIC	LINOLEIC	CARBO-HYDRATE	CAL-CIUM	IRON	VITAMIN A VALUE	THIA-MINE	RIBO-FLAVIN	NIACIN VALUE	ASCOR-BIC ACID
	Cal.	Gm.	Gm.	Gm.	Gm.	Gm.	Gm.	Mg.	Mg.	I.U.	Mg.	Mg.	Mg.	Mg.
MEAT, POULTRY, FISH:														
Beef, 3 ounces, without bone, cooked:														
Chuck, lean and fat, braised	245	23	16	8	7	Tr.	0	10	2.9	30	0.04	0.18	3.5	...
Hamburger, regular, broiled	245	21	17	8	8	Tr.	0	9	2.7	30	0.07	0.18	4.6	...
Steak, sirloin, lean and fat, broiled	330	20	27	13	12	1	0	9	2.5	50	0.05	0.16	4.0	...
Roast, 3 ounces	375	17	34	16	15	1	0	8	2.2	70	0.05	0.13	3.1	...
Chicken, 3 ounces:														
Canned, boned	170	18	10	3	4	2	0	18	1.3	200	0.03	0.11	3.7	3
Flesh only, broiled	115	20	3	1	1	1	0	8	1.4	80	0.05	0.16	7.4	...
Clams, raw, meat only, 3 ounces	65	11	1	...	...	...	2	59	5.2	90	0.08	0.15	1.1	8
Crab meat, canned or cooked, 3 ounces	85	15	2	...	...	...	1	38	0.7	...	0.07	0.07	1.6	...
Haddock, fried, breaded, 3 ounces	140	17	5	1	3	Tr.	5	34	1.0	...	0.03	0.06	2.7	2
Heart, beef, braised, 3 ounces	160	27	5	...	...	...	1	5	5.0	20	0.21	1.04	6.5	1
Lamb, leg roast, cooked, 3 ounces	235	22	16	9	6	Tr.	0	9	1.4	...	0.13	0.23	4.7	...
Liver, beef, fried, 2 ounces	130	15	6	...	...	...	3	6	5.0	30,280	0.15	2.37	9.4	15
Oysters, raw, 1 cup	160	20	4	...	...	...	8	226	13.2	740	0.33	0.43	6.0	...
Pork loin or chops, cooked, 3 ounces without bone	310	21	24	9	10	2	0	9	2.7	0	0.78	0.22	4.7	...
Pork, cured ham, cooked, 3 ounces without bone	245	18	19	7	8	2	0	8	2.2	0	0.40	0.16	3.1	...
Pork luncheon meat, canned, spiced, 2 ounces	165	8	14	5	6	1	1	5	1.2	0	0.18	0.12	1.6	...
Salmon, canned, pink, 3 ounces	120	17	5	1	1	Tr.	0	167	0.7	60	0.03	0.16	6.8	...
Sardines, canned in oil, drained solids, 3 ounces	175	20	9	...	...	...	0	372	2.5	190	0.02	0.17	4.6	...
Shrimp, canned, 3 ounces	100	21	1	...	...	...	1	98	2.6	50	0.01	0.03	1.5	...
Tuna, canned in oil, drained, 3 ounces	170	24	7	2	1	1	0	7	1.6	70	0.04	0.10	10.1	...
FATS, OILS, RELATED PRODUCTS:														
Bacon, medium fat, broiled or fried, 2 slices	90	5	8	3	4	1	1	2	0.5	0	0.08	0.05	0.8	...

Food	Food energy (cal.)	Protein (g)	Fat (g)	Saturated (g)	Oleic (g)	Linoleic (g)	Carbohydrate (g)	Calcium (mg)	Iron (mg)	Vitamin A (I.U.)	Thiamin (mg)	Riboflavin (mg)	Niacin (mg)	Ascorbic acid (mg)
Butter, 1 tablespoon	100	Tr.	12	6	4	Tr.	Tr.	3	0	470				0
Lard, 1 tablespoon	115	0	13	5	6	1	0	0	0	0	0	0	0	0
Margarine, 1 tablespoon	100	Tr.	12	2	6	3	Tr.	3	0	470				0
Oil, corn, 1 tablespoon	125	0	14	1	4	7	0	0	0		0	0	0	0
Oil, cottonseed, 1 tablespoon	125	0	14	4	3	7	0	0	0		0	0	0	0
Oil, olive, 1 tablespoon	125	0	14	2	11	1	0	0	0		0	0	0	0
Oil, safflower, 1 tablespoon	125	0	14	1	2	10	0	0	0		0	0	0	0
Oil, soybean, 1 tablespoon	125	0	14	2	3	7	0	0	0		0	0	0	0
Salad dressings, 1 tablespoon:														
French	65	Tr.	6	1	1	3	3	2	0.1					
Mayonnaise	100	Tr.	11	2	2	6	Tr.	3	0.1	40	Tr.	0.01	Tr.	Tr.
SUGARS, SWEETS:														
Candy, 1 ounce:														
Caramels	115	1	3	2	1	Tr.	22	42	0.4	Tr.	0.01	0.05	0.1	Tr.
Chocolate, milk, plain	145	2	9	5	3	Tr.	16	65	0.3	80	0.02	0.10	0.1	Tr.
Fudge, plain	115	1	4	2	1	Tr.	21	22	0.3	Tr.	0.01	0.03	0.1	Tr.
Marshmallows	90	1	Tr.				23	5	0.5	0	0	Tr.	Tr.	0
Chocolate syrup, thin type, 1 fluid ounce	90	1	1			Tr.	24	6	0.6	Tr.	0.01	0.03	0.2	0
Honey, 1 tablespoon	65	Tr.	0				17	1	0.1	0	Tr.	0.01	0.1	Tr.
Jams, marmalades, preserves, 1 tablespoon	55	Tr.	Tr.				14	4	0.2	Tr.	Tr.	0.01	Tr.	Tr.
Molasses, cane, 1 tablespoon:														
Light	50						13	33	0.9		0.01	0.01	Tr.	
Blackstrap, 3rd extraction	45						11	137	3.2		0.02	0.04	0.4	
Sugar, 1 tablespoon:														
Granulated, cane or beet	40	0	0				11	0	Tr.	0	0	0	0	0
Brown	51	0	0				13	12	0.5	0	Tr.	Tr.	Tr.	0
MISCELLANEOUS:														
Beverages, carbonated, cola type, 1 cup	97	0	0				24			0	0	0	0	0
Bouillon, 1 cube	5	1	Tr.				Tr.							
Gelatin dessert, plain, 1 cup	140	4	0				34						Tr.	0
Sherbet, 1 cup	260	2	2				59	31	Tr.	120	0.02	0.06	Tr.	4
Yeast:														
Baker's, dry, active, 1 pkg.	20	3	Tr.				3	3	1.1	Tr.	0.16	0.38	2.6	Tr.
Dried brewer's, 1 tablespoon	25	3	Tr.				3	17	1.4	Tr.	1.25	0.34	3.0	Tr.

Weight—height tables for ages 7 to 17*

| | MALES | | | | FEMALES | | | |
| | AVERAGE WEIGHT Pounds | RANGE IN WEIGHT Pounds | AVERAGE HEIGHT Inches | RANGE IN HEIGHT Inches | AVERAGE WEIGHT Pounds | RANGE IN WEIGHT Pounds | AVERAGE HEIGHT Inches | RANGE IN HEIGHT Inches |
AGE Years								
7	52.5	45.4– 59.6	48.2	46.0–50.4	51.2	43.7– 58.7	47.9	45.7–50.1
8	58.2	49.5– 66.9	50.4	48.1–52.7	56.9	47.5– 66.3	50.0	47.7–52.3
9	64.4	54.6– 74.2	52.4	50.0–54.8	63.0	51.9– 74.1	52.0	49.6–54.4
10	70.7	59.2– 82.2	54.3	51.8–56.8	70.3	57.1– 83.5	54.2	51.6–56.8
11	77.6	64.5– 90.7	56.2	53.6–58.8	79.0	63.5– 94.5	56.5	53.7–59.3
12	85.6	69.8–101.4	58.2	55.3–61.1	89.7	71.9–107.5	59.0	56.1–61.9
13	95.6	77.4–113.8	60.5	57.3–63.7	100.3	82.3–118.3	60.6	58.0–63.2
14	107.9	87.8–128.0	63.0	59.6–66.4	108.5	91.3–125.7	62.3	59.9–64.7
15	121.7	101.1–142.3	65.6	62.5–68.7	115.0	98.8–131.2	63.2	60.9–65.5
16	131.9	113.0–150.8	67.3	64.5–70.1	117.6	101.7–133.5	63.5	61.3–65.7
17	138.3	119.5–157.1	68.2	65.6–70.8	119.0	103.5–134.5	63.6	61.4–65.8

*From *Basic Body Measurements of School Age Children*, Office of Education, U. S. Department of Health, Education, and Welfare. The ranges given include the cases which fell within the middle two-thirds of those in the sample.

Desirable weights for ages 25 and over*

| | MALES** | | | | FEMALES*** | | |
HEIGHT Ft. In.	SMALL FRAME Lbs.	MEDIUM FRAME Lbs.	LARGE FRAME Lbs.	HEIGHT Ft. In.	SMALL FRAME Lbs.	MEDIUM FRAME Lbs.	LARGE FRAME Lbs.
5 4	118–126	124–136	132–148	5 0	96–104	101–113	109–125
5 5	121–129	127–139	135–152	5 1	99–107	104–116	112–128
5 6	124–133	130–143	138–156	5 2	102–110	107–119	115–131
5 7	128–137	134–147	142–161	5 3	105–113	110–122	118–134
5 8	132–141	138–152	147–166	5 4	108–116	113–126	121–138
5 9	136–145	142–156	151–170	5 5	111–119	116–130	125–142
5 10	140–150	146–160	155–174	5 6	114–123	120–135	129–146
5 11	144–154	150–165	159–179	5 7	118–127	124–139	133–150
6 0	148–158	154–170	164–184	5 8	122–131	128–143	137–154
6 1	152–162	158–175	168–189	5 9	126–135	132–147	141–158
6 2	156–167	162–180	173–194	5 10	130–140	136–151	145–163
6 3	160–171	167–185	178–199	5 11	134–144	140–155	149–168
6 4	164–175	172–190	182–204	6 0	138–148	144–159	153–173

*Metropolitan Life Insurance Company, New York.
**In indoor clothing, wearing shoes with 1-inch heels.
***In indoor clothing, wearing shoes with 2-inch heels. For girls between 18 and 25, subtract 1 pound for each year under 25.

bibliography

General books on foods, nutrition, and meal management

Alexander, Marie M. and Frederick J. Stare, M.D., YOUR DIET: HEALTH IS IN THE BALANCE. New York: The Nutrition Foundation, 1966.

Bogert, L. Jean, George M. Briggs, and Doris Howes Calloway, NUTRITION AND PHYSICAL FITNESS, 8th ed. Philadelphia: W. B. Saunders Company, 1966.

Christakis, George, M.D. and Robert K. Plumb, OBESITY. New York: The Nutrition Foundation, 1966.

CONSUMERS ALL: THE YEARBOOK OF AGRICULTURE 1965. Washington, D.C.: USDA.

Cooper's NUTRITION IN HEALTH AND DISEASE, 15th ed., edited by Helen S. Mitchell et al. Philadelphia: J. B. Lippincott Company, 1968.

Flanagan, Geraldine L., THE FIRST NINE MONTHS OF LIFE. New York: Simon & Schuster, Inc., 1962.

FOOD FOR US ALL: THE YEARBOOK OF AGRICULTURE 1969. Washington, D.C.: USDA.

FOOD: THE YEARBOOK OF AGRICULTURE 1959. Washington, D.C.: USDA.

Griswold, Ruth M., THE EXPERIMENTAL STUDY OF FOODS. Boston: Houghton Mifflin Company, 1962.

Guyton, Arthur C., TEXTBOOK OF MEDICAL PHYSIOLOGY, 3rd ed. Philadelphia: W. B. Saunders Company, 1966.

HANDBOOK OF FOOD PREPARATION, 6th ed. Washington, D.C.: American Home Economics Association, 1971.

Hill, Mary M., FOOD CHOICES: THE TEEN-AGE GIRL. New York: The Nutrition Foundation, 1966.

Kilander, Holger F., HEALTH FOR MODERN LIVING, 2nd ed. Englewood Cliffs, N.J.: Prentice-Hall, Inc., 1965.

Kinder, Faye, MEAL MANAGEMENT. New York: The Macmillan Company, 1962.

McCollum, E. V., THE HISTORY OF NUTRITION. Boston: Houghton Mifflin Company, 1957.

McHenry, Earl W., FOODS WITHOUT FADS: A COMMON SENSE GUIDE TO NUTRITION. Philadelphia: J. B. Lippincott Company, 1960.

——————— and G. H. Beaton, BASIC NUTRITION. Philadelphia: J. B. Lippincott Company, 1963.

McLean, Beth Bailey, MEAL PLANNING AND TABLE SERVICE. Peoria, Ill.: Charles A. Bennett Company, 1967.

Martin, Ethel A., NUTRITION IN ACTION. New York: Holt, Rinehart & Winston, Inc., 1965.

Mayer, Jean, OVERWEIGHT: CAUSES, COST, AND CONTROL. Englewood Cliffs, N.J.: Prentice-Hall, Inc., 1968.

Nickell, Paulena and Jean Muir Dorsey, MANAGEMENT IN FAMILY LIVING, 4th ed. New York: John Wiley and Sons, 1967.

The Nutrition Foundation, PRESENT KNOWLEDGE IN NUTRITION. New York: The Nutrition Foundation, Inc., 1967.

Peet, Louise J., YOUNG HOMEMAKER'S EQUIPMENT GUIDE, 3rd ed. Ames, Iowa: Iowa State University Press, 1967.

PROTECTING OUR FOOD: THE YEARBOOK OF AGRICULTURE 1966. Washington, D.C.: USDA.

Sherman, Henry C. and Caroline S. Lanford, ESSENTIALS OF NUTRITION, 4th ed. New York: The Macmillan Company, 1957.

Stevenson, Gladys T. and Cora Miller, INTRODUCTION TO FOODS AND NUTRITION. New York: John Wiley and Sons, 1960.

Taylor, Clara Mae and Orrea Florence Pye, FOUNDATIONS OF NUTRITION, 6th ed. New York: The Macmillan Company, 1966.

Troelstrup, Arch W., CONSUMER PROBLEMS AND PERSONAL FINANCE, 3rd ed. New York: McGraw-Hill Book Company, 1965.

U. S. Bureau of the Census, STATISTICAL ABSTRACT OF THE UNITED STATES, 1967. Washington, D.C.: U. S. Government Printing Office, 1967.

Vail, Gladys, Ruth M. Griswold, Margaret M. Justin, and Lucile O. Rust, FOODS, 5th ed. Boston: Houghton Mifflin Company, 1967.

White, Ruth Bennett, YOU AND YOUR FOOD, 3rd ed. Englewood Cliffs, N.J.: Prentice-Hall, Inc., 1971.

Wohl, Michael G. and Robert S. Goodheart, MODERN NUTRITION IN HEALTH AND DISEASE, 4th ed. Philadelphia: Lea & Febiger, 1968.

Wright, Carlton E., FOOD BUYING. New York: The Macmillan Company, 1962.

USDA bulletins and pamphlets*

BUDGETS

A GUIDE TO BUDGETING FOR THE FAMILY, Home and Garden Bulletin No. 108, 1970.

A GUIDE TO BUDGETING FOR THE YOUNG COUPLE, Home and Garden Bulletin No. 98, 1964.

CONSUMER GUIDANCE

FAMILY FOOD BUYING GUIDE, Home Economics Research Report No. 37, Agricultural Research Service, 1970.

FOOD GUIDE FOR THE YOUNG COUPLE, Home and Garden Bulletin No. 85, 1967.

---

*Unstarred publications are free. Starred (*) publications 1 copy free, more must be purchased. All may be obtained from the Superintendent of Documents, Government Printing Office, Washington, D.C. 20402. Return address should include ZIP code.

FOOD MAKES THE DIFFERENCE: IDEAS FOR ECONOMY-MINDED FAMILIES, USDA Pamphlet No. 934, 1969.

FOOD MAKES THE DIFFERENCE: IDEAS FOR FAMILIES USING DONATED FOODS, USDA Pamphlet No. 935, 1969.

FRUIT IN FAMILY MEALS: A GUIDE FOR CONSUMERS, Home and Garden Bulletin No. 125, 1968.

HOW TO BUY BEEF ROAST, Home and Garden Bulletin No. 146, 1968.

HOW TO BUY BEEFSTEAKS, Home and Garden Bulletin No. 145, 1968.

HOW TO BUY CANNED AND FROZEN VEGETABLES, Home and Garden Bulletin No. 167, 1969.

HOW TO BUY EGGS, Home and Garden Bulletin No. 144, 1968.

HOW TO BUY POULTRY, Home and Garden Bulletin No. 157, 1968.

HOW TO USE USDA GRADES IN BUYING FOOD—DAIRY PRODUCTS, POULTRY, FRUITS AND VEGETABLES, EGGS, MEAT, Consumer and Marketing Service Pamphlet No. 708, no date.

NUTRITION: FOOD AT WORK FOR YOU, USDA Publication No. GS-1, 1968.

PROCEEDINGS OF NUTRITION EDUCATION CONFERENCE—EFFECTIVE COMMUNICATIONS, Miscellaneous Publication No. 1075, 1967.

TOWARD THE NEW, A REPORT ON BETTER FOODS AND NUTRITION FROM AGRICULTURAL RESEARCH, Agriculture Information Bulletin No. 341, 1970.

FOOD PRESERVATION

FREEZING COMBINATION MAIN DISHES, Home and Garden Bulletin No. 40, 1970.

FREEZING MEAT AND FISH IN THE HOME, Home and Garden Bulletin No. 93, 1966.

HOME CANNING OF FRUITS AND VEGETABLES, Home and Garden Bulletin No. 8, 1967.

HOME FREEZING OF FRUITS AND VEGETABLES, Home and Garden Bulletin No. 10, 1967.

HOME FREEZING OF POULTRY, Home and Garden Bulletin No. 70, 1970.

HOW TO MAKE JELLIES, JAMS, AND PRESERVES AT HOME, Home and Garden Bulletin No. 56, 1967.

MAKING PICKLES AND RELISHES AT HOME, Home and Garden Bulletin No. 92, 1970.

PRESSURE CANNERS—USE AND CARE, Home and Garden Bulletin No. 30, 1964.

PLANNING BALANCED MEALS

APPLES IN APPEALING WAYS, Home and Garden Bulletin No. 161, 1969.

BAKING FOR PEOPLE WITH FOOD ALLERGIES, Home and Garden Bulletin No. 147, 1968.

BEEF AND VEAL IN FAMILY MEALS: A GUIDE FOR CONSUMERS, Home and Garden Bulletin No. 118, 1967.

CEREALS AND PASTA IN FAMILY MEALS: A GUIDE FOR CONSUMERS, Home and Garden Bulletin No. 150, 1968.

CHEESE IN FAMILY MEALS: A GUIDE FOR CONSUMERS, Home and Garden Bulletin No. 112, 1966.

EGGS IN FAMILY MEALS: A GUIDE FOR CONSUMERS, Home and Garden Bulletin No. 103, 1969.

FAMILY FARE: FOOD MANAGEMENT AND RECIPES, Home and Garden Bulletin No. 1, 1968.

FAMILY MEALS AT LOW COST, Program Aid No. 472, 1965.

FOOD FOR FAMILIES WITH SCHOOL CHILDREN, Home and Garden Bulletin No. 13, 1963.

FOOD FOR FAMILIES WITH YOUNG CHILDREN, Home and Garden Bulletin No. 5, 1968.

LAMB IN FAMILY MEALS: A GUIDE FOR CONSUMERS, Home and Garden Bulletin No. 24, 1967.

MEAT, POULTRY—CARE TIPS FOR YOU, Home and Garden Bulletin No. 174, 1970.

MEAT, POULTRY—CLEAN FOR YOU, Home and Garden Bulletin No. 173, 1969.

MEAT, POULTRY—LABELED FOR YOU, Home and Garden Bulletin No. 172, 1969.

MEAT, POULTRY—STANDARDS FOR YOU, Home and Garden Bulletin No. 171, 1969.

MEAT, POULTRY—WHOLESOME FOR YOU, Home and Garden Bulletin No. 170, 1969.

*MILK IN FAMILY MEALS: A GUIDE FOR CONSUMERS, Home and Garden Bulletin No. 127, 1967.

*NUTRITIVE VALUE OF FOODS, Home and Garden Bulletin No. 72, 1970.

NUTS IN FAMILY MEAL: A GUIDE FOR CONSUMERS, Consumer Service Bulletin No. 176, 1970.

PORK IN FAMILY MEALS: A GUIDE FOR CONSUMERS, Home and Garden Bulletin No. 160, 1969.

*POULTRY IN FAMILY MEALS: A GUIDE FOR CONSUMERS, Home and Garden Bulletin No. 110, 1967.

*VEGETABLES IN FAMILY MEALS: A GUIDE FOR CONSUMERS, Home and Garden Bulletin No. 105, 1969.

FOOD AND NUTRITION GUIDES

CALORIES AND WEIGHT: THE USDA POCKET GUIDE, Home and Garden Bulletin No. 153, 1968.

COMPOSITION OF FOODS—RAW, PROCESSED, PREPARED, Agriculture Handbook No. 8, 1963.

CONSERVING THE NUTRITIVE VALUE IN FOODS, Home and Garden Bulletin No. 90, 1965.

EAT A GOOD BREAKFAST . . . TO START A GOOD DAY, USDA Publication No. L-268, 1967.

FAMILY FOOD BUYING, A GUIDE FOR CALCULATING AMOUNTS TO BUY, COMPARING COSTS, Home Economics Research Report No. 37, 1969.

FAMILY FOOD STOCKPILE FOR SURVIVAL, Home and Garden Bulletin No. 77, 1969.

FOOD FOR FITNESS . . . A DAILY FOOD GUIDE, USDA Publication No. L-424, 1967.

*FOOD FOR FITNESS . . . A DAILY FOOD GUIDE, wall chart, 1958.

FOOD GUIDE FOR OLDER FOLKS, Home and Garden Bulletin No. 17, 1969.

A GUIDE TO GOOD EATING, USDA Leaflet.

MONEY-SAVING MAIN DISHES, Home and Garden Bulletin No. 43, 1969.

NUTRITIVE VALUE OF FOODS, Home and Garden Bulletin No. 72, 1964.

POTATOES IN POPULAR WAYS, Home and Garden Bulletin No. 55, 1967.

CARE AND STORAGE OF FOOD

HOME CARE OF PURCHASED FROZEN FOODS, Home and Garden Bulletin No. 69, 1967.

HOME FREEZERS—THEIR SELECTION AND USE, Home and Garden Bulletin No. 48, 1960.

KEEPING FOOD SAFE TO EAT: A GUIDE FOR HOMEMAKERS, Home and Garden Bulletin No. 162, 1969.

*RECIPE FLIERS ON FOOD FOR THRIFTY FAMILIES, Packet B-1, 1967.

STORING PERISHABLE FOODS IN THE HOME, Home and Garden Bulletin No. 78, 1965.

WHAT TO DO WHEN YOUR FREEZER STOPS, Leaflet No. 321.

EQUIPMENT

BELTSVILLE ENERGY-SAVING KITCHEN, DESIGN NO. 2, Leaflet No. 463, 1963.

BELTSVILLE ENERGY-SAVING KITCHEN, DESIGN NO. 3, Leaflet No. 518, 1963.

THE BELTSVILLE KITCHEN-WORKROOM WITH ENERGY-SAVING FEATURES, Home and Garden Bulletin No. 14, 1966.

QUALITY AND CONSUMPTION OF OUR DIETS

DIETARY LEVELS OF HOUSEHOLDS IN THE UNITED STATES, SPRING 1965, Household Food Consumption Survey 1965–66, Report No. 6, Agricultural Research Service, 1969.

Page numbers in *italics* refer to illustrations, and numbers in **boldface** refer to recipes.